Obstetric and
Gynecological Emergencies

Obstetric and Gynecological Emergencies

Deepti Goswami MD, MRCOG
Professor
Department of Obstetrics and Gynecology
Maulana Azad Medical College and
Lok Nayak Hospital, New Delhi

Sangeeta Bhasin MD
Chief Medical Officer NFSG
Department of Obstetrics and Gynecology
Maulana Azad Medical College and
Lok Nayak Hospital, New Delhi

Swaraj Batra MS, FICOG
Director Professor and Head
Department of Obstetrics and Gynecology
Maulana Azad Medical College and
Lok Nayak Hospital, New Delhi

Foreword
Kamla Sharma

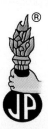

JAYPEE BROTHERS MEDICAL PUBLISHERS (P) LTD

New Delhi · Panama City · London

Jaypee Brothers Medical Publishers (P) Ltd.

Headquarter
Jaypee Brothers Medical Publishers (P) Ltd
4838/24, Ansari Road, Daryaganj
New Delhi 110 002, India
Phone: +91-11-43574357
Fax: +91-11-43574314
Email: jaypee@jaypeebrothers.com

Overseas Offices

J.P. Medical Ltd.,
83 Victoria Street London
SW1H 0HW (UK)
Phone: +44-2031708910
Fax: +02-03-0086180
Email: info@jpmedpub.com

Jaypee-Highlights Medical Publishers Inc.
City of Knowledge, Bld. 237, Clayton
Panama City, Panama
Phone: 507-317-0160
Fax: +50-73-010499
Email: cservice@jphmedical.com

Website: www.jaypeebrothers.com
Website: www.jaypeedigital.com

Inquiries for bulk sales may be solicited at: jaypee@jaypeebrothers.com

This book has been published in good faith that the contents provided by the authors contained herein are original, and is intended for educational purposes only. While every effort is made to ensure a accuracy of information, the publisher and the authors specifically disclaim any damage, liability, or loss incurred, directly or indirectly, from the use or application of any of the contents of this work. If not specifically stated, all figures and tables are courtesy of the authors. Where appropriate, the readers should consult with a specialist or contact the manufacturer of the drug or device.

Publisher: Jitendar P Vij
Publishing Director: Tarun Duneja
Cover Design: Seema Dogra

Obstetric and Gynecological Emergencies
First Edition: **2012**

ISBN 978-93-5025-509-4

Printed at Sanat Printers, Kundli.

Contributors

Anjali Tempe
Director Professor
Department of Obstetrics and Gynecology
Maulana Azad Medical College and
Lok Nayak Hospital, New Delhi

Anju Bhalotra
Professor
Department of Anesthesiology
Maulana Azad Medical College and
Lok Nayak Hospital, New Delhi

Ashok Kumar
Professor
Department of Obstetrics and Gynecology
Maulana Azad Medical College and
Lok Nayak Hospital, New Delhi

Asmita Patil
Assistant Professor
Department of Physiology
Lady Hardinge Medical College, New Delhi

Asmita Rathore
Director Professor
Department of Obstetrics and Gynecology
Maulana Azad Medical College and
Lok Nayak Hospital, New Delhi

Avantika Gupta
Resident
Department of Obstetrics and Gynecology
Maulana Azad Medical College and
Lok Nayak Hospital, New Delhi

Binni Makkar
Senior Resident
Department of Obstetrics and Gynecology
Maulana Azad Medical College and
Lok Nayak Hospital, New Delhi

Chandan Dubey
Assistant Professor
Department of Obstetrics and Gynecology
Maulana Azad Medical College and
Lok Nayak Hospital, New Delhi

Deepti Goswami
Professor
Department of Obstetrics and Gynecology
Maulana Azad Medical College and
Lok Nayak Hospital, New Delhi

Deepti Verma
Resident
Department of Obstetrics and Gynecology
Maulana Azad Medical College and
Lok Nayak Hospital, New Delhi

Devender Kumar
Associate Professor
Department of Obstetrics and Gynecology
Maulana Azad Medical College and
Lok Nayak Hospital, New Delhi

Dinesh Dhanwal
Professor
Department of Medicine
Maulana Azad Medical College and
Lok Nayak Hospital, New Delhi

Garima Sharma
Resident
Department of Obstetrics and Gynecology
Maulana Azad Medical College and
Lok Nayak Hospital, New Delhi

Gauri Gandhi
Director Professor
Department of Obstetrics and Gynecology
Maulana Azad Medical College and
Lok Nayak Hospital, New Delhi

Gunjan
Resident
Department of Obstetrics and Gynecology
Maulana Azad Medical College and
Lok Nayak Hospital, New Delhi

Gunjan Manchanda
Specialist
Department of Anesthesiology
Maulana Azad Medical College and
Lok Nayak Hospital, New Delhi

Krishna Agarwal
Associate Professor
Department of Obstetrics and Gynecology
Maulana Azad Medical College and
Lok Nayak Hospital, New Delhi

Latika Sahu
Professor
Department of Obstetrics and Gynecology
Maulana Azad Medical College and
Lok Nayak Hospital, New Delhi

Madhavi M Gupta
Associate Professor
Department of Obstetrics and Gynecology
Maulana Azad Medical College and
Lok Nayak Hospital, New Delhi

Manoj Sharma
Professor
Department of Radiotherapy
Maulana Azad Medical College and
Lok Nayak Hospital, New Delhi

Minu
Senior Resident
Department of Obstetrics and Gynecology
Maulana Azad Medical College and
Lok Nayak Hospital, New Delhi

Mumtaz Khan
Senior Specialist
Department of Obstetrics and Gynecology
Maulana Azad Medical College and
Lok Nayak Hospital, New Delhi

Muntaha
Senior Resident
Department of Obstetrics and Gynecology
Maulana Azad Medical College and
Lok Nayak Hospital, New Delhi

Nargis Begum
Senior Research Fellow
Department of Obstetrics and Gynecology
Maulana Azad Medical College and
Lok Nayak Hospital, New Delhi

Neha Gupta
Senior Resident
Department of Obstetrics and Gynecology
Maulana Azad Medical College and
Lok Nayak Hospital, New Delhi

Neha Singh
Senior Resident
Department of Obstetrics and Gynecology
Maulana Azad Medical College and
Lok Nayak Hospital, New Delhi

P K Rathore
Director Professor
Department of ENT
Maulana Azad Medical College and
Lok Nayak Hospital, New Delhi

Parul Rathore
Senior Resident
Department of Obstetrics and Gynecology
Maulana Azad Medical College and
Lok Nayak Hospital, New Delhi

Poonam Sachdeva
Specialist
Department of Obstetrics and Gynecology
Maulana Azad Medical College and
Lok Nayak Hospital, New Delhi

Pranay Ghosh
Senior Resident
Department of Obstetrics and Gynecology
Maulana Azad Medical College and
Lok Nayak Hospital, New Delhi

Pushpa Mishra
Senior Medical Officer
Department of Obstetrics and Gynecology
Maulana Azad Medical College and
Lok Nayak Hospital, New Delhi

Rachna Sharma
Specialist
Department of Obstetrics and Gynecology
Maulana Azad Medical College and
Lok Nayak Hospital, New Delhi

Raksha Arora
Director Professor
Department of Obstetrics and Gynecology
Maulana Azad Medical College and
Lok Nayak Hospital, New Delhi

Raktima Anand
Director Professor and Head
Department of Anesthesiology
Maulana Azad Medical College and
Lok Nayak Hospital, New Delhi

Rashmi Jain Gupta
Specialist
Department of Clinical Pathology
Maulana Azad Medical College and
Lok Nayak Hospital, New Delhi

Reena
Resident
Department of Obstetrics and Gynecology
Maulana Azad Medical College and
Lok Nayak Hospital, New Delhi

Renu Tanwar
Associate Professor
Department of Obstetrics and Gynecology
Maulana Azad Medical College and
Lok Nayak Hospital, New Delhi

Reva Tripathi
Director Professor
Department of Obstetrics and Gynecology
Maulana Azad Medical College and
Lok Nayak Hospital, New Delhi

Sangeeta Bhasin
Chief Medical Officer NFSG
Department of Obstetrics and Gynecology
Maulana Azad Medical College and
Lok Nayak Hospital, New Delhi

Sangeeta Gupta
Professor
Department of Obstetrics and Gynecology
Maulana Azad Medical College and
Lok Nayak Hospital, New Delhi

Sanjay Sharma
Senior Resident
Department of Medicine
Maulana Azad Medical College and
Lok Nayak Hospital, New Delhi

Saritha Shyamsunder
Specialist
Department of Obstetrics and Gynecology
Maulana Azad Medical College and
Lok Nayak Hospital, New Delhi

Savita Dagar
Senior Resident
Department of Obstetrics and Gynecology
Maulana Azad Medical College and
Lok Nayak Hospital, New Delhi

Seema
Resident
Department of Obstetrics and Gynecology
Maulana Azad Medical College and
Lok Nayak Hospital, New Delhi

Shakun Tyagi
Assistant Professor
Department of Obstetrics and Gynecology
Maulana Azad Medical College and
Lok Nayak Hospital, New Delhi

Shalini Jathuria
Resident
Department of Obstetrics and Gynecology
Maulana Azad Medical College and
Lok Nayak Hospital, New Delhi

Shikha Sharma
Chief Medical Officer
Department of Obstetrics and Gynecology
Maulana Azad Medical College and
Lok Nayak Hospital, New Delhi

Shonali Chandra
Resident
Department of Obstetrics and Gynecology
Maulana Azad Medical College and
Lok Nayak Hospital, New Delhi

Shweta Tahlan
Resident
Department of Obstetrics and Gynecology
Maulana Azad Medical College and
Lok Nayak Hospital, New Delhi

Siddarth Ramji
Director Professor (Pediatrics) and
Head, Department of Neonatology,
Maulana Azad Medical College and
Lok Nayak Hospital, New Delhi

Sudha Prasad
Director Professor
Department of Obstetrics and Gynecology
Maulana Azad Medical College and
Lok Nayak Hospital, New Delhi

Swaraj Batra
Director Professor and Head
Department of Obstetrics and Gynecology
Maulana Azad Medical College and
Lok Nayak Hospital, New Delhi

Usha Manaktala
Director Professor
Department of Obstetrics and Gynecology
Maulana Azad Medical College and
Lok Nayak Hospital, New Delhi

Vandana K Benwal
Resident
Department of Obstetrics and Gynecology
Maulana Azad Medical College and
Lok Nayak Hospital, New Delhi

Vertika Verma
Resident
Department of Obstetrics and Gynecology
Maulana Azad Medical College and
Lok Nayak Hospital, New Delhi

Vidhi Choudhary
Senior Resident
Department of Obstetrics and Gynecology
Maulana Azad Medical College and
Lok Nayak Hospital, New Delhi

Vijay Zutshi
Consultant
Department of Obstetrics and Gynecology
Maulana Azad Medical College and
Lok Nayak Hospital, New Delhi

YM Mala
Professor
Department of Obstetrics and Gynecology
Maulana Azad Medical College and
Lok Nayak Hospital, New Delhi

Foreword

It gives me great pleasure in writing the foreword for this book 'Obstetric and Gynecological Emergencies' being brought out at the fourteenth Practical Course in Obstetrics and Gynecology by the Department of Obstetrics and Gynecology, Maulana Azad Medical College.

An appropriate and timely action by the residents while dealing with obstetric and gynecological emergencies will save life. The distinguished faculty at MAMC has drawn heavily on their vast clinical experience and in-depth scientific knowledge in compiling this comprehensive yet explicit discussion on different emergency case scenarios as seen in the casualty.

The book constitutes 43 chapters spread out over 400 pages and is divided into three sections. Each chapter is well laid out and written in an easy-to-understand format.

The book is written with focus on practical and academic needs of both postgraduate students and practicing consultants. It provides a convenient source of information and a practical guideline for ready reference in the management of challenging emergency situations in the casualty.

I congratulate and compliment the efforts put in by the Faculty members and the Editors in bringing out this excellent practical discourse on emergency management of common obstetric and gynecological conditions and I am sure it will prove to be of great use to everyone.

Dr Kamla Sharma
Ex-Director Professor and
Head of Department
Obstetrics & Gynecology,
Maulana Azad Medical College,
New Delhi

Preface

Once again, the faculty at Maulana Azad Medical College has come together to combine their extensive scientific knowledge and vast clinical experience to bring forth this book on *Obstetric and Gynecological Emergencies*.

Though the management of emergency situations in medical practice remains the same everywhere, the speciality of Obstetrics and Gynecology stands apart for two reasons. First, it is the only speciality in which a single emergent event can threaten the lives of two individuals, the mother and her fetus. Second, it is the only speciality where an otherwise completely healthy woman may succumb purely to a pregnancy related complication.

The resident doctor posted in the casualty, who is the first person to face such a situation, needs to be aware of the varying emergency clinical presentations she might encounter and how to proceed towards a diagnosis so that prompt corrective action can be taken. This book was conceptualized with this thought in mind.

We have constructed a collection of nearly 100 true case scenarios as one sees them in the casualty, the main objective being to provide a convenient source of information in the 'emergency hour.

It has been divided into three sections, the first dealing with commonly encountered emergency situations in Obstetrics, the second dealing with emergency situations in Gynecology and the third dealing with situations common to both Obstetrics and Gynecology.

We have included chapters on postpartum collapse, cardiopulmonary resuscitation, diabetic ketoacidosis, newborn resuscitation and medicolegal issues related to Obstetrics and Gynecology written by experts in these fields. The editors are grateful to them for their clinical and intellectual inputs.

This book is a coordinated effort by all the contributors. The opportunity to edit it has not only been a challenge but also an enjoyable learning experience for us. We hope you will find the content as enlightening as we have found it.

With humility, we offer our sincere thanks to all our patients ... for without patients, how can a doctor treat.

Deepti Goswami
Sangeeta Bhasin
Swaraj Batra

Contents

SECTION II: GYNECOLOGICAL EMERGENCIES

SECTION III: EMERGENCIES COMMON TO OBSTETRICS AND GYNECOLOGY

Plate 1

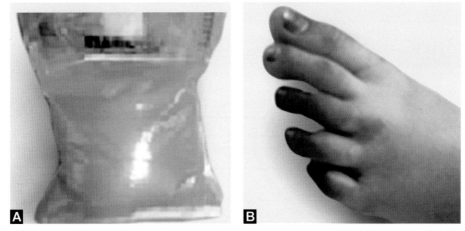

Figures 38.3A and B: Organs affected due to sepsis A) Pyuria, B) Gangrene of toes

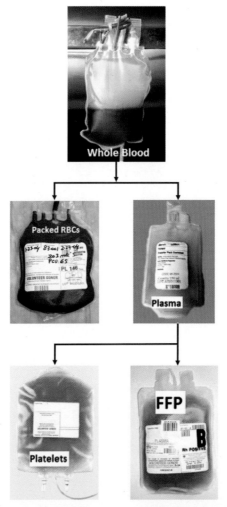

Figure 41.2A: Separated blood components

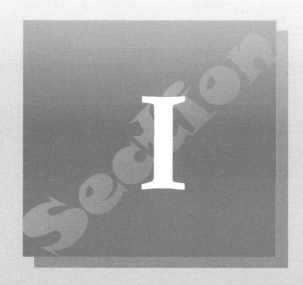

Obstetric Emergencies

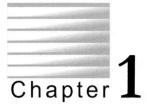

Chapter 1

Ectopic Pregnancy

Sudha Prasad, Pranay Ghosh

INTRODUCTION

Implantation of a fertilized ovum in an area other than the endometrial lining of the uterus is known as ectopic pregnancy. The incidence of ectopic pregnancy has increased from 4.5/1000 in 1970 to 19.7/1000 in 1992 in the West.[1,2] Ruptured ectopic pregnancy remains an important cause of maternal death. However, due to early diagnosis and treatment after the advent of transvaginal ultrasonography (USG) and beta subunit of human chorionic gonadotropin (β-hCG) tests, the incidence of rupture and case fatality has declined.

Pregnancies in the fallopian tube are commonest accounting for 97 percent of ectopic pregnancies: 55 percent occur in ampulla, 25 percent in isthmus, 17 percent in fimbria, and 3 percent in the abdominal cavity, ovary and cervix.[3] If a woman of reproductive age group presents with abdominal pain, vaginal bleeding, syncope or hypotension, ectopic pregnancy should be suspected. The clinical symptom triad of ectopic pregnancy includes amenorrhea, irregular bleeding per vaginum and lower abdominal pain. A pregnancy testing should be done and if the patient is pregnant, an ultrasound evaluation should be performed. If the results of USG are indeterminate, the serum β-hCG concentration should be measured. Serial measurement of β-hCG and progesterone concentrations may be useful when the diagnosis is in doubt. The management options for ectopic pregnancy include expectant management, medical treatment and surgery. Advances in surgical and medical treatment for ectopic pregnancy have allowed the incorporation of minimally invasive or noninvasive treatment.

Risk Factors for Ectopic Pregnancy[4-6]

- History of PID
- Previous tubal surgery
- Previous ectopic pregnancy
- History of infertility
- History of *chlamydial* or *gonococcal cervicitis*
- Documented tubal abnormality
- Tubal ligation
- Current IUD use
- *In utero* DES exposure

CASE SCENARIO-1

Mrs A, a 30-year-old nulliparous lady, presented with 6 weeks amenorrhea and vaginal spotting. On examination, her vitals were stable and the abdomen was soft and non tender. Per vaginum (P/V) examination revealed a bulky uterus with a tender left adnexal mass. Urine pregnancy test was positive.

> **Comments:** A diagnosis of ectopic tubal pregnancy should be considered as the patient is presenting with the classical symptoms of amenorrhea and vaginal spotting and an adnexal mass on vaginal examination.

Differential Diagnosis will Include

- Ruptured corpus luteal cyst or follicle
- Ovarian torsion
- Pelvic inflammatory disease
- Tubo-ovarian abscess
- Acute appendicitis
- Spontaneous or threatened abortion.

POINTS TO BE NOTED IN HISTORY

- Documentation of risk factors is an important part of history taking
- Abdominal pain—nature, duration, intensity of pain, aggravating or relieving factors and any history of syncopal episodes
- History of preceding amenorrhea—ectopic pregnancy is most common in women of reproductive age who present with approximately seven weeks after amenorrhea. However, a history of preceding amenorrhea may not be there and some patients may confuse vaginal spotting for a normal menstrual cycle
- Vaginal bleeding—duration, amount and association with passage of clots or fleshy tissue suggestive of products of conception (which may be seen in spontaneous abortion)
- History of fever—this may be present in case of pelvic inflammatory disease or tubo-ovarian abscess.

> **History in this case:** A woman in reproductive age group presenting with a history of amenorrhea and vaginal bleeding. No associated history of fever, urinary or bowel complaints.

POINTS TO BE NOTED IN EXAMINATION

General Examination

General examination pallor blood pressure (BP) and respiratory rate and vitals including temperature and pulse.

Cardiovascular and Respiratory System Examination

Abdominal Examination

Abdominal tenderness, signs of intraperitoneal hemorrhage including guarding, rigidity and rebound tenderness, bowel sounds.

Pelvic Examination

Per Speculum (P/S) Examination

- Cervical os: Whether open or closed
- Bleeding: Amount and site of bleeding
- Whether any products of conception seen or not

Per Vaginum (P/V) Examination

- Cervical motion tenderness
- Uterine size and position: Uterus may be normal in size or slightly bulky in case of a tubal ectopic
- Palpable adnexal mass: Suggestive of a tubal ectopic pregnancy, tubo-ovarian mass or a corpus luteal cyst.

> **Examination in this case:**
> Pulse – 88/min, Temp – 98.4°F, BP- 116/84 mm Hg, RR – 18/min
> General physical examination- unremarkable
> Abdominal examination - the abdomen was soft and non tender, no signs of intraperitoneal hemorrhage
> P/S - os closed, slight bleeding from the os
> P/V- uterus bulky, tender left adnexal mass nearly 2×2 cm

Diagnosis

Left unruptured tubal ectopic pregnancy

INVESTIGATIONS

Blood Investigation

Hemogram, Blood group KFT, LFT

Ultrasound Imaging

Ultrasound imaging is the diagnostic test of choice in a case of suspected ectopic pregnancy. Transvaginal ultrasound findings suggestive of ectopic pregnancy are given in Table 1.1:[7]

Ectopic pregnancy should be suspected when the patients β-hCG level is more than 6,500 IU/L and the transabdominal scan does not show an intrauterine gestational sac or when the transvaginal sonography does not show an intrauterine gestational sac and the β-hCG level is more than 1,500 IU/L.

β-Human Chorionic Gonadotropin Measurement

β-hCG is detectable in urine and blood as early as 1 week before an expected menstrual period. However, a single measurement of β- hCG is not very informative. In a normal viable pregnancy, the first trimester β-hCG concentration doubles about every 2 days. An increase of at least 66 percent over 48 hours has been used as a cut-off for viability.[8] Ectopic pregnancy may present with rising, falling or plateau of β-hCG levels, thus requiring serial estimation. In a non-viable pregnancy, a subnormal increase in β-hCG concentration is seen. However, a doubling of serum levels over 48 hours does not rule out ectopic pregnancy. Similarly, falling levels confirm nonviability but do not rule out ectopic pregnancy.

Table 1.1: Transvaginal ultrasound findings suggestive of ectopic pregnancy	
Finding	*Likelihood Ratio*
Ectopic cardiac activity	100 (diagnostic)
Ectopic gestational sac	23
Ectopic mass and fluid in POD	9.9
Fluid in POD	4.4
Ectopic mass	3.6
No intrauterine gestational sac	2.2
Normal adnexal region	0.55
Intrauterine gestational sac	0.07

Progesterone Measurement

Serum progesterone levels can detect pregnancy failure and patients with suspected ectopic pregnancy, but it cannot distinguish ectopic pregnancy from spontaneous abortion. Sensitivity for diagnosis of ectopic pregnancy is low (15 %), i.e. 85 percent of patients with ectopic pregnancy will have normal serum progesterone levels.[7]

Progesterone estimation can identify 2 subgroups of patients—stable patients with serum progesterone level above 22 ng/mL, who have a high likelihood of a viable intrauterine pregnancy and patients with levels of 5 ng/mL or less, who almost certainly have a nonviable pregnancy. Invasive testing (e.g. D&C) can be withheld till further testing in the former patients but offered to the latter group, as can the treatment with methotrexate.

Diagnostic Uterine Curettage

If chorionic villi are not detected on uterine curettage, ectopic pregnancy should be suspected. However, curettage should be only considered when β-hCG levels are falling, or when the levels are elevated and ultrasonography does not show intrauterine pregnancy. Chorionic villi are present in obtained curettage and are confirmed when the tissue floats in saline which is indicative of spontaneous abortion although it is not 100 percent accurate. It should be supported by histopathological examination and the above said β-hCG estimation.

Culdocentesis

It is a diagnostic tool for identifying intraperitoneal bleeding which involves insertion of an 18-gauge spinal needle attached to a 50 mL syringe into the cul-de-sac and aspiration of unclotted blood from the cul-de-sac. However, it does not provide information whether the blood is from an ectopic pregnancy or any other cause of intraperitoneal bleeding.

Laparoscopy

Laparoscopy remains the gold standard in detection of ectopic pregnancy and allows visualization of the pelvis and other peritoneal organs. It allows the assessment of the unaffected fallopian tube and additional information like the presence of intraperitoneal adhesions or endometriosis. The diagnostic performance of various diagnostic tests is summarized in Table 1.2.

Investigations in this case:
- Blood group with Rh testing : B+
- Hemogram with hematocrit and complete blood count : Hb - 11.2 gm%, Hct - 34%, TLC - 11,200
- Renal and liver function tests – Normal
- Urine (albumin, sugar and microscopy) – Normal
- β-hCG : 1410 IU/L
- USG : Left sided adnexal mass suggestive of tubal ectopic pregnancy, intrauterine pseudogestational sac

---

Treatment: This patient should be offered medical management.

A patient presenting with an unruptured ectopic pregnancy can be offered expectant or medical management depending on β-hCG levels, size of ectopic mass and other criterion discussed below.

EXPECTANT MANAGEMENT

An ideal patient for expectant management is the one having β-hCG level less than 1,000 IU/L and declining, an ectopic mass less than 4 cm, no fetal heartbeat and is willing for follow-up. (grade C recommendation). Women managed expectantly should be followed twice weekly with serial hCG measurements and weekly by transvaginal sonography to ensure a rapidly decreasing β-hCG level

Table 1.2: Diagnostic tests for detecting ectopic pregnancy		
Diagnostic test	*Sensitivity (%)*	*Specificity (%)*
TVS with β-hCG >1,500 IU/L	67-100	100
Inappropriate rise of β-hCG	36	63-71
Single progesterone level to distinguish ectopic from nonectopic pregnancy	15	>90
Single progesterone level to distinguish pregnancy failure from viable intrauterine pregnancy	95	40

and a reduction in the size of the mass by seven days. Thereafter, weekly β- hCG and TVS examination are advised till levels are less than 20 IU/L (Level III evidence). Expectant management is between 47 and 82 percent effective in managing ectopic pregnancy.[9]

MEDICAL MANAGEMENT

Methotrexate, a folic acid antagonist which inhibits DNA synthesis in actively dividing cells including trophoblasts, is the drug of choice. It is given as single dose regime or as variable dose regime (Table 1.3). Success rate in properly selected patients is up to 94 percent. Other therapeutic agents include hyperosmolar glucose, prostaglandins and mifepristone.

The criteria for starting methotrexate in treatment of ectopic pregnancy are:[10]

- Hemodynamic stability
- Pre-treatment β-hCG level less than 15,000 IU/L
- Absence of ultrasound evidence of fetal cardiac activity
- Gestation less than 6 weeks
- Tubal diameter of less than 3 cm with tubal serosa intact.

Table 1.3: Methotrexate therapy for primary treatment of ectopic pregnancy [11]	
Regimen	*Follow-up*
Single dose regime Methotrexate 50 mg/m²	Measure β-hCG levels. Days 4 and 7 • If difference is >15%, repeat weekly until undetectable • If difference is <15% , repeat methotrexate dose and begin new day 1 • If fetal cardiac activity present day 7, repeat Methotrexate dose, begin new day 1 • Surgical treatment if β-hCG levels not decreasing or fetal cardiac activity persists after 3 doses of methotrexate
Variable dose regime Methotrexate 1 mg/kg I/M days 1,3,5,7 Leukovorin 0.1 mg/kg I/M days 2,4,6,8	Continue alternate day injections until β-hCG levels decrease 15% in 48 hours, or 4 doses of methotrexate is given, then weekly β-hCG until undetectable

*The levels of β- hCG generally increase by 4th day of administration of methotrexate injection.

The overall success rate is greater with multiple-dose therapy than with single-dose therapy (93% vs. 88%); however single-dose therapy is less expensive and has a lower rate of side effects. Less intensive monitoring is required and no folinic acid rescue is required with single-dose therapy. Patients who are Rh –ve require administration of Rh (D) immunoglobulin (50 µg).

Contraindications to Methotrexate

Include liver or renal disease, immunodeficiency, breastfeeding, blood dyscrasias, alcohol use, active pulmonary disease and peptic ulcer.

Medical Therapy by Local Injection

Direct injection of methotrexate, prostaglandin F2α, hyperosmolar glucose and potassium chloride into the fallopian tube or the ectopic mass have been attempted. Direct injection of methotrexate has theoretical advantage over systemic therapy, that the concentration of methotrexate at the site of implantation is much higher than in systemic administration. The use of other agents requires further larger trials to establish their safety and efficacy.

CASE SCENARIO-2

A 28 year-old-lady, G3P2L2, presented with pain abdomen for 1 day after a preceding amenorrhea of 7 weeks. On examination, she was significantly pale with pulse 110/min and BP 94/60 mm Hg. Abdominal examination revealed lower abdominal tenderness and abdominal distension with evidence of free fluid (shifting dullness). On vaginal examination, there was cervical motion tenderness and vague fullness in left fornix.

Comment: Ruptured ectopic pregnancy should always be considered in a woman of reproductive age group presenting with hemodynamic instability and signs of intraperitoneal hemorrhage.

Differential Diagnosis

- Ruptured corpus luteal cyst
- Acute abdomen due to surgical causes: acute appendicitis, perforation peritonitis etc.

History in this case:
Patient is a woman in reproductive age group and has presented with amenorrhea, abdominal pain, hemodynamic instability and signs of intraperitoneal hemorrhage.

Examination in this case:
Pulse – 110/min, Temp – 98.4°F, BP- 94/60 mm Hg, RR – 24/min
General physical examination- unremarkable
Abdominal examination – mild lower abdominal tenderness, abdominal distension
P/S - os closed, vagina healthy
P/V- vague fullness in left adnexa with cervical motion tenderness

Diagnosis

Ruptured tubal ectopic pregnancy

Investigations in this case:
- Blood group with Rh testing : A+
- Hemogram with hematocrit and complete blood count : Hb - 8.2 gm%, Hct - 25%, TLC - 9,100/cu mm
- Renal and liver function tests – Normal
- Urine pregnancy test-positive
- Urine (albumin , sugar and microscopy) – Normal
- USG : Free fluid in cul-de-sac and an intrauterine pseudosac (Figure 1.1)

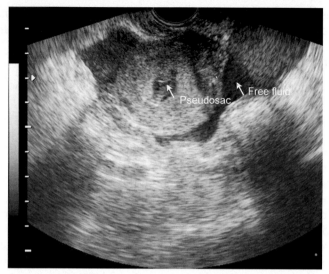

Figure 1.1: USG of patient 2 showing free fluid in cul-de-sac following a ruptured tubal ectopic pregnancy and an intrauterine pseudosac

Treatment

- Vitals should be stabilized by crystalloid and colloid replacement
- Simultaneously, the patient should be prepared for emergency surgery
- Adequate blood should be arranged before commencing surgery.

SURGICAL MANAGEMENT

Surgical management of ectopic pregnancy should be reserved for patients who have contraindications to medical treatment, those in whom medical treatment has failed, those who are hemodynamically unstable or those who refuse medical treatment. Laparoscopy is preferable over laparotomy unless the patient is unstable[12] (grade A recommendation). Laparoscopy is more cost-effective, has a shorter recovery time, less surgical blood loss and less anesthesia requirement. The presence of hemoperitoneum should not preclude the use of laparoscopy.

Indications for Laparotomy in a Case of Ectopic Pregnancy

- The patient is hemodynamically unstable (grade C recommendation)
- Serum β- hCG is >15,000 IU/L
- Failed conservative and medical methods
- Extensive intra-abdominal adhesions.

Conservative tubal surgery is when the tubes are salvaged, e.g. salpingostomy, salpingotomy and fimbrial expression of the ectopic pregnancy.

Radical surgery is defined by salpingectomy. In an unstable patient with hemoperitoneum, when the abdomen is opened, the uterus should be lifted up as it stretches the blood vessels and decreases the bleeding.

Salpingostomy: This procedure is used to remove a pregnancy that is usually less than 2 cm in length and located in the distal part of fallopian tube. A linear incision of nearly 10-15 mm or less is made on the anti-mesenteric border immediately over the ectopic pregnancy. The products are extruded from the incision and can be removed. The incision is left unsutured to heal by secondary intention.

Salpingotomy: It is the same as salpingostomy except that the incision is closed with a suture, usually 7-0 vicryl.

Salpingectomy: Tubal resection can be used for both ruptured and unruptured ectopic pregnancies and can be performed both via laparoscopy and laparotomy. The mesosalpinx is clamped with a succession of clamps as close to the tube as possible. The tube is then excised by cutting a small myometrial wedge at the uterine cornu. Suture loop or bipolar coagulation must be used before cutting the tube.

Follow-up after Conservative Tubal Surgery for Ectopic Pregnancy

There is a difference of opinion regarding follow-up with β-hCG of patients who undergo conservative tubal surgery for ectopic pregnancy:

- Most workers suggest that to avoid undiagnosed persistent ectopic pregnancies, it is necessary to estimate β-hCG prior to surgery and then repeat the measurements at intervals after surgery. A number of different regimes have been suggested to monitor the β-hCG levels.
  - The simplest one is that suggested by Yao and Tulandi who recommended that levels be estimated once seven days after surgery and if the level is higher than expected, the patient should be given a single IM dose of methotrexate.[13]
  - The other follow up protocol involves serum β-hCG estimations before and on at least one occasion within a week of therapy.
- An alternate approach suggests that the hormonal monitoring is not necessary and does not help in detecting retained products. It is suggested that such cases invariably present with abdominal pain which is a much cheaper option than monitoring β-hCG levels (grade B recommendation).

PERSISTENT TROPHOBLAST

Serum β- hCG levels following salpingostomy fall quickly and are expected to be 10 percent of preoperative values by day 12. Persistent ectopic pregnancy (PEP) complicates 5 to 20 percent of salpingostomies. Factors that increase the risk of PEP include:

- Small pregnancies, i.e. < 2cm
- Early therapy, i.e. before 42 menstrual days
- β- hCG values exceeding 3000 IU/L
- Implantation medial to salpingostomy site
  In case of PEP or increasing β-hCG, additional surgical or medical treatment may be required.

HETEROTROPIC PREGNANCY

It refers to coexistence of intra- and extra-uterine pregnancies and is a rare condition (1:30,000). However, with advent of assisted reproductive techniques, the incidence is as high as 0.75 to 1.5 percent of pregnancies. The techniques and medium used for embryo transfer may also be involved.[14]

Abdominal pain, adnexal mass, signs of peritoneal irritation and an enlarged uterus together constitute the major clinical features associated with heterotropic pregnancy.

The majority of heterotropic pregnancies have a single tubal gestation along with an intrauterine pregnancy. The prognosis for a viable intrauterine pregnancy, however, is good, and these combined pregnancies have produced a living child in about 70 percent of cases. A high index of suspicion, repeated ultrasounds, and early intervention are mandatory to salvage the viable intrauterine pregnancy and avoid maternal mortality.[13] Expectant treatment does not seem to have a role in management of a patient with a heterotropic pregnancy as the specific course of the extra-uterine component cannot be monitored with serial β-hCG estimation.

NON-TUBAL ECTOPIC PREGNANCY

Interstitial (Cornual) Pregnancy

A pregnancy developing in the interstitial portion of the oviduct is called interstitial/cornual pregnancy. The transvaginal ultrasonic criteria for interstitial pregnancy are:

- An empty uterine cavity
- A chorionic sac seen separately and >1 cm from the most lateral edge of the uterine cavity
- A thick myometrial layer surrounding the chorionic sac.

Clinical presentation: The gestational sac is better protected in the interstitium as compared to other portions of the tube, *hence the symptoms of interstitial ectopic pregnancies may manifest at a more advanced gestation than tubal ectopic pregnancy.* Since the interstitial area is richly vascularized, rupture usually causes profound and sudden shock.

Management: Cornual resection and repair of defect by laparotomy remains the standard conservative procedure of choice.

Ovarian Pregnancy

Rarely a pregnancy may develop in the ovary. Ovarian pregnancy accounts for less than 3% of all ectopic pregnancies. Spiegelberg criteria for diagnosis include:
- The ipsilateral tube is intact and clearly separate from the ovary
- The gestational sac definitely occupies the normal position of the ovary.
- The sac is connected to the uterus by the uteroovarian ligament.
- Ovarian tissue is definitely demonstrated in the wall of the sac.

Differential diagnosis: Hemorrhage from the corpus luteum, hemorrhagic ovarian cyst.

Clinical presentation: Clinically the condition is difficult to distinguish from tubal pregnancy.

Management: Usually involves surgical excision of the affected ovarian tissue which can be done by laparotomy or by laparoscopy. Medical management with methotrexate has also been reported.

Cervical Pregnancy

A pregnancy may get implanted in the cervical canal below the level of internal os. Rubin's criteria for diagnosis of cervical pregnancy include:
- Cervical glands must be opposite to the placental attachment.
- Placental attachment to the cervix is situated below the entrance of uterine vessels or below the peritoneal reflection on the anterior and posterior uterine surfaces.
- Fetal elements must be absent from the uterus.

Clinical presentation: Patient may present with excessive vaginal bleeding and on examination cervix may appear ballooned up and very soft.

Management: Treatment is surgical and often requires an abdominal hysterectomy. Medical therapy may also be considered for the primary treatment of cervical pregnancy or in addition to surgical therapy.

KEY POINTS

- Diagnosis of ectopic pregnancy should be considered when a woman of reproductive age presents with amenorrhea, abdominal pain and vaginal bleeding.
- A thorough history, clinical examination and investigations are required to establish the diagnosis of ectopic pregnancy
- Documentation of risk factors is an important part of history taking
- Management options for ectopic pregnancy are expectant management, medical management, surgically assisted medical management and surgical management.
- In case of ruptured ectopic pregnancy, patient stabilization with fluids (colloids and crystalloids) is essential and should proceed simultaneously as the patient is being prepared for surgery.

REFERENCES

1. Goldner TE, Lawson HW, Xia Z, Atrash HK. Surveillance for ectopic pregnancy—United States, 1970-1989. MMWR CDC Surveill Summ 1993;42:73-85.
2. Centers for Disease Control and Prevention (CDC). Ectopic pregnancy—United States, 1990-1992. MMWR Morb Mortal Wkly Rep 1995;44:46-8.
3. Della-Giustina D, Denny M. Ectopic pregnancy. Emerg Med Clin North Am 2003;21:565-84.

4. Dart RG, Kaplan B, Varaklis K. Predictive value of history and physical examination in patients with suspected ectopic pregnancy. Ann Emerg Med 1999;33:283-90.

5. Ankum WM, Mol BW, van der Veen F, Bossuyt PM. Risk factors for ectopic pregnancy: a meta-analysis. Fertil Steril 1996;65:1093-9.

6. Mol BW, Ankum WM, Bossuyt PM, van der Veen F. Contraception and the risk of ectopic pregnancy: a meta-analysis. Contraception 1995;52:337-41.

7. BW, Van der Veen F, Bossuyt PM. Implementation of probabilistic decision rules improves the predictive values of algorithms in the diagnostic management of ectopic pregnancy. Hum Reprod 1999;14:2855-62.

8. Dart RG, Mitterando J, Dart LM. Rate of change of serial beta-human chorionic gonadotropin values as a predictor of ectopic pregnancy in patients with indeterminate transvaginal ultrasound findings. Ann Emerg Med 1999;34:703-10.

9. Trio D, Strobelt N, Picciolo C, Lapinski RH, Ghidini A. Prognostic factors for successful expectant management of ectopic pregnancy. Fertil Steril 1995;63:469-72.

10. Lipscomb GH, McCord ML, Stovall TG, Huff G, Portera SG, Ling FW. Predictors of success of methotrexate treatment in women with tubal ectopic pregnancies. N Engl J Med 1999;341:1974-8.

11. Lipscomb GH, Meyer NL, Flynn DE, Peterson M, Ling FW. Oral methotrexate for treatment of ectopic pregnancy. Am J Obstet Gynecol 2002;186:1192-5.

12. Tulandi T, Saleh A. Surgical management of ectopic pregnancy. Clin Obstet Gynecol 1999;42:31-8.

13. Yao M, Tulandi T. Current status of surgical and non-surgical management of ectopic pregnancy. Fertil Steril 1997;67:421-33.

14. Rojansky N, Schenker JG. Heterotopic pregnancy and assisted reproduction: an update. J Assist Reprod Genet 1996;13:594.

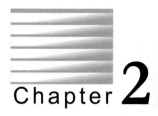

Chapter 2

Hydatidiform Mole

Sangeeta Bhasin

INTRODUCTION

Hydatidiform mole (H. mole) or molar pregnancy is the relatively benign end of the spectrum of gestational trophoblastic disease (GTD), characterized by malformations of the chorionic villi which have the potential to turn malignant.

Grossly, a well developed complete mole appears as a mass of thin walled, translucent, fluid filled vesicles resembling a 'cluster of grapes'. Histologically, it is a conglomeration of enlarged, edematous, avascular and degenerated chorionic villi showing variable amount of proliferation of the syncytial and cytotrophoblast which causes excessive secretion of human chorionic gonadotropin (hCG), chorionic thyrotropin and progesterone. Estrogen production is low due to the absence of fetal supply of precursors.

The incidence varies across the world, ranging between 0.5-2.5 out of 1000 pregnancies. It is 10 times higher in Asia than in Europe and America,[1] and in India, it is seen in 1 in 400 pregnancies.

Risk Factors

- Maternal age less than 15 and more than 35 years with greatest relative risk being in women more than 50 years
- Decreased dietary levels of protein, animal fat and fat soluble vitamin A/carotene
- A past history of molar pregnancy elevates the risk to between 1 to 2 percent.

Types of Hydatidiform Mole (Table 2.1)

- A **complete mole** results from fertilization of an anucleated ovum (having no chromosomes) with a sperm. This then duplicates, giving rise to 46 chromosomes of paternal origin only.
- A **partial mole** results from fertilization of an ovum by 2 sperms giving rise to 69 chromosome of paternal and maternal origin.

CASE SCENARIO-1

A 20-year-old primigravida presents to the gynecology casualty with 3 months of amenorrhea, a history of excessive vomiting and irregular bleeding per vaginum for the last 7-8 days. On direct questioning, she gives a history of vaginal passage of grape like vesicles. On examination, her uterus is 16-18 weeks in size.

> **Comment:** A history of amenorrhea followed by vaginal bleeding with excessive vomiting and vaginal passage of grape like vesicles goes very much in favor of a diagnosis of hydatidiform mole.

Differential Diagnosis

- Threatened abortion with wrong dates
- Multiple pregnancy
- Polyhydramnios
- Co incidental uterine pathology, e.g. fibroid with pregnancy.

POINTS TO BE NOTED IN HISTORY

- Period of amenorrhea—This is usually of short duration (2-3 months) in hydatidiform mole.
- Vaginal bleeding—Note the pattern and amount of bleeding
  - Vaginal bleeding after a variable period of amenorrhea is the most common symptom of hydatidiform mole. It results from separation of molar tissue from the decidua. Bleeding may be continuous or intermittent and may vary from being just a brownish discharge to heavy bleeding significant enough to cause severe anemia.
- A history of vaginal passage of hydropic villi or grape like vesicles is characteristic of hydatidiform mole. Occasionally, the entire mole may be spontaneously expelled at around 16 weeks.
- A history of hyperemesis with associated dehydration and electrolyte imbalance may be seen in 25 percent of patients with hydatidiform mole.
  This results from high hCG levels produced by abnormal trophoblastic proliferation
- A variable degree of lower abdominal pain may be there.
- Pain may be of a dull aching character from distension of the uterus due to concealed hemorrhage. It may be colicky when expulsion starts or sudden and severe when an invasive mole perforates the uterus.
- A history of breathlessness or acute respiratory distress.

Table 2.1: Comparison of complete and partial mole[2]		
	Complete mole	*Partial mole*
Karyotype	Paternal chromosomes only, 46 XX (96%), 46XY (4%)	Diploid paternal and haploid maternal contribution, 69 XXY or 69 XYY
Pathology		
Macroscopic appearance	Whole conceptus is transformed into a bunch of grape like vesicles, no fetal tissue present	Often normal, fetal tissue often present
Microscopic appearance	Diffuse villous edema and trophoblastic proliferation	Focal hydropic villi, variable mild trophoblastic proliferation. Microscopic diagnosis may be difficult.
Clinical		
Diagnosis	Usually diagnosed as molar gestation from clinical and ultrasonographic features. Symptoms-severe and early	Usually diagnosed as missed abortion. Symptoms -often mild
Uterus large for date	25-50 %	<15%
Theca lutein cysts	Seen in 25-30 %	rare
Medical complications	Seen in 10-25 %	rare
Post molar GTN	6.8-20 %	<5 %

- A rare but dramatic symptom of complete mole is Acute Respiratory Distress seen with moles more than 16 weeks size and having high circulating levels of hCG. It may be caused by trophoblastic pulmonary embolization, pulmonary metastases or may result from other contributory factors like severe anemia, toxemia, hyperthyroidism and iatrogenic fluid overload cardiac failure.[3]

Transient left ventricular functional impairment with breathlessness during induction of anesthesia for suction curettage usually resolves within 48 hours with appropriate ventilatory support and use of diuretics.[1]

- A history of tremors or anxiety may point towards hyperthyroidism.
  - Hyperthyroidism may occur due to cross reactivity between hCG and TSH at the TSH receptor site, the high hCG causing an increase in the level of serum free thyroxine. Though lab evidence of hyperthyroidism may be seen in 10 percent of patients, clinical manifestations occur in 1 to 7 percent only. These disappear once the mole is evacuated. Short-term antithyroid therapy may be required to control hyperthyroidism and prevent thyroid storm during molar evacuation.
- A history of quickening will be absent.
- Menstrual history: a history regarding regularity of cycles, cycle length, duration and degree of flow should be taken to rule out the presence of a fibroid.

> **History in this patient:**
> A primigravida with 3 months amenorrhea, excessive vomiting and irregular bleeding per vaginum for 7-8 days. There was a history of passing grape like vesicles per vaginum
> Her menstrual history was 4/30 days, regular

POINTS TO BE NOTED IN EXAMINATION

General Examination

- *Pulse:* Tachycardia may be related to the degree of anemia resulting from bleeding, dehydration resulting from hyperemesis or the presence of hyperthyroidism
- *Blood Pressure:* Early onset preeclampsia is almost pathognomic of hydatidiform mole and may be seen in 26 percent of patients. Although proteinuria, hypertension and hyperreflexia are common, convulsions are rare.[3]
- *Respiratory rate:* Tachypnea/dyspnea may result from acute respiratory distress or high output cardiac failure of severe anemia, hyperthyroidism or toxemia
- Thyroid storm may manifest as hyperthermia, delirium, tachyarrythmia, convulsions, high output cardiac failure or cardiovascular collapse
- Pallor may be out of proportion to the amount of bleeding
- Note icterus, cyanosis, tremors, and edema
- Note signs of cardiac failure

Cardiovascular and Respiratory System Examination

Abdominal Examination

- In more than half the patients, the uterus is larger than gestational age. This is attributed to excessive trophoblast growth as well as distention from blood retained within the endometrial cavity. The uterus corresponds to gestational age in 25 percent and is smaller than gestational age in 25 percent with inactive or dead mole
- The uterus is soft and doughy in consistency and may be difficult to palpate
- No fetal parts are palpable. There are no fetal movements and external ballottement cannot be elicited
- No fetal heart sound is heard

Pelvic Examination

Local External Examination

- Vulval or vaginal metastases may appear as purple hemorrhagic masses which may bleed copiously on touch. These usually disappear spontaneously after evacuation. The presence of metastases does not necessarily imply that invasive mole or choriocarcinoma has developed.[4]

Per Speculum (P/S) Examination

- Look for cervical metastases, condition of cervical os –whether open or closed, presence of vesicles/products of conception at the os, amount of bleeding present.

Per Vaginum (P/V) Examination

- Note uterine size/consistency, absence of internal ballottement.
- Presence of any mass/tenderness in the fornices.

    As a consequence of hyperstimulation by the excessive amount of hCG, the ovaries may contain multiple **theca lutein cysts** varying in size from microscopic to 10 cm or more. They are clinically evident in 25 to 35 percent cases and are associated with high hCG levels >100,000 IU/L. The surface is smooth and yellow and lined with lutein cells. These cysts regress after evacuation of the mole but may sometimes take 2 to 4 months to do so. They generally do not require any intervention unless they cause signs and symptoms of excessive pelvic pressure when they can be decompressed by ultrasound guided aspiration. They may sometimes rupture or undergo torsion/hemorrhage/ infarction and present with an acute abdomen.

    Patients with theca lutein cysts appear to have a higher incidence of malignant sequel after evacuation.[3]

> **Examination in this case**
> The patient was pale (clinically 8 gm% Hb)
> Pulse -100/ min, BP - 100/60 mm Hg, The chest was clear.
> On abdominal examination: abdomen was soft, the uterus was 16 to 18 weeks in size which was much more than the period of amenorrhea, felt soft and doughy with no external ballottement.
> On pelvic examination: the cervix and vagina were healthy, the os was closed with a slight trickle of blood coming through it, uterus was 16-18 weeks in size. There was no internal ballottement. Bilateral fornices were free.

Diagnosis

Hydatidiform mole

The Changing Course of H Mole

- This classical clinical picture of H. Mole has changed over the years. The increased use of high resolution first trimester transvaginal sonography and the availability of accurate hCG testing have brought down the mean gestational age at diagnosis from 16-20 weeks to much less than 12 weeks. Though vaginal bleeding is still the most common symptom, the incidence of increased uterine size, pre eclampsia and hyperemesis has come down to 28 percent, 1.3 percent and 8 percent respectively as compared to 51 percent, 27 percent and 26 percent seen earlier. Severe anemia is seen in less than 10 percent as compared to 50 percent earlier. Hyperthyroidism and respiratory distress are rarely seen.[3]
- The majority of histologically proven complete moles now present with an ultrasound diagnosis of delayed miscarriage or anembryonic pregnancy. Because only 40 to 60 percent of cases may be diagnosed as molar on routine ultrasound, histological examination is necessary to achieve a correct diagnosis. All products of conception from nonviable pregnancies should therefore undergo histological examination irrespective of ultrasound findings.[5]

- The Royal College of Obstetricians and Gynaecologists (RCOG), however, does not recommend routine histological examination of products of conception following therapeutic termination of pregnancy provided fetal parts have been identified on prior ultrasound examination.[6] It has been suggested that a urine pregnancy test or serum hCG concentration should be checked 3 to 4 weeks later to ensure a return to normal range.[7]

MANAGEMENT OF HYDATIDIFORM MOLE

Basic principles of management include
- Confirmation of diagnosis
- Pretreatment evaluation
- Definitive treatment: Suction curettage/hysterectomy
- Post-treatment follow up/surveillance

Confirmation of Diagnosis

- **Passage of vesicular tissue per vaginum** may be the first diagnostic clinical evidence suggesting hydatidiform mole.
- **Ultrasound:**
  - The accuracy of pre-evacuation ultrasound diagnosis of molar pregnancy increases with increasing gestational age, 35 to 40 percent before 14 weeks and 60 percent after 14 weeks.[8]
  - Characteristic ultrasonographic scans of a complete mole show a uterine cavity filled with a heterogenous mass – a typical snow storm appearance of mixed echogenicity representing hydropic villi with intrauterine hemorrhage – without associated fetal development and with or without theca lutein cysts.
  - These features may not be apparent in the early first trimester when intrauterine bleeding has still not occurred and the scan may show a fine vesicular or honeycombed appearance only.
  - The ultrasound diagnosis of a partial mole is more complex and includes both cystic spaces in the placenta and a ratio of transverse to antero posterior dimension of the gestational sac as more than 1.[9]
- **Quantitative serum β hCG testing**
  - Quantitative serum β hCG in hydatidiform mole is much more than expected for gestational age (greater than two multiples of the median), often exceeding 10^5 U/L.
  - Competitive radioimmunoassay using a polyclonal antibody which recognizes all forms of β hCG remains the gold standard assay in the management of GTD. It is sensitive to a level of 1 U/L in serum and 20 U/L in urine and is generally not prone to false positive readings. The amount of hCG produced co-relates with tumor volume, so a value of 5 IU/L corresponds to approximately 10^4-10^5 viable tumor cells. The assay is therefore much more sensitive than the best imaging modality.[4]
  - Findings from recent studies that used a hyperglycosylated hCG assay suggest that a high ratio of this variant to total hCG can detect malignant forms of GTD.[10]
- **Definitive diagnosis is made by histological examination of products of conceptions.** Ploidy status and immunohistochemistry staining for P57 helps in distinguishing partial from complete moles and molar from non molar miscarriage.[7]

Pre-treatment Evaluation

- Baseline investigations
  - Complete hemogram with platelet count
  - Blood group ABO Rh
  - Coagulation profile,

- Liver and renal function tests
- Baseline arterial blood gases (ABG) with consideration of invasive hemodynamic monitoring
- Obtaining baseline hCG levels
- Screening for occult metastatic disease- chest X-ray
  - The most common metastatic appearance on a chest X-ray is multiple discrete rounded lesions, but large and solitary lesions, a military pattern, and pleural effusions can occur.
  - A CT chest is not needed if the chest X-ray is normal since discovery of micrometastasis, which may be seen in about 40 percent of patients, does not affect outcome.[7]
  - CT/ MRI for routinely evaluating liver or brain are not required unless there is evidence of extra uterine disease.[11]
- Screening for hyperthyroidism –T_3, T_4, TSH

Surgical Evacuation

- Suction curettage is the preferred method of evacuation for complete moles irrespective of uterine size and for partial moles where the size of the fetus permits it.
- Medical evacuation of a complete mole should be avoided as also cervical preparation with prostaglandins because of the theoretical concern of potential dissemination and embolization of trophoblastic tissue (through the venous system to the pulmonary vasculature) induced by repeated uterine contractions.[12]
- Suction should be started only after a euvolemic status has been achieved, adequate (at least 2 units) cross-matched blood is available and medical complications like hypertension and hyperthyroidism have been taken care of.
- Large bore intravenous access should be established (preferably at 2 sites).
- The procedure is carried out in the operation theatre under general or regional anesthesia by or under the supervision of a senior surgeon.
- The cervical os is serially dilated up to 12 mm size suction cannula. The cannula is advanced just beyond the internal os and rotated so as to suck out the products. If the uterus is large, the fundus can be massaged gently to assist in involution.
- A gentle sharp curettage is performed after the evacuation is complete and the tissue sent for histopathology in a separate container.
- The use of oxytocin infusion prior to completion of evacuation is not recommended. If there is significant hemorrhage prior to evacuation, surgical evacuation should be expedited and the need for oxytocin infusion weighed against the risk of tumor embolization.[13] If bleeding is severe immediately after suction evacuation, a single dose of ergometrine may stem the hemorrhage.[3]
- Anti D prophylaxis is not required for complete mole but is required for partial mole.

Post Evacuation Follow-Up

16 percent of patients with complete mole and less than 0.5 percent with partial mole may develop persistent trophoblastic disease. It is important that these patients be identified rapidly as nearly all of them can be cured with appropriate chemotherapy. Close and consistent follow-up is therefore essential. The recommendations for post molar follow up are

a. Serial quantitative serum β hCG levels
   - Monitor hCG values 48 hours and then every week after evacuation till a normal value is achieved. After an H mole evacuation, β-hCG usually becomes nomal by 8 to 10 weeks.
   - Subsequently, hCG levels should be determined for 2 more weeks after the first normal level to confirm persistence spontaneous hCG regression
   - Monitor hCG every 1-2 months for a further 6 months from the date of evacuation if hCG has returned to normal within 56 days after the pregnancy event. If hCG has not reverted to normal within 56 days of the pregnancy event, follow up should continue for 6 months from normalization of the hCG value[13]

- The rationale behind monitoring for 6 months after normalization of hCG values is to allow identification of patients who develop post molar GTN after achieving normal hCG values, the vast majority of which do so within 6 months after evacuation

b. Clinical examination
  - Frequent pelvic examinations are performed while hCG levels are elevated
    – to identify development of vaginal metastasis,
    – to monitor size of theca lutein cysts, and
    – to monitor involution of the uterus.

c. Reliable contraception should be practiced for 6 months at least.
  - Barrier contraception should be used till hCG levels revert to normal. After that, combined oral contraceptive (COC) pills can be used. Using COCs before normalization of hCG values increases the risk of developing GTN slightly (1.19 relative risk). Using intrauterine contraceptive device before hCG normalizes may increase the risk of perforation.[13]
  - After completion of surveillance documenting remission for 6 months, pregnancy can be permitted and hCG monitoring discontinued.

d. If anytime during follow-up there are features suggesting residual disease like recurrent or persistent vaginal bleeding/amenorrhea/failure of uterine involution/persistence of ovarian enlargement or if hCG starts rising-
  - Rule out fresh pregnancy
  - Examine thoroughly for evidence of residual disease.
  - Repeat chest X-ray and ultrasound pelvis.

Investigations in this patient:
Hb 7 gm%, TLC 6000/ cu mm, platelets 1.1 lac/cu mm
ABG normal
LFT/ KFT/ coagulation profile/TFT within normal range,
Chest X ray –Normal
Ultrasound abdomen/pelvis showed a heterogenous mass with cystic spaces in the uterine cavity suggestive of H, mole. The endo-myometrial junction was well preserved. No fetus was identified. Both ovaries were normal. Liver, spleen bilateral kidneys were normal. There was no free fluid.
Serum β hCG- 10^5 IU/L
Management in this patient:
The patient was propped up, given oxygen by mask. Two units of packed red cells were transfused. She was then taken up for a suction curettage under general anesthesia. Postevacuation, the patient remained stable. A β hCG was sent 48 hours later which was 10,000 IU/L. She was discharged one week later after contraceptive counseling and advised regular weekly follow-up with hCG.

Complications of Hydatidiform Mole

- Medical complications—Anemia, hyperemesis, hyperthyroidism, pre-eclampsia, coagulopathy, infection
- Complications after evacuation—Uterine perforation, excessive hemorrhage, respiratory distress syndrome
- Thyroid storm may be induced by anesthesia and surgery
- Development of persistent mole

Role of Primary Hysterectomy

- Since the risk of developing gestational trophoblastic neoplasia is increased in women over 40, hysterectomy is a logical treatment option in women who have completed childbearing.
- The uterus is removed with the mole *in situ*. The adnexa may be preserved; theca lutein cysts should be left *in situ* unless torsed/ ruptured/actively bleeding.
- Though hysterectomy reduces the incidence of post-molar malignant sequel from 20 percent after suction curettage to less than 5 percent, it does not completely eliminate the risk; the follow up protocol, is therefore similar to that followed after suction curettage.

Risk Factors for Developing Post-molar GTD

Factors which increase the risk of developing post-molar GTD and hence requiring chemotherapy are:[2]
- Advanced maternal age
- Clinical factors that reflect increased and abnormal trophoblast growth
  - Uterine size more than gestational age
  - Presence of early onset pre-eclampsia/hyperthyroidism
  - Pre-evacuation β hCG more than 10^5 U/L
  - Bilateral theca lutein cysts
  - Developing acute respiratory distress after evacuation
  - Postevacuation uterine hemorrhage/subinvolution
- Oral contraceptives given before hCG falls to normal.

Role of Prophylactic Chemotherapy

Though the use of prophylactic chemotherapy (PC) given as single course Actinomycin D/ Methotrexate- Folinic acid combination at the time of molar evacuation in high-risk molar pregnancies has been found to decrease the incidence of malignant sequel from 47 to 14 percent, the role of PC still remains controversial. The reasons could be:[2]
- Since only 15 percent of patients who develop post molar GTD belong to the high-risk category, (the remaining being in the groups with intermediate or low-risk criteria) basing treatment decisions upon risk factors is not appropriate.
- Since the drugs used for PC are the same that are used as first line treatment therapy, the risk of developing drug resistance remains.
- Since PC does not completely eliminate the risk of post-molar GTD, surveillance with serial hCG is still required.
- The risk of developing persistent tumor is 7.5-20 percent in complete moles and < than 5 percent in partial moles. Hence there is concern regarding the exposure of all patients to potentially toxic chemotherapy.

Currently therefore, the role of prophylactic chemotherapy may be limited to
- patients not compliant to follow up
- where reliable hCG surveillance is not available

Indications for Treatment with Chemotherapeutic Drugs

The risk of post-molar GTD ranges from 3 to 20 percent for partial and complete moles. Criteria used for the diagnosis of post-molar gestational trophoblastic disease are[3,4,7]
- Four values or more of hCG documenting a plateau (+/- 10% of hCG value) over at least 3 weeks: days 1, 7, 14,21
- A rise of hCG of 10 percent or more for 3 values or longer over at least 2 weeks: days 1, 7, 14
- Persistence of hCG 6 months after evacuation even if decreasing.
- Presence of histological evidence of choriocarcinoma.
- Heavy vaginal bleeding or evidence of gastrointestinal or intraperitoneal hemorrhage.
- Evidence of metastasis in liver, brain, GIT or radiological opacities in chest X-ray > 2 cm.

Role of Second Evacuation[14,15]

Up to 30 percent of patients may continue to bleed after evacuation. They may show an elevation of hCG along with presence of vascular molar tissue in the uterine cavity. While there is no clinical indication for the routine use of a second evacuation, it may be recommended in select cases where hCG is less than 5000 IU/L. Its role is, however, controversial. The main advantage is that it will obviate the need for chemotherapy in 10 to 20 percent patients. The use of ultrasound guidance

Table 2.2: Correlation between no. of evacuations and subsequent requirement of chemotherapy	
No. of evacuations	*Patients treated with chemotherapy %*
1	2.4
2	18
3	50
4	81

during the procedure will help to reduce the risk of uterine perforation. Further evacuations are not recommended because of the risk of complications and an increased likelihood of requiring chemotherapy (Table 2.2).

PREGNANCY AFTER HYDATIDIFORM MOLE

- The risk of a molar pregnancy in a woman whose last pregnancy was a complete or partial mole is about 1 percent.
- These women should undergo early ultrasound screening of all pregnancies to exclude recurrent mole More than 98 percent of such women will not have a repeat mole nor are they prone to obstetric complications.
- The placenta (or products of conception) should be sent for histopathological examination for evidence of occult trophoblastic disease.
- After completion of pregnancy, hCG levels should be checked after 6 weeks and 10 weeks to ensure no reactivation of previous molar disease.

CO EXISTENT FETUS AND HYDATIDIFORM MOLE

- The incidence of a twin pregnancy consisting of a normal conceptus and a coexisting complete mole is 0.005 to 0.01 percent of pregnancies.[2]
- A thorough obstetrical ultrasound to assess fetal anatomy, identify nonviable fetuses and fully characterize placental morphology is required. When there is diagnostic doubt about whether the pregnancy is a complete mole with a coexisting normal fetus or a partial mole, invasive testing for karyotyping should be considered.
- The outcome of such pregnancies is poor with a live birth rate of 25 percent. There is increased risk of early fetal loss (40%), premature delivery (36%) and preeclampsia.[13] The issue of increased propensity to develop persistent disease and metastases is controversial.

FALSE POSITIVE hCG LEVELS – THE PHANTOM hCG

Persistent low elevations of hCG may sometimes turn out to be false positive assays. These result from interference with hCG immunoreactive assays caused by nonspecific heterophile antibodies. False positives can be identified by:[2]
- Serial hCG values do not vary substantially inspite of prolonged observation
- Values do not change with therapeutic interventions like surgery or chemotherapy
- More than 5 fold difference is found in hCG results with alternative immunoassays
- Absence of detectable hCG or hCG related molecule immunoreactivity in a parallel urine sample
- Pretreatment of serum with heterophile antibody blocking agent prevents or limits false positives
- Lack of dilutional parallelism when serial dilutions of serum are tested
- Women with false positive results also commonly have falsely elevated results in other unrelated tests like CEA/CA-125/ PSA/TSH

KEY POINTS

- Hydatidiform mole is the benign end of the spectrum of gestational trophoblastic disease
- Serum β hCG is a reliable tumor marker used in the diagnosis and follow up of patients of H. mole
- The clinical presentation and gestational age at diagnosis of molar pregnancy has changed over the years.
- Suction curettage is the preferred method of evacuation irrespective of uterine size.
- Pregnancy should be avoided for at least 6 months after evacuation.
- Regular follow up is essential for the early diagnosis of gestational trophoblastic neoplasia.

REFERENCES

1. Palmer JR. Advances in the epidemiology of gestational trophoblastic disease. J Reprod Med 1994;39:155-62.
2. Hurteau JA. Gestational trophoblastic disease: management of hydatidiform mole. Clin Obstet Gynecol 2003;46:557-69.
3. Soper J, Creasman WT. Gestational Trophoblastic Disease, In: DiSaia PJ, Creasman WT (eds). Clinical Gynecologic Oncology.7th edn. Philadelphia: Saunders Elsevier, 2007. pp. 201-33.
4. Seckl MJ, Newlands ES. Management of Gestational Trophoblastic Disease. In: Gershenson D, McGuire W, Gore M, Quinn MA, Thomas G (eds). Gynecologic Cancer-Controversies in Management. Churchill Livingstone, 2004. pp. 555-73.
5. Royal College of Obstetricians and Gynaecologists. The Management of Early Pregnancy Loss. Green-top Guideline No. 25, 2nd ed. London RCOG; 2006.
6. Royal College of Obstetricians and Gynaecologists. The care of women requesting induced abortion. Evidence based Clinical Guideline No. 7. London RCOG; 2004.
7. Seckl MJ, Sebire NJ, Berkowitz RS. Gestational trophoblastic disease. Lancet 2010;376:717-29.
8. Fowler DJ, Lindsay I, Seckl MJ, Sebire NJ. Routine pre-evacuation ultrasound diagnosis of hydatidiform mole: experience of more than 1000 cases from a regional referral center. Ultrasound Obstet Gynecol 2006;27:56-60.
9. Benson CR, Genest DR, Bernstein MR, Soto Wright V, Goldstein DR, Berkowitz RS. Sonographic appearance of first trimester complete hydatidiform moles. J Ultrasound Obstet Gynecol 2000;16:188-91.
10. Cole LA, Muller CY. Hyperglycosylated hCG in the management of quiescent and chemorefractory gestational trophoblastic diseases. Gynecol Oncol 2010;116:3-9.
11. Gestational Trophoblastic Disease. In: Cunningham FG, Leveno KJ, Bloom SL, Hauth JC, Rouse DJ, Spong CY (eds). Williams Obstetrics. 23rd edn. McGraw Hill, 2010. pp. 257-65.
12. Tidy J, Gillespie AM, Bright N, Radstone CR, Coleman RE, Hancock BW. Gestational Trophoblastic Disease; a study of mode of evacuation and subsequent need for treatment with chemotherapy. Gynecol Oncol 2000;78;309-12.
13. Royal College of Obstetricians and Gynaecologists. The Management of Gestational Trophoblastic Disease. Green-top Guideline No. 38. London RCOG; 2010.
14. Pezeshki M, Hancock BW, Silocks P, Everard JE, Coleman J, Gillespie AM, et al. The role of repeat uterine evacuation in the management of persistent gestational trophoblastic disease. Gynecol Oncol 2004;95:423-9.
15. Savage P, Short D, Fuller S, Seckl MJ. Review of the role of second uterine evacuation in the management of molar pregnancy. Gynecol Oncol 2005;99:251-2.

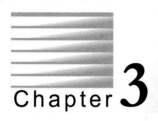

Chapter **3**

Inevitable and Incomplete Abortion

Shakun Tyagi, Parul Rathore

Introduction

Abortion is the expulsion of an embryo or fetus weighing 500 grams or less.[1] This is estimated to be at 20-22 weeks of gestation (154 days) by the WHO. Abortion may be classified as inevitable, incomplete or complete depending on the stage of expulsion of products of conception. In this chapter, discussion will be restricted to inevitable and incomplete abortion.

Etiology of spontaneous abortion is multifactorial. Approximately, 50 to 60 percent of embryos that are spontaneously aborted contain chromosomal anomalies.[2] Endocrine and metabolic factors account for 10 to 15 percent cases of spontaneous abortion. Anatomical factor accounts for 10-15% cases. This includes cervical incompetence, congenital anomalies of uterus, uterine fibroid and uterine adhesions. Other causes are: infections (5% cases), immunological causes (5-10), maternal medical illness and ABO blood group incompatibility. About 40 to 60 percent cases might remain unexplained. Advanced age, extremes of age, stress, and advanced paternal age are independent risk factors for a spontaneous abortion.[3, 4, 5]

INEVITABLE ABORTION

An inevitable abortion involves continuous and progressive dilation of the cervix without expulsion of the products of conception before the period of viability. In this presentation the changes have progressed to a state from where continuation of pregnancy is impossible.

CASE SCENARIO-1

A primigravida, married for 6 months, presents to the casualty with history of two and a half months amenorrhea with cramping pain in lower abdomen and bleeding for 6 hours with history of passage of clots. Pain is felt in the suprapubic region radiating to the back. She has no history of preceding illness, trauma, intercourse or drug intake.

> **Comment:** Any sexually active female patient with amenorrhea followed by abnormal bleeding should be considered to have a pregnancy complication unless proven otherwise.

About 25 to 30 percent of all pregnancies have some bleeding during early pregnancy. Bleeding may subside on its own and the pregnancy may continue as in case of threatened abortion or it may represent a prelude to a sequence of events which may end with abortion.

Differential Diagnosis

- Threatened abortion
- Inevitable abortion
- Incomplete abortion
- Missed abortion
- Hydatidiform mole
- Ectopic pregnancy
- Gynecological causes like pregnancy with CIN, cervical polyp or cancer cervix

POINTS TO BE NOTED IN HISTORY

- Date of last menstrual period: To know the period of gestation
- Bleeding: Details of bleeding should include degree, duration, presence and passage of tissue. Bleeding may be quantified roughly by the number of pads soaked per hour. An average pad absorbs approximately 20 to 30 mL of blood. Quantification of the amount of bleeding is very important because life-threatening hemorrhage may occur during the process of abortion. The presence of blood clots suggests heavy bleeding. The passage of blood clots may be confused with passage of products of conception (POC). Ask for the history of passage of any grape-like vesicles which would be suggestive of hydatidiform mole. History of altered coloured bleeding is suggestive of missed abortion or subchorionic bleed
- Abdominal pain: The pain is usually in the suprapubic area, but complaint of pain in one or both lower quadrants is not uncommon. The pain may radiate to the lower back, buttocks, genitalia, and perineum. If the pain is only on one side, consider an ectopic pregnancy or complications related to coexisting ovarian cyst (rupture, torsion, hemorrhage) as possible causes.
- History of any prior surgical uterine evacuation or foul smelling discharge will have to be enquired to rule out septic abortion or persistent trophoblastic disease
- Also enquire regarding any previous scans during current pregnancy
- Other symptoms such as fever or chills are more characteristic of an infection, such as in a septic abortion. In such a case detailed history suggestive of any gynecological intervention or any systemic infection such as malaria should be taken.
- History of fainting attack with pain lower abdomen with pallor and hypotension in excess of the observed bleeding is suggestive of ruptured ectopic pregnancy.
- History of use of any drugs for any medical disorder or for the purpose of medical abortion should be taken.
- History of any chronic illness such as diabetes, thyroid disease, renal disease and hypertension should be taken.

> **History in this case:** Amenorrhea of two and a half month followed by lower abdominal pain and heavy bleeding (passage of clots) is suggestive of spontaneous abortion (miscarriage).

POINTS TO BE NOTED IN EXAMINATION

General

Estimating the patient's hemodynamic stability is the first step in examination. Obtain orthostatic vital signs- pulse, blood pressure (BP) and respiratory rate (RR). Check for pallor.

Brief general physical and systemic examination is performed followed by abdominal and pelvic examinations.

Cardiovascular and Respiratory System Examination

Abdominal Examination

The abdominal examination helps determine whether or not the state of an acute abdomen is present. If rebound tenderness or abdominal distension is present, ectopic pregnancy should be the primary diagnosis. In case of suspected ectopic pregnancy, pallor is more than the evident blood loss.

Pelvic Examination

Per Speculum (P/S) Examination

In case of heavy vaginal bleeding it is not much informative as cervix and vagina are not well visualized. In the absence of heavy bleeding, the cervix and vagina should be examined carefully. An open cervical os is suggestive of inevitable abortion. If the cervix and vagina are inflamed and there is foul smelling discharge along with history of pain, lower abdomen, suspect septic abortion.

Per Vaginum (P/V) Examination

Check for cervical excitation pain which is suggestive of either ectopic pregnancy or local infection. Check the status of internal os in a multiparous patient. Assess for the position and size of the uterus, whether it corresponds to the period of gestation, uterine or forniceal tenderness and for any adnexal mass.

Size of the uterus can be less than period of gestation in case of:
• Incomplete abortion
• Missed abortion
• Wrong dates

Size of the uterus can be more than period of gestation in case of:
• Wrong date
• Multiple pregnancy
• Fibroid uterus
• Hydatidiform mole
• Retroplacental bleed or clot

> **Examination in this case**
> The patient was pale; Pulse- 126/minute, BP - 94/60 mm Hg.
> Abdominal examination- was normal with soft abdomen.
> Local examination- sanitary pad was completely soaked with blood.
> P/S- cervical os open with POCs protruding through it.
> P/V- os open, POCs felt protruding through os, uterus was soft, enlarged to about 8 to 10 weeks size, non tender, bilateral fornices were free.

Diagnosis

Inevitable abortion

INVESTIGATIONS

• Blood for grouping and cross-matching in case patient presents with heavy bleeding or severe anemia as she may need blood transfusion. Rh typing is important to determine whether anti-D immunoglobulins are required.

- *Hemogram:* It will help document the amount of blood loss and whether anemia is present. If the hemoglobin (<7g/dL) and hematocrit are very low and the patient is symptomatic then blood component (packed cell) transfusions would be warranted. The white blood cell counts will provide evidence regarding infection (elevated counts and a left shift on differential count).
- Bleeding time, clotting time and clot retraction time in cases of excessive hemorrhage. Full coagulation profile with prothrombin time if these investigations are abnormal.
- Urine sugar and albumin examination: Urine ketones should be checked if patient presents with excessive vomiting.
- *Imaging Studies:* Transvaginal sonography should be performed when diagnosis is doubtful to rule out an ectopic pregnancy, retained POC, hematometra or other etiologies.

TREATMENT

The treatment depends on the hemodynamic status of the patient and type of abortion.

In women who present with hemodynamic compromise, hemodynamic stability is established and simultaneously preparations are made for surgical evacuation of the uterus.

- Secure IV access should be established using two 16 gauge cannulae and crystalloids should be administered initially depending on the estimated blood loss.
- Vacuum aspiration has been the method of choice for management of miscarriage where there is an intact intrauterine sac. A cochrane review concluded that vacuum aspiration is superior to sharp curettage, being associated with decreased blood loss and shorter duration of procedure.[6]
- The products of conception should be examined for presence of villi by naked eye and should be subjected to histopathological examination for confirmation of pregnancy and to rule out hydatidiform mole.

> **Treatment in this case:** Patient was resuscitated with IV fluids. Suction evacuation of the uterus was done and POC were sent for histopathological examination.

INCOMPLETE ABORTION

Definition

Failure of early pregnancy when the entire POC are not expelled, instead a part is retained in the uterine cavity; it is defined as incomplete abortion.

CASE SCENARIO-2

A G3P2L2 with 3 months amenorrhea presented to the outpatient clinic with history of pain and bleeding per vaginum for five days. There was history of intake of some abortifacient drug about a week ago followed by passage of some fleshy mass.

> **Comment:** Continued excessive bleeding even after passage of POC should make one suspect incomplete abortion.

Differential Diagnosis

Other causes of first trimester bleeding as discussed earlier
Following points should be noted in history:
As in case of inevitable abortion, history is taken regarding details of bleeding, pain, any prior surgical intervention, fever or any foul smelling discharge.

Examination in this case
Vital signs- stable.
General and systemic examination -unremarkable
Abdominal examination- soft abdomen, bowel sounds present, no guarding, tenderness or rigidity.
P/S- cervical os closed, slight bleeding present.
P/V - No cervical excitation pain, cervical os closed, uterus anteverted, 6 wks in size, soft, mobile and bilateral fornices free.

History and examination help in making the diagnosis to plan further management. In case of incomplete abortion, the size of the uterus is less than the period of gestation.

If cervical excitation pain is present with normal size uterus associated with adnexal mass, a strong possibility of ectopic pregnancy should be considered.

Investigations in this case:
- Blood group and Rh typing- A+
- Hemogram –Hb 9g%
- Urine routine and microscopy- albumin/sugar nil
- USG Pelvis (to check for the contents of the uterus and any adnexal mass) - echogenic contents in the uterine cavity measuring 20mm. Bilateral ovaries were normal. No free fluid in the pelvic cavity.

Treatment in this case: Surgical evacuation of the uterus was performed and POC were sent for histopathological examination.

NON-SURGICAL MANAGEMENT

- Classically all patients with inevitable, missed or incomplete abortion are managed by surgical evacuation of the uterus. Prior vaginal prostaglandin administration in cases of missed abortion and incomplete abortion with closed cervical os is associated with significant reduction in dilatation force, hemorrhage and uterine/cervical trauma.
- Apart from surgical evacuation, women who are not bleeding excessively and are stable can be managed expectantly or by using medical methods. According to the Royal College of Obstetricians and Gynaecologists (RCOG) guidelines for early pregnancy loss, protocols should be developed locally with selection criteria, therapeutic regimens and arrangements for follow-up for various types of abortion. With increasing interest in medical abortion evidence is now available in favour of expectant and medical management for various types of abortion.
- **The drawback of expectant and conservative management is that it can be offered only to those women who can access 24 hour emergency services.**
- **Expectant management**- is an effective and acceptable method to offer to women who are diagnosed with incomplete or inevitable abortion. Women should be counselled that complete resolution may take several weeks and surgical evacuation might be required at a later date. Efficacy depends on the type of miscarriage, duration of follow-up and whether ultrasound or clinical assessment is used for review.
- **Medical methods** – Medical methods are an effective alternative in the management of confirmed first-trimester miscarriage. Various medical methods for uterine evacuation have been described using prostaglandin analogues (misoprostol or gemeprost) with or without antiprogesterone priming (mifepristone). Efficacy rates for these medical methods vary widely from 13 percent to 96 percent depending on the type of miscarriage, sac size, whether follow-up is clinical or involves ultrasound, total dose and route of administration. Higher success rates (70-96%) have been associated with incomplete miscarriage, high dose misoprostol (1200-1400 µg), prostaglandins administered vaginally and clinical follow-up without routine ultrasound.[7,8, 9] Sufficient evidence is available to prove that misoprostol is a safe and effective means of non-surgical uterine evacuation. A single dose of 600 micrograms oral or vaginal misoprostol is recommended in women with a uterine size less than or equivalent to 12 weeks.[10]

Type of abortion	Ultrasound findings	Clinical presentation	Action
	Table 3.1: Brief overview of various types of abortions[16]		
Threatened abortion	Intrauterine pregnancy, i.e. gestation sac with yolk sac; +/- fetal pole and cardiac activity	Bleeding; +/- pain; Speculum/pelvic examination: os closed	Reassure. Follow up depending on symptoms
Inevitable abortion	Intrauterine pregnancy, i.e. gestation sac with yolk sac; +/- fetal pole and cardiac activity	Bleeding; +/- pain; Speculum/pelvic examination: os open	Loss of pregnancy inevitable. Evaluate for amount of bleeding and discuss options for evacuation
Incomplete abortion	Retained products of conception	Bleeding; +/- pain; Speculum/pelvic examination: +/- os open, +/- products at the os	Evaluate for amount of bleeding discuss options
Complete abortion	Empty uterus; or USG appearances showing less than 15 mm in diameter of retained tissue	Minimal bleeding; pain usually absent; Speculum/pelvic examination: os closed	Explain, Reassure and follow up.
Missed abortion/ early fetal demise/ an embryonic pregnancy	CRL > 6 mm, no cardiac activity. Empty gestational sac with mean diameter > 20 mm	Dark coloured altered bleeding; +/- pain	Expectant/medical/ surgical evacuation

The advantages of medical methods over surgical evacuation are better patient acceptability, decreased incidence of pelvic infection, management possible on a day-care and outpatient requirement. An increase in pain, bleeding and possible need for emergency surgical evacuation are negative factors influencing acceptability. To avoid anxiety patients need to be informed that bleeding may continue for 3 weeks after medical uterine evacuation.

A Cochrane review drew the following conclusions regarding the use of medical methods for uterine evacuation[11]:
- Safe and effective medical methods are available.
- Combined regimens are more effective than single agents.
- Dose of mifepristone can be safely lowered to 200 mg without significantly decreasing effectiveness.
- Vaginal misoprostol is more effective than oral and has less side-effect than sublingual or buccal administration.

Contraindications: Medical method should not be offered to the women with hemodynamic instability, evidence of infected retained tissue and persistent excessive bleeding where surgical evacuation of the uterus should be carried out. It is also contraindicated in suspected cases of gestational trophoblastic disease (GTD). [12]

OTHER ASPECTS OF MANAGEMENT

- *Postabortal intrauterine contraceptive device (IUCD):* If the patient is desirous of temporary method of contraception insertion of an IUCD immediately after abortion is safe and practical according to a recent Cochrane review.[13] Although, IUD expulsion rates appear higher in postabortal IUD insertion than after interval insertions, IUD use is higher at six months with immediate than with interval insertion.
- *Postabortal antibiotic:* According to a Cochrane review, there is not enough evidence to evaluate a policy of routine antibiotic prophylaxis to women with incomplete abortion.[14] In the absence of

enough evidence regarding the use of antibiotics post evacuation the local hospital policy should be followed. Either preoperative single dose of ciprofloxacin and metronidazole or post evacuation five dose therapy can be given.

- *Injection Anti-D:* A non-sensitized Rh-negative woman should receive Anti-D antibodies within 72 hours of miscarriage to prevent complications due to Rh isoimmunization during subsequent pregnancy. Injection anti-D immunoglobin (Ig) is administered in a dose of 250 IU up to 19+6 weeks of gestation. Anti-D Ig should be given to all non-sensitised Rh D-negative women who have a spontaneous complete or incomplete miscarriage at or after 12+0 weeks of gestation and those undergoing surgical or medical evacuation of the uterus, regardless of gestation. Anti-D Ig is not required for spontaneous miscarriage before 12+0 weeks of gestation, provided there is no instrumentation.[15] In the market 150 μgm Anti-D is available for Rh-ve women undergoing abortion.

CONCLUSION

Inevitable and incomplete abortion have similar etiologies and might present in a similar clinical fashion except for few basic differences regarding the status of cervical os and whether the patient has already passed any products of conception. Both inevitable and incomplete abortions have similar treatment but final management option will depend on the hemodynamic status of the patient and the method of uterine evacuation that patient accepts. It is important to identify the patients with ectopic pregnancy, septic abortion or GTD who present with first trimester bleeding per vaginum.

KEY POINTS

- Complications related to pregnancy should always be ruled out in a sexually active woman in reproductive age group who presents with abnormal bleeding per vaginum.
- Inevitable abortion and incomplete abortion represent stages in the series of events when products of conception are expelled from the uterine cavity during the process of spontaneous abortion.
- The hemorrhage during inevitable abortion and incomplete abortion can be life threatening if the uterine cavity is not timely evacuated.
- In hemodynamically stable women the management is gradually shifting towards medical methods of uterine evacuation.

REFERENCES

1. Abortion. In : Cunningham FG, Kenneth JL, Bloom SL, Hauth JC, Gilstrap LC III, Wenstrom KD (eds).Williams Obstetrics.22nd edn . India: Mcgraw Hill, 2005. pp. 232-51.
2. Kajii T, Ferrier A, Niikawa N, Takahara H, Ohama K, Avirachan S. Anatomic and chromosomal anomalies in 639 spontaneous abortuses. Hum Genet 1980;55:87-98.
3. Arck PC, Rucke M, Rose M, et al. Early risk factors for miscarriage: a prospective cohort study in pregnant women. Reprod Biomed Online 2008;17:101-13.
4. Maconochie N, Doyle P, Prior S, Simmons R. Risk factors for first trimester miscarriage results from a UK-population-based case-control study. BJOG 2007;114:170-86.
5. Gracia CR, Sammel MD, Chittams J, Hummel AC, Shaunik A, Barnhart KT. Risk factors for spontaneous abortion in early symptomatic first-trimester pregnancies. Obstet Gynecol 2005;106:993-9.
6. Forna F, Gulmezoglu AM. Surgical procedures to evacuate incomplete abortion. Cochrane database Syst Rev 2001;(1):CD001993.
7. Hinshaw HKS. Medical management of miscarriage. In: Grudzinskas JG, O'Brien PMS (eds). Problems in Early Pregnancy: Advances in diagnosis and management. London: RCOG press, 1997.pp. 284-95.
8. el-Refaey H, Hinshaw K, Henshaw R, Smith N, Templeton A. Medical management of missed abortion and an embryonic pregnancy. BMJ 1992;305:1399.

9. Henshaw RC, Cooper K, el-Refaey H, Smith NC, Templeton AA. Medical management of miscarriage: non-surgical uterine evacuation of incomplete and inevitable spontaneous abortion. BMJ 1993;306:894-5.

10. Blum J, Winikoff B, Gemzell-Danielsson K, Ho PC, Schiavon R, Weeks A. Treatment of incomplete abortion and miscarriage with misoprostol. Int J Gynaecol Obstet 2007;99:S186-9.

11. Kulier R, Gülmezoglu AM, Hofmeyr GJ, Cheng LN, Campana A. Medical methods for first trimester abortion. Cochrane Database Syst Rev 2004;(2):CD002855.

12. Ballagh SA, Harris HA, Demasio K. Is curettage needed for uncomplicated incomplete spontaneous abortion? Am J Obstet Gynecol 1998;179:1279-82.

13. Grimes DA, Lopez LM, Schulz KF, Stanwood NL. Immediate postabortal insertion of intrauterine devices. Cochrane Database Syst Rev 2010;(6):CD001777.

14. May W, Gülmezoglu AM, Ba-Thike K. Antibiotics for incomplete abortion. Cochrane Database Syst Rev 2007;(4):CD001779.

15. The Use of Anti-D Immunoglobulin for Rhesus D Prophylaxis. Green-top Guideline No. 22; March 2011; http://www.rcog.org.uk/files/rcog-corp/GTG22AntiD.pdf

16. Cheong Y, Umranikar A. Problems in early pregnancy. In: Luesley DM, Baker PN (eds). Obstetrics and Gynaecology: An Evidence-based Text for MRCOG. 2nd edn. London: Hodder Arnold, 2010. pp. 649-56.

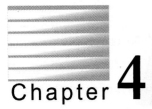

Chapter 4

Septic Abortion

Deepti Goswami

INTRODUCTION

Abortion is fetal loss before 20 weeks of pregnancy. Septic abortion is characterized by infection of the uterus and its contents. It usually follows unsafe abortion or incomplete abortion. Retained products of conception (POC) are a good culture media for the infecting organisms, most common being *E. coli*, streptococci and anaerobes. The infection may spread up and involve myometrium, parametrium, tubes, ovaries and peritoneum.

Unsafe abortion is the one done by person lacking the necessary skills or in an environment lacking the minimal standards of care. Worldwide, one in eight (13%) maternal deaths (i.e. 67,000), are due to unsafe abortion. Somewhere in the world a woman dies every 8 minutes because of an unsafe abortion[1] while another 5 million suffer long-term complications.

Although medical termination of pregnancy (MTP) is legal in India since 1971, largest number of deaths from unsafe abortions occurs here accounting for 8.9 percent of maternal deaths (around 15,000) every year. Sixty to seventy percent of the cases hospitalized with septic abortion report interference by unqualified person.[2-6] Common clinical presentations of septic abortion and their management are discussed here.

CASE SCENARIO-1

A 30-year-old woman G5P4 L4 presented to the emergency with history of 2 months amenorrhea and MTP done 5 days back. She was complaining of high-grade fever for the past 3 days, lower abdominal pain and bleeding per vaginum.

Comments: Diagnosis of septic abortion should be considered since she complained of vaginal bleeding, lower abdominal pain and fever ≥100.4°F for more than 24 hours.

Differential Diagnosis

- Other causes of bleeding in early pregnancy—incomplete abortion, ectopic pregnancy, hydatidiform mole.
- Fever due to other cause like urinary tract infection

POINTS TO BE NOTED IN HISTORY

- History of interference—how, where and by whom was the inference done, use of abortifacients.
- Fever—whether it was associated with chills, general malaise
- Bleeding—duration, amount and presence of clots or pieces of tissue
- Cramping—duration, severity location and any history of fainting (which may be suggestive of ectopic pregnancy)
- Any complaint of dysuria, decreased urinary output
- Any complain of diarrhea, tenesmus (suggest pelvic abscess)
- Past obstetrical and gynecological history.

> **History in this case:**
> History of abortion done with instruments by a doctor at a clinic in village. The next day she developed fever, malaise, mild continuous bleeding with cramping pain per abdomen. No urinary or bowel complaints.

POINTS TO BE NOTED IN EXAMINATION

General

- General condition
- Temperature, pulse, respiratory rate (RR) and blood pressure (BP)
- Pallor, jaundice
- Urinary output <30 mL/hour is a sign of low blood volume seen with shock, hemorrhage, dehydration and can be a sign of renal failure.

Cardiovascular and Respiratory System Examination

Abdominal Examination

- Location and severity of pain
- Tenderness, guarding, rigidity and rebound tenderness
- Presence of free fluid in peritoneal cavity
- Bowel sounds
- Whether the uterus is palpable per abdomen.

Pelvic Examination

Per Speculum (P/S) Examination

- Bleeding: Amount and site of bleeding
- Visible POC are gently removed with an ovum forceps and sent for histopathology
- Cervical os: Whether closed or open
- Cervical discharge: Amount, color and smell. Cervical swab is sent for gram stain, culture and sensitivity.
- Lacerations and foreign matter

Per Vaginum (P/V) Examination

- Uterine size and position: To help avoid uterine perforation during evacuation.
- Tenderness on palpation of the uterus, adnexae or when the uterus is moved (differential diagnosis- ectopic pregnancy)
- Pelvic masses: Suggest presence of tubo-ovarian masses/abscess (differential diagnosis- ectopic pregnancy, ovarian tumor, fibroid).

> **Examination in this case:**
> Pulse—104/min, BP—110/70 mm Hg, Temp—101°F, RR—24/min
> General and systemic examination-unremarkable
> Abdominal examination- unremarkable
> P/S—necrotic foul smelling POC in vagina, mild bleeding from the os.
> P/V—Uterus bulky, soft, os open, POC felt through os, significant tenderness in both fornices, no adnexal mass

Diagnosis

Septic abortion

INVESTIGATIONS

Hemoglobin, hematocrit, complete blood counts, blood group
Kidney and liver function tests
Blood culture should be sent before starting antibiotics. It may be negative in more than 50 percent
of cases of severe sepsis or septic shock
Urine routine and microscopy and culture, cervical swab for culture and sensitivity,
Ultrasonography (USG) of pelvis

> **Investigations in this case:**
> * Hemoglobin—10 g%, hematocrit—30 %
> * Blood group, Rh testing—B+
> * Complete blood count—14,000/cu mm with raised neutrophils
> * Blood urea, serum creatinine, liver function tests—Normal
> * Blood culture was sent
> * Urine—albumin, sugar and microscopy—normal.
> * Cervical swab was for culture and sensitivity.
> * USG—Bulky uterus with retained POC, no adnexal mass/free fluid.

TREATMENT

Intravenous antibiotics and evacuation of the uterus.
  a. *Antibiotics:* Effective against gram-negative, gram-positive, anaerobic organisms and *Chlamydia*
     are used in septic abortion.
  b. *Uterine evacuation:* The retained products of conception should be evacuated under antibiotic
     cover.
     * Vacuum aspiration is avoided if there is prior interference.
     * Oxytocin (20 units in 500 mL of IV fluid) and methylergometrine (0.2 mg IM) are used to
       manage atonic uterus.
     * Intrauterine contraceptive device is not inserted at the time of evacuation.
     * Evacuated POC are sent for histopathology.
  c. *Further management:*
     * Close monitoring for fever, pulse rate, bleeding per vaginum and symptomatic improvement.
     * Antibiotics need to be changed if patient does not improve within 48 hours or if reports
       indicate that the bacteria are resistant.
       If fever persists other causes of fever (typhoid, malaria) should also be investigated.
     * IV therapy is continued until the patient is afebrile for 48 hours and is followed by oral
       treatment. Doxycyclin (100 mg 2 times daily) is given for 14 days.
  d. *Tetanus immunoprophylaxis:*
  e. *Follow-up and contraceptive counseling*
     Anti-D immunoglobulin is given to Rh-negative women; the dose is 50-100 µg for sensitizing
events in first trimester and 300 µg for second trimester.[7]

Treatment in this case:
Ampicillin 1g intravenous (IV) every 6 hours
Gentamicin 80 mg IV every 12 hours
Metronidazole 500 mg IV every 8 hours
Retained POCs were evacuated under antibiotic cover and sent for histopathology
A booster dose of tetanus toxoid 0.5 mL was given

CASE SCENARIO-2

A 28-year-old woman G4 P3L3 was brought to the emergency complaining of acute pain abdomen, bleeding per vaginum and having not passed urine for 12 hour. History of interference by *Dai* to terminate pregnancy of 3 months duration.

Comment: The history suggests unsafe abortion. Development of acute abdomen and decreased urine output soon after the interference should make one suspect intestinal perforation and possibility of renal failure.

Differential Diagnosis

- Ectopic pregnancy
- Acute abdomen due to surgical cause, e.g. acute appendicitis.

Proceed for History and Examination as Discussed in Case 1

History in this case: Interference by *Dai* 2 days back – some abortifacient and instrument was inserted per vaginum. She developed severe pain abdomen with vomiting thereafter and had not passed urine for the past 12 hours.

Examination in this case:
General condition unsatisfactory, extremities warm
Pulse-110/min, BP- 84 systolic, RR-40/min, Temperature-101.4°F
Pallor –significant, no jaundice or cyanosis
Respiratory and cardiovascular examination -tachypnea and tachycardia
Abdominal examination - tenderness with guarding and rigidity, no free fluid, no mass; bowel sounds absent.
P/S – mild bleeding, os open.
P/V- POC felt through os, uterus 12 weeks size, tender, vague fullness in pouch of Douglas.
Patient catheterized- No urine obtained

Diagnosis

Septic abortion with septic shock, generalized peritonitis and suspected renal failure

IMMEDIATE TREATMENT IN SUCH CASES

Management of Shock[8,9]

a. *Universal measures:*
   - Airway should be open
   - Do not give anything orally as patient may vomit and aspirate
   - Keep the patient warm but do not over heat
   - Maintain circulation to vital organs by elevating the legs. Too much elevation is avoided as it will cause blood to collect in the uterus.
b. *Oxygen:* By mask or nasal cannulae at 6 to 8 liters/minute.

c. *Fluids:* Two IV access should be set up with 16–18 gauge needle and blood is collected for investigations. Normal saline or ringer lactate is started at a rate of 1 liter in 20 to 30 minutes; 1 to 3 liters of fluids infused at this rate help stabilize the patient. The rate is adjusted to 1 liter in 6 to 8 hours once the low fluid volume has been corrected, as indicated by systolic BP of at least 100 mm Hg, heart rate under 90 and urine output of at least 100 mL per 4 hours.

d. *Blood transfusion* - To maintain hemoglobin of 7-9 g%.[8]

e. *Vasopressors* are used to maintain mean arterial pressure of at least 65 mm Hg; they are used only after correcting the inadequate intravascular volume. All patients requiring vasopressors should have an arterial line placed as soon as practical if resources are available.
   - Dopamine is started at a rate of 5 to 10 µg/kg/min IV and the infusion is adjusted according to the BP. Some patients may require high doses of up to 20 µg/kg/min.
   - Norepinephrine is started if the patient remains hypotensive despite volume infusion and moderate doses of dopamine. The dose range is 2 to 20 µg/min IV titrated according to hemodynamic response.
   - Epinephrine is used when BP is poorly responsive to norepinephrine or dopamine. The dose range is 1 to 10 µg/min IV titrated according to hemodynamic response.

f. *Inotropes:* Dobutamine is not routinely used in septic shock as it can lower systemic vascular resistance and cause hypotension. It is recommended when cardiac output remains low despite fluid resuscitation and vasopressors.[8] Starting at 1 to 5 µg/kg/min IV the dose is titrated according to hemodynamic response; not to exceed 20 µg/kg/min.

g. *Steroids:* Stress-dose steroid therapy is given only if BP is poorly responsive to fluid and vasopressor therapy. Hydrocortisone 200 mg/day in four divided doses for 7 days or more is recommended for septic shock,[10] not more than 300 mg is given in a day. As patient improves glucocorticoids should be weaned and not stopped abruptly.

h. *Monitoring:* Pulse rate, oxygen saturation, blood pressure, respiratory rate, and input output. Central venous pressure is monitored and maintained at (8–10 cm water) to guide the fluid replacement. Arterial blood is sent for acid base and gas analysis (ABG). The aim is to raise the systemic pH above 7.1 to 7.2; this requires bicarbonate replacement (ABG abnormalities are discussed in a separate chapter in this book).

Investigations in this case:
- Hemoglobin—6g %, hematocrit—18 %
- Blood group, Rh testing –B +
- Complete blood count—18000/cu mm with raised neutrophils
- Blood urea—80 mg%, serum creatinine—2 mg%
- Liver function tests—Normal
- Blood culture was sent before starting the antibiotics.
- X-ray of chest and abdomen (in sitting and lying down position) - gas under diaphragm (suggestive of uterine or gut perforation).
- USG of abdomen and pelvis- enlarged uterus with retained POC, no adnexal mass, free fluid present in pouch of Douglas.

DEFINITIVE MANAGEMENT

a. *Antibiotics:* Should be started at the earliest in such cases.

b. *Stress ulcer prophylaxis* with H2 blockers or proton pump inhibitors. Ranitidine is given 50 mg IV every 8 hours. An alternative is Pentaprozole 80 mg twice daily, as an infusion given over 15 minutes.

c. *Tetanus immunoprophylaxis:* A booster dose of tetanus toxoid is given.

d. *Surgical Management:* In cases with suspected gut/uterine perforation and generalized peritonitis, an urgent laparotomy is required.

Treatment is this case:
- Inj ceftriaxone 2g IV every 12 hour and inj metronidazole 500 mg IV every 8 hours were started
- A booster dose of tetanus toxoid was given
- In view of suspected gut/uterine perforation, patient was taken up for urgent laparotomy.

Preoperative findings:
- Blood stained seropurulent fluid in peritoneal cavity
- 12 week size uterus with retained POC and fundal perforation
- Inflammed tubes and ovaries
- Perforation of small intestine (in ileum).

Procedure done in this case:
- Resection anastomosis of the intestinal injury by the surgeon
- Uterine evacuation under direct guidance-POC sent for histopathology
- Repair of the uterine perforation
- Thorough lavage of the peritoneal cavity with normal saline
- Abdominal closure leaving a drain in peritoneal cavity

FURTHER MANAGEMENT IN SUCH CASES

- Close monitoring in the intensive care unit postoperatively.
- Broad spectrum antibiotics - guided by cervical, urine and blood culture reports -avoid nephrotoxic preparations in cases with renal failure.
- Further blood transfusions according to the hematocrit
- Monitor for development of complications e.g. disseminated intravascular coagulopathy (DIC).
- Renal failure may require dialysis.

OTHER CLINICAL PRESENTATIONS

- *Pelvic abscess:* It presents as fullness or cystic fluctuant mass in posterior fornix. It is drained by posterior colpotomy.
- *Thrombosis and embolisation:* Chemical abortifacients cause coagulation necrosis of the decidua and thrombosis of the intrauterine and parametrial veins which may spread to the pelvic, paravaginal, paracervical, and ovarian veins. This may lead to gangrene of the uterus and other body parts like lower limbs.[11] Patient then requires hysterectomy/surgical amputation of the affected part.
- *Jaundice and hepatic failure:* May occur due to hepatotoxic abortifacients or *Clostridium perfringens* infection (gas gangrene) which causes massive intravascular hemolysis.
- *DIC:* Due to consumptive coagulopathy – requires correction with packed cells and fresh frozen plasma according to the coagulation profile (bleeding time, clotting time, prothrombin time, activated partial thromboplastin time, FDP).
- *Tetanus:* Tetanus immunoprophylaxis involves drainage of pus and removal of foreign material and necrotic tissue. If patient is fully immunized within the last 10 years a booster dose is given. If not or if she is unsure of her vaccination status, both tetanus vaccine and tetanus antitoxin (3000 units) are given using separate needles and syringes and separate sites of administration. Case that has developed tetanus requires intensive management.
- *Gas gangrene:* Prophylactic use of anti gas gangrene serum (dose 8000 units) is recommended in severely infected cases. The diagnosis of gas gangrene is mainly clinical. There is severe pain and tenderness, local edema, skin discoloration, sweet mousy odour, crepitus, fever, tachycardia, and altered mental status. Treatment involves administration of antibiotics (Penicillin G, clindamycin, metronidazole, chloramphenicol, imipenum), and aggressive surgical debridement.
- In cases where pregnancy is associated with rape or in very young girls - screening for sexually transmitted infections and HIV.

PROGNOSIS

Prognosis depends upon the degree of infection present; time elapsed since intervention and presence of complications. In India, 13 to 25 percent of the cases admitted to hospital succumb to complications due to septic shock, hepato-renal failure and DIC.[3,4,6] Late complications include tubal block and infertility, pelvic inflammatory disease and chronic pelvic pain.

PREVENTION

In India most of the women admitted with septic abortion are parous and the reason for abortion in 81 percent of the cases is unwanted pregnancy.[6] Preventive steps therefore include family planning education and access to contraceptive and safe abortion services.[12]

KEY POINTS

- Diagnosis of septic abortion should be considered when a woman of reproductive age presents with vaginal bleeding, lower abdominal pain and fever.
- A thorough clinical and investigative workup is essential to establish the diagnosis and assess severity of illness.
- Early resuscitation of the septic patient is vital.
- Broad spectrum antibiotics should be given intravenously.
- Surgical management involves treatment of source of infection which includes retained products of conception, intestinal injury, pelvic abscess, peritonitis, gas gangrene, or tetanus.
- Indications for laparotomy are presence of pyoperitoneum, intestinal injury, intestinal obstruction, uterine perforation and hemorrhage.
- Complications of renal failure, jaundice, embolization, DIC and endotoxic shock require multidisciplinary involvement.
- Late complications are tubal block, infertility and chronic pelvic pain.

REFERENCES

1. Unsafe abortions: eight maternal deaths every hour. Lancet 2009;374:1301.
2. Duggal R, Ramachandran V. The abortion assessment project—India: key findings and recommendations. Reprod Health Matters 2004;12:122-9.
3. Chatterjee C, Joardar GK, Mukherjee G, Chakraborty M. Septic abortions: a descriptive study in a teaching hospital at North Bengal, Darjeeling. Indian J Public Health 2007;51:193-4.
4. Jain V, Saha SC, Bagga R, Gopalan S. Unsafe abortion: a neglected tragedy. Review from a tertiary care hospital in India. J Obstet Gynaecol Res 2004;30:197-201.
5. Varkey P, Balakrishna PP, Prasad JH, Abraham S, Joseph A. The reality of unsafe abortion in a rural community in South India. Reprod Health Matters 2000;8:83-91.
6. Sood M, Juneja Y, Goyal U. Maternal mortality and morbidity associated with clandestine abortions. J Indian Med Assoc 1995;93:77-9.
7. Clinical guidelines – ICOG Guideline Committee. Guidelines for the use of Anti-D Immunoglobulin for Rh Prophylaxis. 2009. www.fogsi.org/anti_d_immunoglobulin.pdf
8. Dellinger RP, Levy MM, Carlet JM, Bion J, Parker MM, Jaeschke R, et al. Surviving Sepsis Campaign: international guidelines for management of severe sepsis and septic shock: 2008. Crit Care Med 2008;36:296-327.
9. Clinical management of abortion complications: a practical guide. Geneva, World Health Organization, 1994
10. Marik PE, Pastores SM, Annane D, Meduri GU, Sprung CL, Arlt W, et al. Recommendations for the diagnosis and management of corticosteroid insufficiency in critically ill adult patients: consensus statements from an international task force by the American College of Critical Care Medicine. Crit Care Med 2008;36:1937-49.
11. Burnhill MS. Treatment of women who have undergone chemically induced abortions. J Reprod Med 1985;30:610-4.
12. Mathai M. Preventing unsafe abortion in India. Indian J Med Res 2005;122:98-9.

Chapter 5

Hyperemesis Gravidarum

Renu Tanwar

Introduction

Nausea and vomiting are common in pregnancy, occurring in 70 to 85 percent of all gravid women.[1] 50 percent of pregnant women have both nausea and vomiting, 25 percent have nausea only and 25 percent are unaffected.[2]

Definition

A standard definition of hyperemesis gravidarum is the occurrence of more than three episodes of vomiting per day with ketonuria and more than 3 kg or 5 percent weight loss. However, the diagnosis is usually made clinically following the exclusion of other causes.[3,4]

Hyperemesis gravidarum occurs in 0.5 to 2 percent of pregnancies.[5] Studies have found an admission rate of 0.8 percent for hyperemesis gravidarum[6] with an average hospital stay of 2.6 to 4 days.

The peak incidence is at 8 to 12 weeks of pregnancy, and symptoms usually resolve by week 20 in all but 10 percent of patients.[7] If vomiting begins after 9 weeks gestation, other causes should also be considered. Hyperemesis gravidarum can result in weight loss, nutritional deficiencies, and abnormalities in fluids, electrolyte levels, and acid-base balance.

There are two degrees of severity:[8]

Grade 1- Nausea and vomiting without metabolic imbalance.

Grade 2- Pronounced feeling of sickness with metabolic imbalance.

Pathogenesis

The cause of severe nausea and vomiting in pregnancy has not been identified, although some biological, physiological, psychological and sociocultural factors may contribute.

- Hyperemesis may have a **genetic component,** as sisters and daughters of women with hyperemesis have a higher incidence.
- Some theories hold that elevated human chorionic gonadotropin (hCG) or estradiol levels could be causative.
- Some studies have suggested that *Helicobacter pylori* infection may play a role in hyperemesis.[3]
- **Psychological theories** of the etiology are falling out of favor, and **the American College of Obstetrics and Gynecology** warns that attributing vomiting to psychological disorders has likely impeded progress in understanding the true etiology of hyperemesis gravidarum.

Risk Factors for Hyperemesis Gravidarum[9]

- Hyperemesis is associated with nulliparity, obesity, hyperemesis in prior pregnancy, female gestation, multiple gestation, triploidy, trisomy 21, current or prior molar pregnancy, and hydrops fetalis.
- Women with history of motion sickness, migraine headaches, psychiatric illness, pregestational diabetes, being underweight pregestation,[10] hyperthyroidism, pyridoxine deficiency, and gastrointestinal disorders.
- *Transient hyperthyroidism of hyperemesis gravidarum (THHG):* A self limiting transient hyperthyroidism of hyperemesis gravidarum may persist until 18 weeks of gestation and does not require treatment. [11] Assignment of a diagnosis of THHG requires the following[3]
  - Pathological serology results during hyperemesis
  - Negative history of hyperthyroidism before the pregnancy
  - Absence of thyroid antibodies
  Cigarette smoking and maternal age older than 30 years appear to be protective.

CASE SCENARIO-1

A 26-yrs-old primigravida presents to the emergency with the history of amenorrhea 2 months. She is complaining of nausea and vomiting 2 to 3 episodes/day for past 3 days.
Pulse-86/min, blood pressure (BP)-110/70 mm Hg.
Urine examination is negative for albumin, sugar and ketones.

> **Comment:** While nausea and vomiting of pregnancy is the most common cause, other causes may be operative in a few of the cases.

Differential Diagnosis of Vomiting in Pregnancy[9]

- *Pregnancy associated causes:*
  - Multiple pregnancy
  - Trophoblastic disease
  - Pre-eclampsia
- *Gynecological cause:*
  - Twisted ovarian cyst
- *Gastrointestinal cause:*
  Gastritis, cholecystitis, appendicitis, obstruction, peptic ulceration, hepatitis, pancreatitis, fatty liver of pregnancy
  When associated with diarrhea:
  - Food poisoning
  - Gastroenteritis
  - Medications (iron preparations, drug intoxication)
- *Urinary cause:* Urinary tract infection
  When associated with flank pain:
  - Pyelonephritis
  - Nephrolithiasis
- *Neurological cause:* Raised intracranial pressure
  When associated with neurological symptoms:
  - Porphyria
  - Vestibular disorders
- *Ear, nose and throat disease:*
  - Labyrinthitis
  - Meniere's disease
  - Motion sickness

- *Metabolic cause:*
  - Diabetic ketoacidosis
  - Thyrotoxic crisis
  - Addison's disease
- *Psychological cause:*
  - Bulimia nervosa

POINTS TO BE NOTED IN HISTORY

- Period of amenorrhea
- Vomiting—amount, number, contents
- Altered sense of taste, sensitive to odors
- Urine output
- History of fatigue, exhaustion,
- History of headache, epigastric pain, pyrexia, diarrhea, flank pain –to rule out other causes

POINTS TO BE NOTED IN EXAMINATION

General Examination

- Signs of dehydration – decreased skin turgor, postural changes in pulse, blood pressure.
- Acetone like breath
- Weight loss
- Temperature, respiratory rate, pulse, BP
- Pallor, jaundice
- Goitre

Cardiovascular and Respiratory System Examination

Abdominal Examination

- Tenderness –likely indicate another cause
- Whether the uterus is palpable or not

Pelvic Examination

Per Speculum (P/S) Examination

Look for cervical discharge

Per Vaginum (P/V) Examination

Check for uterine size, consistency, position -to confirm pregnancy; and rule out any adnexal mass

INVESTIGATIONS

- Complete blood count
- Liver function tests (LFTs). LFTs can be slightly elevated with hyperemesis gravidarum. (Enzymes <300 U/L, serum bilirubin <4 mg/dL)
- BUN and creatinine, serum electrolyte.
- Hyperthyroidism causing nausea and vomiting is rare, a free T3 and free T4 level should be drawn if this is a concern. Thyroid-stimulating hormone can be suppressed in hyperemesis.
- Serum amylase-to-creatinine ratio if pancreatitis is a concern.
- Urinalysis – may show elevated specific gravity and rule out other causes, e.g. pyelonephritis.
- Urine for albumin, sugar and ketones.
- Imaging—Ultrasonography (USG) to look for molar pregnancy or multiple gestations.

TREATMENT

Treatment is based on the severity of symptoms and should be multimodal in nature.
Initial management (In case scenario -1)
Mild forms of nausea and vomiting:

Dietary and Lifestyle Advice

- Intake of small amounts of fluids and food throughout the day
- Food should be rich in protein and low in fat and acid
- Light snacks, nuts, dairy products , beans, and dry and salty biscuits
- Avoid stress and take rest in the event of incipient nausea
- Emotional support and, if needed, psychosomatic care administered by a psychologist or a medical doctor with training in psychosomatics can be helpful.

Medication

- Tablet Pyridoxine (vitamin B_6)-10 to 25 mg and can be increased to 200 mg 3 to 4 times per day.[12]
- Tablet Doxylamine (antihistamine H1 receptor blocker) 12.5 mg 3 to 4 times per day. It can be used in combination with pyridoxine.[13] The combination is found to be safe with regard to fetal effects.
- Low dose antiemetics- Ondansetron (5 hydroxy tryptamine 3 receptor agonist) is one of the more commonly used and effective drug and has relatively few side effects.[14] Starting dosage is 4 mg, either IV or PO, and that dose may be repeated every 15-30 minutes until symptoms improve.
- Antihistamines and anticholinergics such as meclizine, dimenhydrinate and diphenhydramine have also been shown to be superior to placebo and can be used safely for the treatment of nausea and vomiting in pregnancy.[15]

The above mentioned medicaments may cause dizziness, drowsiness, constipation or dry mouth. More severe adverse effects comprise convulsions, decreased alertness, heartbeat alterations and hallucinations (doxylamine, metoclopramide, diphenhydramine, dimenhydrinate, promethazine). Headache, muscle pain or tremor and fever (prednisolone, prochlorperazine, promethazine, dimen-hydrinate, doxylamine, metoclopramide) may also occur.
Algorithm of pharmacological management[16] of hyperemesis gravidarum is given in Figure 5.1.

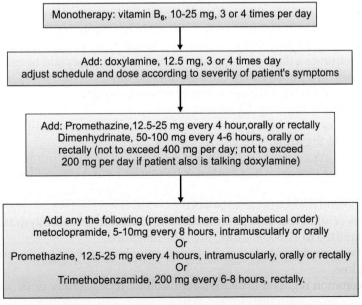

Figure 5.1: Algorithm of pharmacological management

Non-pharmacological Interventions

- Acupressure, especially on the P6 point (Neiguan) on the inside of the wrist.[17,18] There is still minimal experimental evidence that acupuncture is effective in relieving the symptoms of hyperemesis gravidarum.
- Ginger has a mild effect in ameliorating nausea and vomiting without negative effects on the fetus.[19] Available data show that ginger has no apparent teratogenic potential and can be used safely up to a daily dose of 1 gram.

CASE SCENARIO-2

Primigravida with 3 months amenorrhea presents to the emergency with complaints of excessive (8-10) vomiting for last 5 days. She also gives history of inability to tolerate even liquids, weakness and decreased urine output for last 1 day

> **Comment:** This patient has more severe symptoms and requires hospitalization and treatment under supervision.

> **Examination in this case:**
> Patient is dehydrated with low volume pulse-100/min and BP-90/70 mm Hg.
> Urine test done for ketones-moderate

Diagnosis

Hyperemesis gravidarum

Investigations

Investigations to be sent as discussed earlier.

Management

Hospitalization: When a patient cannot tolerate liquids without vomiting and has not responded to outpatient management or has developed severe dehydration or ketonuria then hospitalization, for evaluation and treatment is recommended.[2]

Maintaining hydration or, in the case of severe dehydration achieving quick and sufficient rehydration, is the most important intervention. No study has compared different fluid replacement for nausea and vomiting of pregnancy. Treatment should be continued until vomiting ceases or occurs less than three times a day. Subsequent food reintroduction should be carried out gradually.

- Volume and electrolyte replacement (at least 3 liters/day),
  - Normal saline or Lactated Ringer solution is recommended
  - Dextrose solutions may stop fat breakdown.
  - Continue treatment until the patient can tolerate oral fluids and until test results show little or no ketones in the urine.
- Thiamine- 100 mg intravenous (IV) daily for 2-3 days followed by intravenous multi vitamins is recommended for women who requires intravenous hydration and have vomited for more than 3 weeks.
- Correction of potential electrolyte imbalance
- Administration of vitamins and parenteral administration of carbohydrate and amino acid solutions (about 8400 to 10,500 kJ/day) are recommended.
- Steroids have been considered a last resort in patients who require enteral or parenteral nutrition due to weight loss.
  - The most common regimen is methylprednisolone 16 mg, orally or IV, every 8 hours for 3 days.

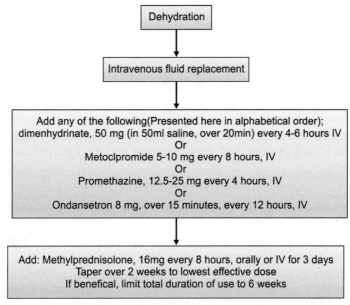

Figure 5.2: Algorithm of Management[16]

- Patients who do not respond within 3 days are not likely to respond.
- For those who do respond, the course may be tapered over 2 weeks.
- Some recent studies have demonstrated an association between oral clefts and methylprednisolone use in the first trimester.[2]
- The current recommendation is that corticosteroids be used with caution and avoided before 10 weeks' gestation. (Figure 5.2)

Additional Strategies

The principal criterion for introducing additional strategies is persistent weight loss.

Enteral Feeding Via Nasogastric Tube

- Well tolerated in pregnancy
- More cost effective
- *Helicobacter pylori* testing may be performed
- In the event of a positive result, H2 blockers (for example, cimetidine) or proton pump inhibitors (for example, omeprazol) can be added to infusions[8]

Total Parenteral Nutrition

- Total parenteral nutrition (TPN) may be useful in highly refractory cases in order to ensure a sufficient calorie intake.
- To date, no fetal or maternal benefit has been found in PICC (peripheral inserted central catheter) lines in comparison to serial peripheral catheters and the use of central catheters is only recommended in exceptional cases.[9]
- Complications could be infections and thrombosis or endocarditis.

PREVENTION

- Taking a multivitamin at the time of conception may decrease the severity of nausea and vomiting of pregnancy.

- Early treatment of nausea and vomiting of pregnancy is recommended to prevent progression to hyperemesis gravidarum.

PROGNOSIS

Nausea and vomiting during pregnancy is self limiting and is usually resolved by around 20 weeks gestation. Hyperemesis gravidarum may be associated with more serious complications including Mallory-Weiss syndrome (acute increase in esophageal pressure due to vomiting) and esophageal rupture (due to severe vomiting), pneumothorax, peripheral neuropathy, coagulopathy, Wernicke's encephalopathy (due to lack of thiamine), pre-eclampsia and fetal growth retardation.[12]

KEY POINTS

- Treatment of hyperemesis should be multimodal, ranging from dietary to psychosomatic counseling or psychoanalytic therapy
- Administration of antiemetic drugs may be necessary, as well as IV fluid replacement, food administration via nasogastric or parenteral routes in severe cases
- General practitioners and obstetricians should ensure that they are well informed about this condition so that they are able to provide advice, counseling and effective medication to pregnant women and thus prevent the exacerbation of symptoms.

REFERENCES

1. Bottomley C, Bourne T. Management strategies for hyperemesis. Best Pract Res Clin Obstet Gynaecol 2009;23:549-64.
2. American College of Obstetrics and Gynecology. ACOG (American College of Obstetrics and Gynecology) Practice Bulletin: nausea and vomiting of pregnancy. Obstet Gynecol 2004;103:803-14.
3. Golberg D, Szilagyi A, Graves L. Hyperemesis gravidarum and *Helicobacter pylori* infection: a systematic review. Obstet Gynecol 2007;110:695-703.
4. Gadsby R, Barnie-Adshead AM, Jagger C. Pregnancy nausea related to women's obstetric and personal histories. Gynecol Obstet Invest 1997;43:108-11.
5. Goodwin TM. Hyperemesis Gravidarum. Obstet Gynecol Clin N Am 2008;35:401-17.
6. Fell DB, Dodds L, Joseph KS, Allen VM, Butler B. Risk factors for hyperemesis gravidarum requiring hospital admission during pregnancy. Obstet Gynecol 2006;107:277-84.
7. Lacroix R, Eason E, Melzack R. Nausea and vomiting during pregnancy: A prospective study of its frequency, intensity, and patterns of change. Am J Obstet Gynecol 2000;182:931-7.
8. Mylonas I, Gingelmaier A, Kainer F. Nausea and vomiting in pregnancy. Dtsch Arztebl 2007;104:A1821-26.
9. Jueckstock JK, Kaestner R, Mylonas I. Managing hyperemesis gravidarum: a multimodal challenge. BMC Med 2010;8:46.
10. Cedergren M, Brynhildsen J, Josefsson A, Sydsjö A, Sydsjö G. Hyperemesis gravidarum that requires hospitalization and the use of antiemetic drugs in relation to maternal body composition. Am J Obstet Gynecol 2008;198:412.e1-5.
11. Glinoer D. The regulation of thyroid function in pregnancy: pathways of endocrine adaptation from physiology to pathology. Endocr Rev 1997;18:404-33.
12. Sheehan P. Hyperemesis gravidarum—assessment and management. Aust Fam Physician 2007;36:698-701.
13. Neutel CI, Johansen HL. Measuring drug effective by default: the case of Bendectin. Can J Public Health 1995;86:66-70.
14. World MJ. Ondansetron and hyperemesis gravidarum. Lancet 1993;341:185.
15. Leathem AM. Safety and efficacy of antiemetics used to treat nausea and vomiting in pregnancy. Clin Pharm 1986;5:660-8.
16. Levichek Z, Atanackovic G, Oepkes D, Maltepe C, Einarson A, Magee L, et al. Nausea and vomiting of pregnancy. Evidence-based treatment algorithm. Can Fam Physician 2002;48:267-8, 277.
17. de Aloysio D, Penacchioni P. Morning sickness control in early pregnancy by Neiguan point acupressure. Obstet Gynecol 1992;80:852-4.
18. Shin HS, Song YA, Seo S. Effect of Nei-Guan point (P6) acupressure on ketonuria levels, nausea and vomiting in women with hyperemesis gravidarum. J Adv Nurs 2007;59:510-9.
19. Portnoi G, Chng LA, Karimi-Tabesh L, Koren G, Tan MP, Einarson A. Prospective comparative study of the safety and effectiveness of ginger for the treatment of nausea and vomiting in pregnancy. Am J Obstet Gynecol 2003;189:1374-7.

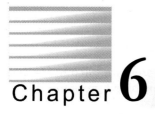

Chapter **6**

Hypertensive Emergencies in Pregnancy

Swaraj Batra, Savita Dagar, Seema

INTRODUCTION

Hypertensive emergencies are important causes of maternal mortality in our country. Hypertensive disorders complicate 5 to 10 percent of all pregnancies of which pre-eclampsia and eclampsia constitutes 70 percent and chronic hypertension 30 percent. Pre-eclampsia/ eclampsia is a multiorgan disorder in pregnancy and is an important cause of maternal and fetal morbidity and mortality. Three percent of severe preeclamptics will develop eclampsia if not given magnesium sulfate prophylaxis versus 0.3% of those who receive it. Twelve percent of women with severe pre-eclampsia- eclampsia develop HELLP syndrome (hemolysis, elevated liver enzyme and low platelets). Recurrence of pre-eclampsia in subsequent pregnancy is more likely if it developed before 30 weeks (70%) as against 25 percent risk if it developed at term in the previous pregnancy. HELLP syndrome recurs in 2 to 19 percent cases. These patients run more risk of developing chronic hypertension later in life.

Classification of Hypertension During Pregnancy (National High BP Education Programme (2000))[1]

Blood pressure (BP) should be recorded twice at 6 hours interval

Transient hypertension: The development of elevated BP during pregnancy or in the first 24 hours postpartum without other signs of pre-eclampsia or pre-existing hypertension (a retrospective diagnosis).

- *Pre-eclampsia-eclampsia:* Increased BP accompanied by proteinuria, edema, or both usually occurring after 20 weeks of gestation (or earlier with trophoblastic diseases such as hydatidiform mole or hydrops).
- *Chronic hypertension:* Hypertension (BP≥140/90 mm Hg) that is present and observable before pregnancy or that is diagnosed before the 20th week of gestation. It is also diagnosed if hypertension is diagnosed for the first time during pregnancy and persists beyond 42 days postpartum. The causes are - essential hypertension, renal diseases, thyrotoxicosis, pheochromocytoma, connective tissue disorders.
- *Pre-eclampsia superimposed on chronic hypertension:* Chronic hypertension (defined above) with increases in BP (30 mm Hg systolic, 15 mm Hg diastolic, or 20 mm Hg mean arterial pressure) together with appearance of proteinuria or generalized edema.

PRE-ECLAMPSIA

Criteria for Diagnosis of Pre-eclampsia

- *Hypertension:* Systolic blood pressure ≥140 mm Hg or diastolic blood pressure ≥90 mm Hg that occurs after 20 weeks of gestation in a woman with previously normal blood pressure.
  and
- *Proteinuria:* Urinary excretion of ≥300 mg of protein in a 24-hour specimen.
- *With or without Edema:* Generalized edema or weight gain of at least 5lb in 1 week.

Diagnostic Criteria for Severe Pre-eclampsia

- Blood pressure ≥160 mm Hg systolic or ≥110 mm Hg diastolic on two occasions at least 6 hours apart while the patient is on bed rest.
- Proteinuria ≥5000 mg in a 24-hour collection, or ≥3+ on two random urine samples collected at least 4 hours apart.
- Oliguria defined as <500 mL per 24 hours.
- Cerebral or visual disturbances
- Pulmonary edema or cyanosis
- Epigastric or right upper quadrant pain
- Impaired liver function
- Thrombocytopenia
- Intrauterine fetal growth restriction (IUGR)

Predisposing Factors for Pre-eclampsia

- Primigravida, teenaged or elderly
- Family h/o hypertension, pre-eclampsia
- Multiple pregnancy, obesity
- Diabetes, pre-existing hypertension, renal disease, connective tissue disorder
- Hydatidiform mole, severe Rh incompatibility

CASE SCENARIO-1

A 24-years-old unbooked primigravida, seven and half months pregnant, has come to the antenatal clinic/ casualty with history of massive swelling of feet for 2 weeks and headache and vomiting for one day. There is no other relevant history. On examination grade 3 pedal edema is present and her BP is 180/120 mm Hg; urine albumin is 3+. On abdominal examination uterus is 30 weeks, corresponding to the period of amenorrhea, liquor is adequate and fetal heart sound (FHS) is present. Uterus is relaxed and not tender. No other positive findings.

> **Comment:** Diagnosis of severe pre-eclampsia should be considered because her BP is > 160/110 mm Hg at 30 weeks gestation, urine albumin is 3+ and grade 3 pedal edema is present. She is complaining of headache and thus there is risk of impending eclampsia.

POINTS TO BE NOTED IN HISTORY

1. Booked or unbooked: First trimester records can help in diagnosis with information regarding weight gain (excessive weight gain >5 lb in a month, tightening of ring etc, are pointer of fluid retention), base line BP and gestational age.
2. Age and parity: Pre-eclampsia often affects young primigravidas and teenagers; whereas older women >35 of age are at greater risk of chronic hypertension with superimposed preeclampsia or eclampsia.
3. Race and ethnicity: Africans are more susceptible than Caucasians
4. History of high BP in present pregnancy, its duration and treatment if any.

5. Ask about symptoms of severe headache, visual disturbances, epigastric pain and vomiting, respiratory difficulty, decreased urine output, excessive weight gain.
6. History of seizures, any history of seizure disorder prior to pregnancy, and in previous pregnancy.
7. History of hypertension in family, in previous pregnancy or pre-pregnancy high blood pressure: If there is history of gestational hypertension in previous pregnancy, there are more chances of developing hypertension in this pregnancy.
8. History of diabetes, thyroid disorder, drug intake and thromboembolism should be elicited. Both hypothyroidism and hyperthyroidism are associated with hypertension. History of thrombophilia, connective tissue disorder, anti phospholipid syndrome, renal diseases, and chronic hypertension should be noted.

> **History in this case:** Unbooked primigravida at seven and half month gestation with complains of headache, vomiting and swelling of feet. Earlier gestation and prepregnancy BP records are not available and there is no relevant family history or history of high BP, diabetes and seizures.

Points to be noted in Examination

- Senior obstetric staff should be involved in the assessment and management of women with severe pre-eclampsia and eclampsia.
- Diagnosis is based primarily on the level of BP and the presence of proteinuria. Clinicians should be aware of the potential involvement of other organs when assessing maternal risk, including placental diseases with fetal manifestation.
- When checking BP, the woman should be rested and sitting at a 45 degree angle. The BP cuff should be of the appropriate size and should be placed at the level of the heart. Korotkoff phase 5 is the appropriate measurement of diastolic blood pressure.
- Assessment of proteinuria- The usual screening test is visual dipstick assessment. A 2+ reading can be taken as evidence of proteinuria. A more accurate test is boiling method or either a spot urine protein creatinine ratio or ideally 24-hour urine protein.
- General physical assessment- check for temperature, pulse, radio-femoral delay (in coarctation of aorta) pallor, jaundice, cyanosis, pedal edema, respiratory rate, oxygen saturation.
- Cardiovascular system (CVS) – Check for the signs of congestive cardiac failure like basal crepitations and raised jugular venous pressure (JVP), dyspnea and tachypnea.
- Central nervous system (CNS) - if patient is drowsy, check for neck rigidity, tendon reflexes for hyper excitable state, pupils (whether equal and reactive to light).
- Abdominal examination – Assess for any tenderness in epigastrium or right hypochondrium. Liver, spleen and renal angles should be palpated.
- Obstetric examination: Assessment of fundal height, presentation, estimated fetal weight, Fetal Heart Sound (FHS). Fundal height less than period of gestation is associated with IUGR or wrong dates. Fundal height more than period of gestation is associated with abruptio placenta, twins, polyhydramnios or wrong dates. Assess uterine tone and contractions.
- Per-vaginal (PV) examination: It is done if termination of pregnancy is desired. Bishop's cervical scoring is noted and cephalopelvic disproportion (CPD) is excluded.

> **Examination in this case:**
> - BP -180/120, Urine albumin- 3+
> - General and systemic examination - unremarkable
> - Abdominal examination – unremarkable
> - Obstetric Examination – Fundal height 30 week, corresponding to period of amenorrhea cephalic presentation, Uterus- relaxed, non- tense, non-tender, FHS- 140/min, regular.

Diagnosis

Severe pre-eclampsia with impending eclampsia.

Table 6.1(a): Differential diagnosis of edema feet and proteinuria in pregnancy
Causes of edema feet
Physiological edema of pregnancy- due to pressure of gravid uterus on inferior vena cava and due to decreased interstitial colloid oncotic pressure seen in pregnancy.   Anemia, hypoproteinemia   Preeclampsia, eclampsia   Congestive cardiac failure   Nephrotic syndrome

Table 6.1(b)
Grading of edema
Grade 1: up to ankle   *Grade 2:* pretibial, up to knee   *Grade 3:* at two independent sites- sacral, pretibial   *Grade 4:* anasarca

Table 6.1(c)
Causes of proteinuria
Contamination with blood   Urinary tract infection   Renal disorder   Connective tissue disorders   Orthostatic proteinuria

Table 6.1(d)
Grading of proteinuria
Grade 1: Trace to +1: 0.3 to 1g/ L   *Grade 2:* +2: up to 2g/ L   *Grade 3:* +3 : 2-5 g/ L   *Grade 4:* > 5g/ L

Test for Proteinuria

Heat and acetic acid test: Fill ¾th of test tube with urine, boil upper part of urine. Boiled part may become cloudy. Add 5 drops of glacial acetic acid. Turbidity clears if it is due to phosphates. Severity of turbidity signifies amount of proteinuria. Test may be falsely positive if urine is alkaline, contaminated with ammonia, chlorhexadine or vaginal discharge.

Quantitative testing is done by Esbach's albuminometer.

MANAGEMENT

Seizure prophylaxsis, management of hypertension to avoid complications and prompt delivery are the mainstay in management of severe pre-eclampsia.

The principles of therapy are –

1. Admission to the labor room/intensive care unit.
2. Prevention of convulsions.

3. Control of acute severe hypertension and to maintain an optimal BP level that minimizes maternal cerebrovascular risks but does not compromise uteroplacental circulation.
4. Investigations.
5. Monitory and fluid management.
6. Further management—Immediate delivery or expectant management depending on period of gestation to maximize the gestational age of the fetus.
7. Management of complications.

1. Admit in Labor Room/Obstetric Intensive Care Unit

• Patient should be lying on a railed cot.
• Good nursing care should be available.

2. Prevention of Convulsions

Magnesium Sulfate: The MAGPIE trial[2] concluded that women with imminent eclampsia are the best candidates to receive magnesium prophylaxis. Magnesium sulfate reduces the risk of eclampsia by 50%. Since the risk of convulsions is more during labor and delivery, the prophylaxis is usually continued during labor and for 24 hours postpartum (Table 6.2).

Mechanism of action: It exerts a specific anticonvulsant action on the cerebral cortex by inhibiting the release of acetylcholine from pre-synaptic vesicles at the neuromuscular junction and blockage of N-methylaspartate (NMDA) receptors.

Therapeutic level – 4-7m Eq/L
Loss of patellar reflexes 10 mEq/L
Respiratory paralysis & arrest ≥ 12mEq/L

Effect on uterus: The inhibition of uterine activity by magnesium sulfate is dose dependent and is observed at levels of at least 8-10mEq/L. This explains why no uterine effect is clinically seen when magnesium is used for prophylaxis and treatment of eclampsia.

Fetal effects: It is not associated with any significant neonatal compromise. It causes a clinically insignificant decrease in fetal heart rate variability.

Antidote: 10% calcium gluconate 1 gm IV given over 10 minutes to reverse mild-to-moderate respiratory depression.

3. Treatment of Hypertension

Treatment of hypertension is indicated to reduce complications of hypertension when diastolic BP is above 100 mm Hg. Aim is to control acute severe hypertension and to maintain an optimal BP that minimizes maternal cerebrovascular risks without compromising uteroplacental circulation.

Table 6.2: Dosage schedule of magnesium sulfate for severe pre-eclampsia and eclampsia

Continuous intravenous infusion
• Loading dose – 4-6 gm of magnesium sulfate diluted in 100 ml of IV fluid administered over 15-20 min.
• Maintenance dose – 2 gm/hour in 100 mL of IV maintenance infusion.
• Discontinue after 24 hours of delivery

Intermittent intramuscular injections (Pritchard regimen)
• Loading dose – 4 gm of 20% solution of magnesium sulfate given intravenously at a rate not exceeding 1 gm/min. (Add 8 ml of 50% magnesium sulfate to 12 ml of normal saline = 4gm in 20 ml= 20% of solution).
  Follow promptly with 10 gm of 50% magnesium sulfate solution intramuscular (IM). One half i.e. 5 gm injected deeply in the upper quadrant of both buttocks.
• Maintenance dose- Every 4 hour, give 5 gm of 50% solution of magnesium sulfate IM injected deeply in the upper quadrant of alternate buttocks, but only after ensuring that:
  – The patellar reflexes are present
  – Respiratory rate>15/min
  – Urine output in the previous 4 hours exceeded 100 ml or 25 ml/hour.
• Discontinue after 24 hours of delivery

- Anti-hypertensives are started if BP is > 150/100 mmHg.
- Labetalol (oral or intravenous), hydralazine (IV) or nifedepine (oral) are used for acute management of severe hypertension (Table 6.3). Maintain on oral therapy after BP comes down.
- Chronic hypertensives should continue antihypertensives and drugs contraindicated in pregnancy like ACE inhibitors are to be replaced.
- Maintain systolic BP 130-150 mm Hg and diastolic BP 90-105 mm Hg.

Maintenance Dose of Antihypertensives for Control of BP

Tablet Labetalol: 100-200 mg BD
Tablet Alpha methyl Dopa: 250 mg TDS to 500 mg QID. It is an alpha adrenergic blocker. It is the most widely used drug for long term control of BP and has slow onset of action.
Tablet Nifedipine: 10 to 30 mg Orally

Table 6.3: Anti Hypertension Drugs. (NHBPEP, 2000)			
Drug (FDA risk)	*Dosage for acute BP control*	*Advantage*	*Side- effects*
Hydralazine(C)	5 mg IV or IM then 5 to 10 mg every 20-40 minutes; Once BP is controlled repeat every 3 hoursMaximum 5 doses can be given. Consider another drug if no response with 20 mg IV or 30 mg IMFor infusion : 0.5 -1.0 mg/hr Maximum dose: 10 mg/hr	Immediate onset of action	• Maternal hypotension, placental abruption and oliguria and fetal heart rate abnormalities are more as compared to other drugs. • Side effects such as headache nausea, vomiting mimic symptoms of deteriorating preeclampsia. • It has an unpredictable effect & a prolonged duration of action which can lead to a precipitous hypotension
Labetalol(C)	10-20 mg IV then 20 to 80 mg every 20-30 minutes Maximum dose: 220 mg For Infusion: 1-2 mg/ min	• It is the first line of treatment due to lower incidence of maternal hypotension and other side effects • Easier to titrate • More predictable dose response • No reflex tachycardia • Decreases systemic vascular resistance without reducing total peripheral blood flow.	Contraindicated in asthma and congestive heart failure.
Nifedipine(C)	Oral tablets recommended only 10-30 mg oral, repeat in 45 minutes if needed Maximum dose: 120 mg/day	Early onset of action	• Fetal distress & sudden maternal hypotension • An interaction between nifedipine and magnesium sulfate can cause profound muscle weakness, maternal hypotension and fetal distress.

4. Investigations

Investigations to be sent in such cases and the results in this case are given below:
- Complete blood count with peripheral blood smear: Hb - 13 gm %, TLC-14,000/mm^3, DLC- P70 L25 E2 M3, Platelet Count- 1.2 lacs/mm^3
- Coagulation profile: Prothrombin time- normal
- Liver function tests (LFT)- S. Bilirubin- 1.0mg/dL, ALT- 75 U/L, AST- 86 U/L, ALP- 236 U/L
- Renal function tests – Blood urea- 40mg/dL, S. creatinine- 1.0 mg/dL, S. uric acid- 6mg/dL
- Blood grouping and typing- O positive
- Urine routine and microscopy, culture and sensitivity: urine albumin 3+
- 24 hour urine collection for protein (3gm/L) and creatinine clearance, protein creatinine ratio >1.
- Fundus examination – normal.

5. Monitoring and Fluid Management

- BP measurement by mercury sphygmomanometer is ideal. BP should be checked every 15 minutes and continuous monitoring is done until the woman is stabilized and then every 30 minutes. Once BP is <170/110 mm Hg 6 hourly BP monitoring is done.
- Pulse oximeter to monitor oxygen saturation.
- Close input- output charting is essential. A catheter with an hourly urometer is advisable in oliguria. Avoid fluid overload to prevent pulmonary edema and IV fluids should be limited to 80 ml/hour.
- Urine albumin is checked every four hours.
- FHS monitoring 1 hourly.
- Fundal height and girth four hourly.
- Fundoscopy
- Blood tests (complete blood count, LFT, KFT) should be repeated at least twice weekly when the results are normal but more often if the clinical condition changes or if there are abnormalities.

6. Further Management and Delivery

- Give betamethasone (corticosteroids) 12 mg. in two doses 12 hr apart for fetal lung maturity if gestation is <34 weeks.
- One has to decide between immediate delivery (Table 6.4) and expectant management depending on period of gestation to maximize the gestational age of the fetus. Expectant management in attempted for very preterm fetus. It should be done in a tertiary care centre under strict vigilance

Table 6.4: Indications for immediate delivery	
Maternal indications	*Fetal indications*
Impending eclampsia/eclampsia	Poor biophysical score (4/8)
Pregnancy beyond 37 completed weeks and beyond 34 weeks in patient controlled on antihypertensives or severe preeclampsia cases.	Reversed flow in umbilical artery or ductus venosus and increased MCA >2 standard deviations for gestational age.
Hemodynamically unstable	
Rapidly worsening maternal status or HELLP syndrome.	
Oliguria	
Intrauterine fetal death (IUD)	
Pulmonary edema	
Cortical Blindness	
Cerebrovascular accident	
Fundus grade 3 and 4 changes	

as benefits may be less than complications of eclampsia, abruption, disseminated intravascular coagulation (DIC), renal failure etc. If BP does not settle or investigations reveal HELLP syndrome labor is induced (provided there is no obstetrical contraindication for vaginal delivery) irrespective of baby being preterm.

Expectant Management

After control of acute condition if it is decided to manage the patient conservatively then patient is advised bed rest in left lateral position (increases placental circulation and renal circulation), diet adequate in proteins, no extra salt, iron, and folic acid. She should be monitored in hospital. Maintain toxemia chart and monitor fetus. If BP settles and patient improves, pregnancy is continued till 34 week and then terminated.

Toxemia Chart

Maternal Monitoring:
- Once BP< 170/110 mm Hg, BP charting is done 6 hourly, for higher BP continuous monitoring is required.
- Urine albumin twice daily
- Input output chart daily
- Fundal height, girth twice weekly
- Blood biochemistry twice weekly
- Fundoscopy at time of admission and to be repeated if develops severe preeclampsia
- Weight: monitor twice weekly.

Fetal Monitoring:
- Daily fetal movement record
- Ultrasonography– fetal biometry, placental localization, amniotic fluid index (AFI) and placental grading, fetal weight.
- Non stress test (NST) – daily
- Biophysical profile (BPP) – twice weekly or more frequently
- Doppler (umbilical artery and middle cerebral artery) – in IUGR. Baseline and then twice weekly or daily depending upon the findings
- Amniocentesis for confirmation of lung maturity, if premature termination of pregnancy is required

Planning Delivery

- The decision to deliver should be made once the patient is stable.
- If the fetus is < 34 weeks of gestation and delivery can be deferred, corticosteroids should be given and after 24 hours the benefits of conservative management should be reassessed.
- Conservative management at very early gestations may improve perinatal outcome but must be carefully balanced with maternal well being.
- The mode of delivery should be determined after considering the presentation of the fetus and the fetal condition, together with likelihood of success of induction of labor. If bishop scoring of cervix is unfavorable, dinoprostone gel is instilled or oxytocin augmentation in higher concentrations is done to prevent fluid overload.
- The third stage should be managed with 5 units oxytocin given IM or slowly IV. Erogmetrine is not used to prevent PPH, as it can further increase the BP.
- Evaluate hematocrit if BP falls as even small blood loss can cause hemoconcentration in these cases. Prompt IV fluid and intensive monitoring is required in such cases but with caution as vigorous fluid replacement can also cause pulmonary edema.
- Vaginal delivery is generally preferred, but if gestation is <32 weeks, cesarean section is more likely as the success of induction is reduced. It should be noted that cesarean section in severe-preeclampsia/eclampsia has higher morbidity and mortality than vaginal delivery.
- Cesarean section may be required if fits are uncontrolled, not responding to anticonvulsant treatment for 8 hours and for other obstetrical indications.

Management of Preeclampsia/Eclampsia in Post-Partum Period

- Continue magnesium sulfate for 24 hrs after delivery or last seizure, whichever is later.
- Anti- hypertensive should be continued after delivery according to the BP and are tapered slowly. BP should be reviewed after 3 months. Methyldopa is avoided in post-partum period as it is secreted in milk and atenolol, labetalol or nifedipine are used.
- Forty four percent cases of eclampsia present post-partum up to 7 days after delivery, so women with signs and symptoms suggestive of impending eclampsia should be carefully monitored and BP should be kept below 150/100mm of Hg.
- Women with hypertension and proteinuria persisting at 6 weeks postpartum may have renal disease or chronic hypertension and should be investigated further.
- Oral contraceptive pills are avoided till BP is elevated.

7. Management of Complications

Complications of preeclampsia are listed below. Management of these complications needs to be individualized and may require multidisciplinary involvement.
- Eclampsia, HELLP syndrome
- Uteroplacental—Abruptio, IUGR, fetal demise, postpartum hemorrhage, prematurity, asphyxia
- Neurological – Eclampsia, cerebral edema, cerebral hemorrhage, hypertensive encephalopathy
- Cardiovascular – Severe hypertension, cardiac failure, pulmonary edema, shock.
- Renal – Oliguria, renal failure
- Hepatic – Hepatocellular dysfunction, subcapsular hematoma, hepatic rupture.
- Hematological: Hemolysis, thrombocytopenia, DIC.
- Eye complications: Blurring of vision, blindness. Scotoma or diplopia can take place. Fifteen percent of patients can have blindness which may be due to involvement of visual cortex of the occipital lobe, the lateral geniculate nuclei and retina due to ischemia or infarction. Retinal detachment may occur. Vision usually returns to normal within a week.

PREVENTION OF PRE ECLAMPSIA

- Identify high-risk cases- multiple pregnancy, molar pregnancy, chronic hypertension, diabetes, hydramnios, history of preeclampsia - eclampsia and hydrops.
- Do screening by BP, urine albumin, weight gain especially after 20 week of pregnancy.
- Tests like Doppler, roll over test etc are not useful for large scale screening.
- Prophylactic medication for prevention of preeclampsia
  - Calcium supplementation- 2 gm/day can prevent preeclampsia in patients with low calcium levels.
  - Low dose aspirin (75 mg/day) can help in cases with previous history of preeclampsia, eclampsia, IUGR or lupus anticoagulant (from 14 – 36 weeks).

ECLAMPSIA

Stages of an Eclamptic Fit

a. *Premonitory stage (30 seconds):* Twitching of limbs, rolling of eyes, turning of head on one side, patient may become unconscious.
b. *Tonic phase (15-30 sec):* Body goes in spasm, respiration ceases, opisthotonus present, tongue protrudes between teeth and cyanosis may be present.
c. *Clonic phase (1 minute):* Muscles contract and relax and patient throws fits, blood stained frothy secretions come from nose and mouth. Tongue can be traumatized during fits.
d. *Phase of coma or sleep:* Eclampsia may be followed by psychosis rarely which responds to antipsychotic medications. Sometimes status epilepticus can occur when convulsions are occurring one after another continuously and may require general anesthesia to control them.

CASE SCENARIO-2

A 19-years-old primigravida, eight months pregnant has come to the casualty with history of seizures 2 hours back and headache and vomiting for one day.

On examination she has grade 3 pedal edema, BP- 190/110 mm Hg and urine albumin- 3+.

On abdominal examination uterus is 30 weeks, corresponding to period of amenorrhea, liquor is adequate and FHS is present. Uterus is relaxed and not tender. No other positive findings. While examining and taking brief history patient was given loading dose of magnesium sulfate. Patient threw a seizure in casualty.

> **Comment:** Until other causes of seizures are excluded, all pregnant women with convulsions should be considered to have eclampsia. 30% patients may not have high BP.

Differential Diagnosis

MRI or CT skull can help in diagnosis of CNS causes of convulsions.

- Epilepsy
- Intracranial tumors
- Meningitis and encephalitis
- Poisoning
- Hypertensive encephalopathy
- Uremic convulsions
- Cysticercosis
- Ruptured cerebral aneurysm

> **History in this case:** Young primigravida at 8 month of gestation with headache,vomiting, pedal edema and seizures

Immediate Management

- Place patient in lateral decubitus position to prevent aspiration. The bed rails should be elevated to prevent maternal injury and padded tongue blade should be inserted between teeth to avoid injury to the tongue during convulsion.
- Such a patient should not be left alone.
- IV access is established and blood samples are collected for investigations.
- Loading dose of magnesium sulfate is given for control of seizures Repeat bolus dose of 2 gm magnesium sulfate administered for recurrent seizure (Table 6.2).
- Intravenous labetalol or oral nifedipine is given to control BP (Table 6.3).
- Pulse oximeter to check oxygen saturation.
- Keep airway clean and patent by frequent oral suctioning.
- Give oxygen by mask at 8-10 liters/minute, if convulsion occurs or pulse oximeter shows hypoxia.
- Patient is catheterized, urine albumin is checked.
- Prevent further convulsion by keeping dim lights and minimal noise.
- If convulsions persist, intubation may be needed to protect airway and for oxygenation.

Examination and Approach to Diagnosis

Once anti-seizure prophylaxis is given, brief history regarding number and duration of fits is noted from relative. Quick general physical examination and abdominal examination is done in a similar manner as described in case scenario 1, particularly:

- Neck rigidity is excluded
- In a comatosed patient pupils are checked for inequality and response to light
- Chest is auscultated for signs of failure and for excluding pulmonary edema and aspiration.

Examination in this case:
- General condition unsatisfactory.
- Patient drowsy but conscious and oriented ,no neck rigidity, pupils equally responding to light.
- *Pulse:* 110/ min, BP= 190/110 mm Hg, Respiratory Rate- 30/min.
- Temperature- 98.4° F, Oxygen saturation (SPO$_2$) 99% at room air
- Bilateral lung fields—clear
- CVS—Tachycardia
- Abdominal examination – Fundal height- 30 week, cephalic presentation, FHS-136/min, regular. Uterus-relaxed, non-tense, non-tender No epigastric/right hypochondrial tenderness.
- PV – os closed, uneffaced, firm, posterior, vertex at brim, pelvis adequate
- Urine albumin - 3+

Diagnosis: Eclampsia

Investigation in this case:
- Hb - 13 gm %, TLC-14,000/mm^3, DLC- P70 L25 E2 M3, Platelet Count- 1.2 lacs/mm^3
- Prothrombin time- normal
- Liver function test- S. Bilirubin- 1.0mg/dL, ALT- 75 U/L, AST- 86 U/L, ALP- 236 U/L
- Kidney function test- Blood urea- 40mg/dL, S. creatinine- 1.0 mg/dL, S. uric acid- 6mg/dL
- Urine routine and microscopy: albumin 3+
- Fundus examination – Grade I hypertensive changes

Further Monitoring and Management

- Patient is kept nil orally and on IV 5% dextrose drip
- If possible do continuous monitoring of pulse rate, BP, SPO$_2$, respiratory rate
- Temperature is recorded 4 hourly
- Patient is catheterized, input/output chart is maintained 1 hourly
- Control of convulsion- loading dose of magnesium sulfate is followed by maintenance dose for 24 hours post delivery or 24 hours after last seizure, whichever is later
- Intermittent administration of an antihypertensive agent to lower blood pressure and to keep it below 150/100 mm Hg
- Avoidance of diuretics unless there is obvious pulmonary edema, limitation of intravenous fluid administration unless fluid loss is excessive and avoidance of hyperosmotic agents
- Investigations are repeated as needed
- Parenteral antibiotics like ampicillin and gentamicin are started if lungs are congested
- FHS is closely monitored and should be checked after the fits. There can be fetal bradycardia, which recovers in 3-5 minutes. This is due to maternal hypotension and lactic academia. If it persists for >10 minute abruption may be there and immediate delivery may be considered
- The woman's condition will always take priority over fetal condition.

Delivering the Patient

- Delivery of fetus is the active cure. Once patient is stabilized, plan should be made to deliver her.
- Pregnancy is terminated by induction with PG E2 gel followed by oxytocin in case of poor Bishop score or artificial ruptures of membrane and oxytocin, if there are no contraindications for vaginal delivery.
- Second stage of labor is shortened by outlet forceps if necessary.
- Methyl ergometrine is avoided in 3rd stage of labor.
- If fits are not controlled in 8 hours time and patient is primigravida and taking time to deliver, cesarean section may be needed. Caesarian section can be done under general anesthesia or epidural block. Intubation may be difficult due to laryngeal edema. Patient should be stabilized and observed for 24 hrs in the high dependency unit before shifting to the ward.

Other Anticonvulsant Regimes Described for Control of Seizures in Eclampsia

- Lean's Diazepam Therapy- 20mg Diazepam IV slowly and 40 mg in 5% dextrose slowly. Respiratory depression should be watched.
- Phenytoin Therapy – 10mg/kg IV slowly, then 200 mg orally BD. Continued for 48 hrs after delivery IV or orally.
- Lytic Cocktail regime
  - Chlorpromazine (50mg) + Promethazine (25mg) IM along with Chlorpromazine (25mg) and Pethidine (100mg) IV in 20 ml of 5% dextrose solution slowly.
  - 100 mg pethidine in 500 ml of 10% dextrose drip slowly at a rate 20-30 drops/min. Drip is continued for 24hrs after convulsion.

Prognostic Factors of Eclampsia

- Poor outcome when total number of fits is >10
- Quick delivery results in better prognosis
- Postnatal fits-poor prognosis
- Coma and features of brain edema-poor prognosis.
- Fatal supratentorial herniation-poor prognosis.
- Any hypertension in pregnancy is marker of increased risk of cardiovascular morbidity and mortality in future. Risk of chronic hypertension is increased by 5 times and stroke by 9-10%. There is four times increased risk of renal failure.

Causes of Maternal Death in Eclampsia

- Cerebral hemorrhage
- Hyperpyrexia due to pontine hemorrhage
- Asphyxia due to aspiration, pulmonary edema and bronchopneumonia
- Renal failure
- DIC and postpartum shock

HELLP SYNDROME

It is defined as constellation of hemolysis, hepatic dysfunction, and low platelet count in a patient with preeclampsia. Proteinuria may not be present in 10-15% of the patients [3], 10% cases have eclampsia[4]. Sibai et al[5] defined laboratory abnormalities for diagnosing HELLP:

- Hemolysis on peripheral smear – evidence of schistocytes, burr cells and helmet cells.
- Hepatic dysfunction-elevated bilirubin > 1.2 mg/dL, or elevated lactate dehydrogenase (LDH)> 600 U/L; an aspartate aminotransferase (AST/ALT)> 70 IU/L; (which are greater than 2 standard deviations of normal)
- Low platelets is defined as count <100,000/mm³ this is the main and earliest coagulation abnormality present in all women with HELLP syndrome. In class I, platelets are < 50,000. In class II, between 50,000 – 1,00,000 and in class III, between 1,00,000 – 1,50,000

Management

The diagnosis of HELLP syndrome is an indication for termination of pregnancy after stabilizing the mother. Expectant management can be considered in patients with <32 weeks pregnancy in a tertiary care center only. Prolonging the latency period beyond 48 hours from the time of diagnosis is controversial and can lead to risk of abruption placentae, pulmonary edema, acute renal failure, eclampsia, maternal and perinatal death. Because only a limited prolongation of pregnancy is expected and there is no difference in fetal survival, expectant management of HELLP syndrome is not continued beyond 24-48 hours required for optimizing maternal and fetal status.

The additional measures to be taken are as follows: Platelet transfusion in patients with platelet count<20,000/mm³ or any evidence of significant bleeding. If a cesarean section is planned, platelet count should be at least 50,000/mm³.

- Steroid therapy – Dexamethasone 10mg IV is given every 6 hours for 2 doses followed by 6 mg IV every 6 hours for 2 additional doses. For patients with profound thrombocytopenia(<20,000/ mm³) or central nervous system dysfunction, dexamethasone 20 mg IV is given every 6 hours for up to 4 doses. It improves laboratory and clinical parameters and reduces the need for maternal transfusion of blood products by significantly improving platelet count but it has not been shown to improve maternal or perinatal outcome. Katz et al (2008) found no advantage with dexamethasone.[6]
- Closely monitor the coagulation profile i.e. platelet count, prothrombin time, APTT and if found deranged on serial investigations, DIC is suspected. To confirm specific test like- D- dimer and fibrin degradation product (FDP) estimation should be done. Fresh frozen plasma is transfused to correct the coagulation profile. Platelet concentrate are transfused as discussed earlier. ALT, AST and platelet usually normalize within three days after delivery

Differential Diagnosis of HELLP Syndrome

Hepatitis, cholecystitis, pyelonephritis, autoimmune and thrombotic thrombocytopenic purpura, gastroenteritis, hemolytic uremic syndrome, Acute fatty liver of pregnancy.

OTHER COMPLICATIONS

Hepatic Hemorrhage

Hepatic hemorrhage with hematoma may present as acute surgical emergency with pain in right hypochondrium and features of intra abdominal bleeding with patient in shock and laparotomy may be life saving. It has high maternal mortality of 30%. Subcapsular liver hematoma can complicate 16% cases of HELLP syndrome (2000)[3.]

Pulmonary Edema

Aspiration is excluded before a diagnosis of pulmonary edema is made.

Causes of pulmonary edema – a) increased pulmonary capillary permeability b) Cardiogenic edema c) combination of both. Invasive monitoring is initiated in renal diseases and associated cardiac diseases. Volume expansion can lead to pulmonary edema. Fluid should not be given more than 60-125ml/hour. Propped up position, diuretics, positive pressure ventilation and urgent delivery may be indicated to control it.

CNS Involvement

Intracranial hemorrhage: The patient is usually admitted with coma following headache and convulsions. There is presence of motor and sensory deficit and focal neurological signs. CT scan shows hypodense areas.

Hypertensive encephalopathy: The patient presents with severe headache, visual disturbances, nausea, vomiting, confusion or coma. MRI shows involvement of subcortical white matter of occipital lobes.

Management: Aggressive treatment of BP i.e. lowering of mean arterial BP (MAP) by 25% over 30-60 minutes or to 110 mmHg. Reduce intracranial pressure with the help of osmotic agents like mannitol. Manage in consultation with neurologist.

Renal Involvement

Oliguria i.e. urinary output <30 mL/hour is common in severe preeclampsia. One liter of ringer lactate solution is given over 12 hours at a rate 85ml/hr to maintain urine output of >100 mL/hour. In renal dysfunction initial loading dose can be safely given and maintenance dose needs alteration. If urine output is <100 mL/hr despite this, CVP monitoring is done. Serum creatinine levels are monitored. Dialysis may be needed and patient is managed in consultation with urologist. An

Flow chart 6.1: Management of oliguria

```
                        ┌─────────────────────┐
                        │  Intial value of CVP │
                        └─────────────────────┘
              ┌───────────────────┼───────────────────────┐
        ┌───────────┐      ┌───────────┐           ┌───────────┐
        │ <4 mm Hg  │      │ <4-8 mm Hg│           │ <8 mm Hg  │
        └───────────┘      └───────────┘           └───────────┘
              │                  │                        │
    ┌──────────────────┐  ┌──────────────────┐   ┌──────────────────────┐
    │50 ml colloid over│  │Expectant         │   │Signs of pulmonary     │
    │5min              │  │management        │   │edema                  │
    └──────────────────┘  └──────────────────┘   └──────────────────────┘
              │                  │                        │
       ┌────────────┐      ┌────────────┐          ┌────────────────┐
       │Urine output│      │Urine output│          │20 mg frusemide │
       └────────────┘      └────────────┘          └────────────────┘
```

increase in urine output after delivery is a good prognostic sign. Proteinuria and edema usually disappear within a week and BP normalizes within a few days to 2 weeks after delivery.

Eye Involvement

It may be in the form of cortical blindness, retinal detachment or papilledema. However, quick recovery after delivery is the rule. Papilledema is an indication of termination of pregnancy.

Uteroplacental Complications

Deliver the patient and do the post partum management.

PATHOPHYSIOLOGY

Pathophysiological changes in different organs in preeclampsia/eclampsia are a result of vasospasm, endothelial injury and ischemia

Organ	Histopathology/anatomical changes	Biochemical /pathological complication
Kidney	Glomerular endotheliosis blocking the filteration barrier (endothelial cells are swollen) Glomeruli enlarged, bloodless and capillary loops dilated and contracted. Homogenous subendothelial deposits of protein and fibrin like material. Increased excretion of urinary podocyte cells responsible for proteinuria.	Elevated serum creatinine, uric acid Elevated urinary sodium Increased tubular absorption of calcium, uric acid Proteinuria Acute renal failure

Contd...

Contd...

Liver	Rarely acute tubular necrosis Periportal thrombi, necrosis. Hepatic infarction accompanied with hemorrhagic areas Subcapsular hematoma due to infarction and hemorrhage Subcapsular hematoma can be identified on CT/MRI	Elevated ALT, AST jaundice, HELLP syndrome
Brain	Intracerebral hemorrhage, cortical and subcortical petechial hemorrhage, subcortical edema, non hemorrhagic areas of softening Microscopic lesion-fibrinoid necrosis of arterial wall, perivascular microinfarcts and hemorrhage	Headache, scotoma Convulsions, blindness Cerebral edema, Posterior reversible encephalopathy syndrome
Visual changes	Areas involved are occipital lobe, lateral geniculate nuclei, retina Retina-ischemia, infarction, detachment	Scotoma, blurred vision Diplopia, blindness
Uteroplacental perfusion	Defects in trophoblastic invasion and placentation, increased syncytial knots, fibrinoid degeneration, cytotrophoblast proliferation, infarction, villous necrosis and retroplacental hematoma Vasospasm of uteroplacental vessels Abnormal waveform of uterine artery	Preeclampsia syndrome IUGR
Circulatory system and blood	Endothelial cell injury, vasospasm, increased vascular reactivity to various agents, hemoconcentration, extracellular fluid increases, peripheral smear shows schistocytosis, spherocytosis and reticulocytosis. This is due to microangiopathic hemolysis caused by endothelial disruption with platelet adherence and fibrin deposition	Multiorgan involvement, decreased blood volume, fluid retention and edema
Coagulopathy	Low grade coagulopathy, decreased platelet count, increased platelet specific protein and thromboplastin. Endothelium released factors are increased like fibronectin type 1, plasminogen activator inhibitor. Excess intravascular thrombin, antithrombin 3 complexes and increased degradation products	DIC
Endocrine	Increase in vascular sensitivity to angiotensin II, catecholamines and vasopressin. This abnormal sensitivity is acquired between 17 week of gestation and the clinical onset of gestational hypertension. In patients with gestational hypertension, endothelial cell damage causes increased platelet activation which in turn releases thromboxane A2. The increased ratio of thromboxane to prostacyclin increases vascular tone and thereby blood pressure.	Hypertension

KEY POINTS

- Preeclampsia is diagnosed when pregnant patient has hypertension and proteinuria with or without edema after 20 week of pregnancy.
- Preeclampsia with convulsion is known as eclampsia.
- Prediction, screening and diagnosis is mainly clinical.
- Treatment of severe preeclampsia/eclampsia is seizure prophylaxis, antihypertensive drugs and delivery.
- Main risks to fetus are prematurity and birth asphyxia.
- Exact pathophysiology is unknown but endothelial cell injury; vasospasm and fibrinolysis are important components affecting multiple organs.
- Oral contraceptives should be avoided till BP is elevated.

REFERENCES

1. Report of the National High Blood Pressure Education Program Working Group on High Blood Pressure in Pregnancy. Am J Obstet Gynecol 2000;183:S1-S22.
2. Altman D, Carroli G, Duley L, Farrell B, Moodley J, Neilson J, Smith D; Magpie Trial Collaboration Group. Do women with pre-eclampsia, and their babies, benefit from magnesium sulfate? The Magpie Trial: a randomised placebo-controlled trial. Lancet 2002;359:1877-90.
3. Haddad B, Barton JR, Livingston JC, Chahine R, Sibai BM. Risk factors for adverse maternal outcomes among women with HELLP (hemolysis, elevated liver enzymes, and low platelet count) syndrome. Am J Obstet Gynecol 2000;83:444-8.
4. Keiser S, Owens M, Parrish M: HELLP syndrome II. Concurrent eclampsia in 70 cases. Abstract No 781, 29th Annual meeting of Society for Maternal Fetal Medicine, January 26-31, 2009.
5. Sibai BM, Ramadan MK, Chari RS, Friedman SA. Pregnancies complicated by HELLP syndrome (hemolysis, elevated liver enzymes, and low platelets): subsequent pregnancy outcome and long-term prognosis. Am J Obstet Gynecol 1995;172:125-9.
6. Katz L, de Amorim MM, Figueiroa JN, Pinto e Silva JL. Postpartum dexamethasone for women with hemolysis, elevated liver enzymes, and low platelets (HELLP) syndrome: a double-blind, placebo-controlled, randomized clinical trial. Am J Obstet Gynecol 2008;198:283.e1-8.

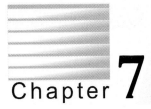

Chapter 7

Cardiac Failure in Pregnancy

Anjali Tempe, Pushpa Mishra, Gunjan

INTRODUCTION

The incidence of heart disease in India is less than 1 percent. Rheumatic heart disease is still common due to low socio-economic status, lack of hygiene and nonavailabilty of medical care and accounts for the majority of heart diseases in pregnancy.

The incidence of cardiac disorders and acute pulmonary edema in pregnancy is reported to be 1 percent and 1 in 500-1000 respectively in the Western centers.[1] In Brazil, maternal mortality rate was 2.7 per 1000 pregnancies complicated by heart disease.[1] In the USA, cardiac disorders accounted for 7.6 percent of severe obstetrical morbidities diagnosed during hospitalization for deliveries. In the West, cardiogenic pulmonary edema accounts for less than half of the cases of acute pulmonary edema. However, in India majority of cases of pulmonary edema are due to cardiac lesions and valvular lesions are the most common among them.

Physiological Changes in Cardiovascular System in Pregnancy (Table 7.1)

- Hypervolemia[2]
- Decreased blood viscosity[3]
- Increased cardiac output
- Decreased systemic vascular resistance
- Increased heart rate[4]
- Decreased pulmonary vascular resistance
- Increased pulmonary capillary wedge pressure
- Increased left ventricular stroke volume
- Decreased central venous pressure
- Decreased colloid oncotic pressure[5]

In healthy pregnant women, the cardiac performance remains unchanged because increased blood volume and cardiac output are compensated by decreased vascular resistance with increased pulse rate.

Pathophysiology of Cardiac Failure in Pregnancy

Cardiac failure is a clinical syndrome rather than specific diagnosis, in which an abnormality of cardiac structure or function is responsible for the inability of the heart to eject or fill the blood at a

Table 7.1: Hemodynamic changes in normal pregnancy at term compared to nonpregnant status		
Parameters	Nonpregnant	Change(%) in pregnancy at term
Cardiac output (L/min)	4.3~0.9	+44
Heart rate (Beat/min)	71~10	+17
Systemic vascular resistance (dynes/cm/sec²)	1530~520	-21
Pulmonary vascular resistance (dynes/cm/sec²)	199~47	-35
Pulmonary capillary wedge pressure (mm Hg)	6.3~2.1	+18
Left ventricular stroke work index (g/m/m²)	41~8	+17
Colloid oncotic pressure (mm Hg)	20.8~1.0	-14

rate commensurate with the requirement of the metabolising tissue.[6] It is an imprecise term used when heart cannot maintain the cardiac output adequately or does so only at the expense of elevated filling pressure.

Different Types of Heart Failure

- Right, left and biventricular failure
- Systolic and diastolic failure
- High output and low output failure
- Forward (due to inadequate cardiac output) and backward failure (due to pulmonary and systemic venous congestion)
- Acute and chronic heart failure

All forms of heart diseases may lead to heart failure. Heart failure is frequently, but not always, caused by a defect in myocardial contraction; it may result from primary abnormality in heart musculature, i.e. cardiomyopathies, viral myocarditis, coronary atherosclerosis, congenital, valvular and hypertensive heart disease, acute hypertensive crisis, rupture of aortic valve leaflet, endocarditis or with a massive pulmonary embolism.[6]

Other causes of heart failure in pregnancy: Besides heart disease, the other causes of heart failure in pregnancy are hypertensive disorders, tocolytic therapy, septicemia, hemorrhage and anemia.

Heart failure results in a constellation of clinical manifestations including circulatory congestion, dyspnea, fatigue and weakness. In the mildest form of heart failure, cardiac output is adequate at rest but inadequate when metabolic demands are increased, i.e. during exercise or some other form of stress. Clinical features depend upon nature of heart disease, type of failure and neural endocrine changes.

Management depends upon accurate clinical diagnosis. Cardiac patients in pregnancy may need medical ICU care or high dependency care and require expert management from a team of doctors including obstetrician, anesthesiologist, cardiologist, pulmonologist and pediatrician due to the problems faced by the patient peculiar to heart disease like cardiac failure, pulmonary edema, thromboembolic episodes etc.

CASE SCENARIO-1

Mrs. X, 25 years of age, married for 1 year, primigravida with 32 weeks period of gestation presented to the casualty with the complaints of breathlessness on slightest exertion and obvious respiratory distress for the last one month with bilateral swelling over feet which was progressively increasing. There was no history of any intake of medicines or previous hospitalization.

Comment: The presenting features are highly suggestive of cardiac failure and pulmonary congestion in this case.

Differential Diagnosis

Differential diagnosis in such a case would be:
- Valvular heart disease of rheumatic origin causing pulmonary edema.
- Congestive cardiac failure due to anemia or hypertension.
- Cardiomyopathy.
- Any respiratory disease causing cor pulmonale.
- Rarely connective tissue diseases and thyrotoxicosis.
- Other reasons like tocolytic therapy and septicemia in the West (though rare in India)

POINTS TO BE NOTED IN HISTORY

- A detailed history of duration of her symptoms of breathlessness, since when her physical activities are limited and how much in terms of New York Heart Association Classification (NYHA).

> **New York Heart Association Functional Classification of Heart Disease:[7]**
> **Class I:** No limitation of physical activity
> **Class II:** Slight limitation of physical activity
> **Class III:** Marked limitation of physical activity
> **Class IV:** Dyspnea at rest

- History of cough, hemoptysis, chest pain, palpitation, syncope earlier in this pregnancy, night sweats or getting up in night (air hunger) are suggestive of cardiac disease.
- History of petechial hemorrhage, osler nodes, splenomegaly (in infective endocarditis), cyanotic spells, squatting episodes (in congenital heart disease).
- History of urinary and bowel symptoms to rule out other differential diagnosis of edema and breathlessness like renal disease, anemia.
- History of antenatal care and if a multigravida, history of hypertension in previous pregnancy to rule out hypertension in pregnancy as a cause of cardiac failure.
- History of cold intolerance or hyperthermia to rule out thyrotoxicosis.
- History of chronic ill health, malnutrition, socioeconomic status etc to rule out anemia.
- If she is a known case of heart disease then treatment history in the form of antibiotics, cardiac drugs, history of any surgical intervention like balloon mitral valvotomy, open valve replacement.
- History of any thromboembolic event previously with history of anticoagulant medication.
- *Obstetric History:* Any history related to previous pregnancy, postpartum period, any obstetric complications, any history suggestive of failure in previous pregnancy.
- *Past History:* History suggestive of rheumatic heart disease like fever with sore throat, multiple joints pain in childhood, subcutaneous nodules, involuntary movements, etc. History of tuberculosis, hypertension, diabetes mellitus, hypercholesterolemia, blood transfusion, deep vein thrombosis, pulmonary embolism, previous cardiac event or cardiac surgery.
- *Family History:* History of tuberculosis, hypertension, diabetes mellitus, thromboembolic disease or any history of congenital heart disease.
- *Personal History:* History of cigarette smoking, alcohol intake, drug abuse, bowel and bladder habits, sleep pattern, contraception history.
- *Dietary History:* Total calorie intake with reference to carbohydrate, protein and fat intake.

> **Important history in this case:** Primigravida with 32 weeks period of gestation with breathlessness on slightest exertion, palpitation and bilateral pedal edema and is suggestive of NYHA grade III-IV cardiac disease.

POINTS TO BE NOTED IN EXAMINATION

General Examination

- Built, nutrition, height, weight, body mass index.
- Temperature, pulse rate, blood pressure (BP), respiratory rate (RR), grade of NYHA confirmation.
- Pallor, cyanosis, clubbing, icterus, tongue, teeth, gums and tonsils.
- Jugular venous pressure (JVP), thyroid, trachea, lymph nodes in neck, neck veins.
- Edema- pedal, periorbital, vulval, abdominal.

Cardiovascular Examination

- *Inspection:* It should include precordium, apex impulse, other pulsations, dilated veins, scar, etc. In heart failure, apex beat is shifted to left markedly (as apex beat shifts to left slightly in normal pregnancy).
- *Palpation:* It includes confirmation of findings of inspection like apex beat, left parasternal heave, thrills and other pulsations.
- *Percussion:* Borders of heart and lower sternal resonance (in women because of breast, tissue is difficult to elicit).
- *Auscultation:* All cardiac areas should be auscultated for murmur to know the type of lesion (MS/MR/AS/AR) or septal defects (ASD/VSD) etc. and area of murmur best heard is to be noted. The important findings in different areas are:
  - Accentuated first heart sound with mid diastolic murmur with presystolic accentuation (suggestive of mitral stenosis, which is most common).
  - Ejection systolic murmur and click in aortic stenosis.
  - Early diastolic murmur and Austin flint murmur in aortic regurgitation.
  - Pansystolic murmur in mitral regurgitation.
  - Loud P2 (suggestive of pulmonary hypertension).

Respiratory System Examination

- *Inspection:* It includes shape of chest, respiratory movements, respiratory rate, scar, any visible pulsation etc.
- *Palpation:* The findings of inspection including chest movements, tactile vocal fremitus, any tenderness to be confirmed.
- *Percussion:* To know about resonance, any abnormal dullness.
- *Auscultation:* Auscultation of both lungs to be done meticulously to find out any fine crepitations at the lung bases or any added sounds like rhonchi, wheeze or rales particularly in patients who are in cardiac failure.

Abdominal Examination

- *Inspection:* On inspection there should be comment upon any distension of abdomen, gravid status, umbilicus, scar marks, hernial sites, any visible peristalsis, and abdominal movements in all quadrants.
- *Palpation:* To look for symphysio fundal height, abdominal girth, obstetric grips to know about lie, presentation, position and attitude, adequacy of liquor and estimated fetal weight. Palpation for hepatosplenomegaly is a must in a case of heart disease.
- *Auscultation:* Fetal heart sounds for fetal well-being.

INVESTIGATIONS

Investigations should be done to confirm the diagnosis of patients who are undiagnosed and un-investigated earlier in the pregnancy and there is strong suspicion of heart disease with or without valvular lesions.

1. *Blood routine examination:* Hemogram, liver function test, kidney function test, serum electrolytes (must if patient is taking diuretics), coagulation profile (to be done if patient is on anticoagulant therapy).
2. *Chest X-ray:* Done very rarely in pregnancy or should be done with abdominal shield if necessary. It may show enlarged cardiac silhouette. It can also show prominent vascular margins with aortic knuckle and congestion.
3. *Electrocardiogram (ECG):* It should be done to know left ventricular hypertrophy and axis deviation. This investigation however cannot help in diagnosis of a lesion.
4. *Echocardiography and Doppler:* This is mandatory and very important investigation for diagnosis and management. It gives information regarding:
   • Nature and site of lesion,
   • Ventricular function
   • Diameter of valves
   • Opening and closing of valves
   • Left ventricular ejection fraction
   • Any vegetations/clots/pericardial effusion
   • Cardiomyopathies/calcification
   • In operative cases-function of replaced valve.
5. *Arterial blood gas analysis (ABG):* It can be particularly useful in severely ill patients and in congenital cyanotic heart disease to diagnose right to left shunts.
6. *Central venous pressure monitoring (CVP):* It can be used for intravenous fluid management, but in pregnant patient oral route should be preferred over parenteral route for fluid intake. However CVP monitoring would be important in a critically ill patient.
7. *Pulse oximetery:* Used for oxygen saturation monitoring of operated/critically ill patients.
8. *Pulmonary artery catheter (SWAN-GANZ):* PA catheter has got very limited role in obstetric practice and generally is not used in pregnant patient. It is indicated rarely for hemodynamic monitoring of a severely ill patient.[5]

MANAGEMENT

General Measures

a. The management depends upon patient's general condition. It involves a team of doctors at tertiary level including obstetrician, cardiologist, pediatrician, anesthesiologists and rarely cardiac surgeons with ICU care or high dependency unit care.
b. Bed rest.
c. Oxygen by mask at rate of 6 L/min for adequate ventilation.
d. Propped up position/lateral decubitus position.
e. Vital charting (pulse and respiratory rate half hourly or even more frequently in critically ill patients and temperature and BP two hourly).
f. Strict intake and output monitoring.
g. Intermittent chest auscultation for crepitations.
h. Adequate pain relief and sedation: Inj morphine 2 to 4 mg slow intravenous (IV) may be given. Availability of opioid antagonist, naloxone should be confirmed for resuscitation of newborn, if patient is in labor.

Medications

a. *Diuretics:* Inj. Furosemide can be given in dose of 20 to 40 mg IV 8 hrly to decrease the preload and pulmonary edema.[8] It can be used in maximum doses of 200 mg/24 hour.

b. *Beta blockers:* If failure is precipitated by tachycardia, beta blocker agents are preferred.[9] Most commonly used drugs are atenolol, labetalol, propanalol and metoprolol. They act as beta receptor blockers, decrease the heart rate, force of contraction and cardiac output. Atenolol can be used in doses of 25 to 100 mg/day while labetalol is used in doses of 300 to 600 mg/day in divided doses.

c. *Vasodilators:* An important part of treatment of patient with heart failure, specifically used in hypertensive heart diseases. Most commonly used are Hydralazine and Nitroglycerine. Hydralazine is arterial vasodilator and can be used in the dose of 25 to 50 mg in divided doses.

d. *Digoxin:* It is used due to its ionotropic effects. Indicated in heart failure and maternal arrhythmia. It is started with a loading dose of 1.0 to 1.5 mg orally in 24 hour period. Maintenance dosage is usually 0.25 mg daily.

e. *Antibiotic Prophylaxis:*
   - According to the new guidelines of the American College of Obstetricians and Gynecologists (2008), American College of Cardiology and American Heart Association, antibiotic prophylaxis is not recommended for all patients.
   - If required inj Ampicillin 2.0 gm IV, Cefazoline or Ceftriaxone 1gm is given IV 30 to 60 min before procedure.
   - Patients who are allergic to penicillin are given inj Vancomycin 1 gm IV 12 hourly or inj Clindamycin 600 mg IV 8 hourly.[10]
   - However in India, because of the hygienic conditions of patients in the labor room and lower socioeconomic status, it would be wiser to follow the previous recommendations unless proved otherwise by substantial data.

Interventional Measures

a. *Balloon mitral valvotomy:* It is usually done after the patient's status has improved by medical therapy with cardiology consultation. It is mostly undertaken if the mitral valve area is less than 1 cm^2.

b. *Open valvotomy and valve replacement:* These two procedures are rarely undertaken in pregnancy as it involves the use of cardiopulmonary bypass and fetal compromise may occur due to that. However, it may be undertaken rarely with termination of pregnancy by a cesarean section at reasonable maturity of fetus.

Management of Labor

It is advisable for patient with heart failure to deliver vaginally. Morbidity and mortality rate after cesarean section will be higher due to complications of anesthesia and operative intervention. The other important points regarding the management are:
- General measures (as mentioned above).
- Adequate pain relief, although intravenous analgesics provide satisfactory pain relief, continuous epidural analgesia is recommended. Analgesics most commonly used are morphine, tramadol etc.
- Restrict intravenous fluid to less than 75 mL/hour.
- Avoid bolus oxytocin and ergot compounds.
- Prevention of thromboembolism by pneumatic compression stockings or prophylactic anticoagulant therapy.
- Avoid undue prolongation of second stage of labor. Prophylactic forceps can be used when patient is not delivering for more than half hour in second stage in labor.
- Watch for sign and symptoms of cardiac failure in postpartum period.

PERIPARTUM CARDIOMYOPATHY

Introduction and Pathophysiology

Peripartum cardiomyopathy (PPCM) is a rare cause of heart failure that affects women late in pregnancy or in early postpartum period. Incidence varies widely within a range of 1:3000 to 1:15000 deliveries in United States, 1:1000 in South Africa and 1:1000 in Haiti. *It is associated with high mortality rates of 18 to 50 percent.*

The other etiological factors seem to be myocarditis[15], obesity, hypertension and undetected ventricular hypertrophy. Dilated cardiomyopathy is also detected in HIV infection and clinically silent mitral stenosis.

Risk Factors for PPCM

- Age >30 years
- African race
- Multiparity
- Twin pregnancy
- History of pre-eclampsia or eclampsia
- Postpartum hypertension
- Maternal cocain use and
- 4 weeks of tocolytic therapy.

Diagnosis of PPCM

It is a diagnosis of exclusion. The condition is mainly because of systolic dysfunction of heart.
- Earlier the diagnostic criteria were:
  - Development of heart failure in last month of pregnancy or within 5 months of delivery.[11]
  - Absence of identifiable causes of heart failure.[12]
  - Absence of recognisable heart disease before last month of pregnancy.[12]
- Later on from 1999 the diagnostic criteria are based on echocardiography:[13]
  - Ejection fraction of < 45%, fractional shortening of < 30% of heart muscles, or both
  - End diastolic left ventricular dimention of >2.7 cm/m^2 of body surface area.[13]

Lately diastolic dysfunction is also recognised as a cause of heart failure, representing up to 50 percent of all heart failure patients with similar dire prognosis. In PPCM, diastolic dysfunction could be a successive phenotype of systolic dysfunction. A study done by Hilfiker-Kleiner, et al showed that 16-KDA cleavage product of prolactin is seen in abundance in PPCM patients and this seems to be the major culprit for development of PPCM[16], so bromocriptine may be advocated for management.

Signs and Symptoms

- Dyspnea is a universal feature.
- Cough, orthopnea, palpitation, paroxysmal nocturnal dyspnea, chest pain, hemoptysis and abdominal pain.
- Hallmark finding is impressive cardiomegaly and echocardiographic findings.

CASE SCENARIO-2

A 38-year-old female, G3P2L2 with 8 month amenorrhea presented to casualty with complaints of palpitation and breathlessness for 4 days, which is progressively worsening. She has no history of heart disease earlier or in this pregnancy. She is taking regular antenatal care. On examination, she has signs and symptoms of congestive cardiac failure.

History

The important points in history can help rule out other causes of heart failure like
- History suggestive of anemia- low socioeconomic class, nutritional status, worm infestations
- Cardiac symptoms suggestive of undetected rheumatic heart disease or any other cardiac lesion
- History of hypertension in earlier or present pregnancy and treatment taken
- History of chronic respiratory disease like tuberculosis, COPD
- History of viral fever in recent past to rule out viral myocarditis
- History of heat intolerance or thyroid supplementation to rule out thyrotoxicosis
- In the absence of any suggestive history a fair suspicion of PPCM can clinch the diagnosis.

Examination

Look for signs and symptoms to identify the causes of heart failure like:
- Built, nutrition, height, weight, body mass index
- Pallor, cyanosis, clubbing, icterus, tongue, teeth, gums and tonsils
- JVP, thyroid, lymph nodes in neck, neck veins
- Edema-Pedal, periorbital, vulval, abdominal etc.
- Temperature, pulse rate, BP, respiratory rate
- A thorough respiratory and cardiovascular system examination.

Investigation

- *Echocardiography:* It is the main stay of diagnosis. An apparently healthy pregnant woman without any history of heart disease with suggestive echo findings would be generally a case of PPCM after other causes have been ruled out.
- *Chest X-ray:* Marked cardiomegaly with signs of congestive cardiac failure.

Management

The management is mainly symptomatic and includes:
a. *Bed rest.*
b. *Diuretics*—To decrease preload.
c. *Vasodilators*—To reduce afterload.
d. *Digitalis*—For ionotropic effects, unless complex arrhythmias are present.
e. *Anticoagulant therapy*—Prophylactic heparin can be used to prevent associated thromboembolism which is common.
f. *Immunosuppressive therapy* can be considered if the myocardial biopsy indicates myocarditis and there is no improvement after two week of standard therapy.
g. *Extracorporeal Membrane Oxygenation* has been reported to be life saving in women with fulminant cardiomyopathy.[16]

Prognosis

The prognosis in these patients is guarded and especially poor in those with low left ventricular ejection fraction. In a study by Fett and co-workers, who performed 6 monthly echocardiogram in 116 pregnant patients with PPCM, 28 percent of the patients recovered within 6 month postpartum (i.e. left ventricular ejection fraction > 50%) and 3/4th of these patients took more than 12 months to attain this level.[17] Those patients who attain normal ventricular function within 6 months time have a good prognosis, but those who don't, have high morbidity and mortality rates.

Women who recover from PPCM are at a high risk for recurrence in subsequent pregnancy. About 20 percent of patients may develop heart failure in next pregnancy; higher percentage will show left ventricular dysfunction. Women with persistent ventricular dysfunction should be advised to avoid pregnancy. The other complications are pulmonary embolism, cerebral ischemic stroke and rarely heart transplantation may be needed.

Obstetric Outcome with PPCM

Patient can be allowed to deliver vaginally. The cesarean rates are higher than normal due to possible higher incidence of advanced maternal age, hypertension, twin pregnancy etc.[19] There is an entity called Peripartum antenatal cardiomyopathy (PACM) which is detected earlier in pregnancy, not in later months.[18] The clinical picture and prognosis is the same but an increased rate of premature deliveries and more fetal compromise is noted.[18]

HYPERTROPHIC CARDIOMYOPATHY

This is another form of cardiomyopathy which is hypertrophic. It may be familial or sporadic (*Idiopathic hypertrophic subaortic stenosis*). It is caused by mutation in group of genes that encode proteins of the cardiac sarcomere. Inheritance is autosomal dominant, genetic screening is complex and not currently available.

Diagnosis is established by echocardiographic identification of a hypertrophied and non dilated left ventricle in the absence of other cardiovascular condition. Symptoms are similar to other cardiomyopathies. Pregnancy is well tolerated but congestive cardiac failure is more common.

Management

- Management is similar to that for aortic stenosis
- Strenuous exercise is prohibited.
- Abrupt positional changes are avoided to prevent reflex vasodilatation and decreased preload.
- Diuretics and drugs causing diuresis are generally not used. If symptoms develop, i.e. angina, drugs like beta blockers and calcium channel blockers can be used.
- The route of delivery is determined by obstetrical indication.
- Spinal analgesia is contraindicated and epidural analgesia is controversial.[19]

KEY POINTS

- Pregnant women are more vulnerable to develop cardiac failure and pulmonary edema due to circulatory changes peculiar to pregnancy.
- Pulmonary edema in pregnancy is caused by heart disease, hypertensive disorders, anemia, septicemia, tocolytic therapy, etc. In India, valvular lesions due to rheumatic heart disease is the most common cause.
- Management in antenatal period consists of medical management (diuretics, α blockers, digoxin) and supportive measures.
- Vaginal delivery is allowed unless there is an obstetric indication for cesarean.
- Management during labor involves adequate pain relief, restriction of IV fluids and monitoring for signs and symptoms of cardiac failure.
- The patient should be watched for signs and symptoms of cardiac failure for one week in the postpartum period.
- Peripartum cardiomyopathy is a rare cause of heart failure (without any apparent cause) affecting women in late pregnancy and early postpartum period. It is a diagnosis of exclusion. Echocardiography is confirmatory.

REFERENCES

1. Avila WS, Rossi EG, Ramires JA, et al. Pregnancy in patients with heart disease: experience with 1,000 cases. Clin Cardiol 2003;26:135-42.

2. Pritchard JE. Changes in the blood volume during pregnancy and delivery. Anesthesiology 1965;26:393-9.
3. Huisman A, Aarnoudse JG, Heuvelmans JH, et al. Whole blood viscosity during normal pregnancy. Br J Obstet Gynaecol 1987;94:1143-9.
4. Stein PK, Hagley MT, Cole PL, Domitrovich PP, Kleiger RE, Rottman JN. Changes in 24-hour heart rate variability during normal pregnancy. Am J Obstet Gynecol 1999;180:978-85.
5. Clark SL, Cotton DB, Lee W, et al. Central hemodynamic assessment of normal term pregnancy. Am J Obstet Gynecol 1989;161:1439-42.
6. Mann DL. Heart failure and Cor Pulmonale. In: Kasper DL, Braunwald E, Fauci AS, Hauser SL, Longo DL, Jameson JL, Loscalzo J (eds). Harrison's principles of internal medicine. 17th edn. New York: McGraw-Hill, 2008.pp.1443.
7. Criteria Committee, New York Heart Association. Diseases of the heart and blood vessels. Nomenclature and criteria for diagnosis. 6th ed. Boston: Little, Brown, 1964:114.
8. Siva A, Shah AM. Moderate mitral stenosis in pregnancy: the hemodynamic impact of diuresis. Heart 2005; 91:e3.
9. al Kasab SM, Sabag T, al Zaibag M, et al. Beta-adrenergic receptor blockade in the management of pregnant women with mitral stenosis. Am J Obstet Gynecol 1990;163:37-40.
10. American College of Obstetricians and Gynecologists Committee on Obstetric Practice. ACOG Committee Opinion No. 421, November 2008: antibiotic prophylaxis for infective endocarditis. Obstet Gynecol 2008;112:1193-4.
11. Rogers FJ, Cooper S. Peripartum heart failure caused by left ventricular diastolic dysfunction. J Am Osteopath Assoc 2010;110:87-90.
12. Demakis JG, Rahimtoola SH, Sutton GC, et al. Natural course of peripartum cardiomyopathy. Circulation 1971;44:1053-61.
13. Hibbard JU, Lindheimer M, Lang RM. A modified definition for peripartum cardiomyopathy and prognosis based on echocardiography. Obstet Gynecol 1999;94:311-6.
14. Hilfiker-Kleiner D, Kaminski K, Podewski E, et al. A cathepsin D-cleaved 16 kDa form of prolactin mediates postpartum cardiomyopathy. Cell 2007;128:589-600.
15. Felker GM, Thompson RE, Hare JM, et al. Underlying causes and long-term survival in patients with initially unexplained cardiomyopathy. N Engl J Med 2000;342:1077-84.
16. Smith IJ, Gillham MJ. Fulminant peripartum cardiomyopathy rescue with extracorporeal membranous oxygenation. Int J Obstet Anesth 2009;18:186-8.
17. Fett JD, Sannon H, Thélisma E, Sprunger T, Suresh V. Recovery from severe heart failure following peripartum cardiomyopathy. Int J Gynaecol Obstet 2009;104:125-7.
18. Elkayam U, Akhter MW, Singh H, et al. Pregnancy-associated cardiomyopathy: clinical characteristics and a comparison between early and late presentation. Circulation 2005;111:2050-5.
19. Camann WR, Thornhill ML. Cardiovascular disease. In: Chestnut DH (ed). Obstetric Anesthesia: Principles and Practice. 2nd edn. St. Louis: Mosby, 1999. pp. 776.

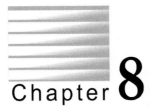

Chapter 8

Acute Asthmatic Attack in Pregnancy

Mumtaz Khan

INTRODUCTION

Bronchial asthma is a potentially serious airways disease characterized by chronic airway inflammation, with increased airway responsiveness to a variety of stimuli, and airway obstruction that is partially or completely reversible. It is the most common respiratory disease complicating pregnancy with an incidence of approximately 8 percent.[1, 2]

The diagnosis is confirmed by demonstrating airway obstruction on spirometry that is at least partially reversible, (>12% increase in FEV_1 (forced expiratory volume in 1 second) following bronchodilator - inhalation of β_2 agonists (salbutamol).[3] Measurement of PEFR (peak expiratory flow rate) could also be the basis for diagnosis. The PEFR should be measured in the morning, immediately on waking up and before use of bronchodilators and again at bedtime, 5 to 10 minutes after use of bronchodilators. A variability of more than 20 percent baseline is diagnostic for asthma.[4,5]

Mild and moderate asthma if properly managed has excellent pregnancy outcomes both for mother and the baby. Severe and poorly controlled asthma is associated with higher maternal morbidity and mortality and predisposes to complications like prematurity, pre-eclampsia, fetal growth restriction and increased incidence of cesarean section.[6] Acute asthmatic attack in pregnancy is a life threatening emergency needing multidisciplinary management approach.

CASE SCENARIO

A 30-year-old G2P1 with 34 weeks pregnancy presents with acute onset of breathlessness since half an hour.

Comments: When such a patient is brought to the emergency she requires to be attended immediately. First aid measures must start at once while simultaneous history taking and examination is done to reach a diagnosis.

Symptoms of asthma include difficulty in breathing/shortness of breath, tightness in the chest, cough associated with wheezing and production of sputum. These symptoms may worsen at night and may be precipitated by exposure to certain allergens, exercise or infections.

Differential Diagnosis

For patients presenting for the first time with breathlessness in pregnancy, besides asthma, one should consider the various **differential diagnosis**:-
- *Heart disease:* Any history of dyspnea on exertion, previous history of heart disease, h/o fever, persistent cough, pain in chest and other relevant history.

- *Hypertension:* Ask about history of swelling over body and feet, history of high BP records. Pulmonary edema which may complicate a pre-existing heart disease or hypertension.
- *Anemia*
- Dyspnea of pregnancy is differentiated from asthma by the absence of cough, wheeze, chest tightness and airway obstruction.
- Pneumonia/pneumonitis
- Bronchitis.
- Pneumothorax
- Pulmonary embolism
- Adult respiratory distress syndrome(ARDS)
- Anaphylaxis/allergic reaction
- Gastroesophageal reflux.
- Postnasal drip leading to chronic cough

FIRST AID MEASURES

- Keep the patient propped up in bed and give humidified oxygen 40 to 60 percent
- Put an intravenous (IV) cannula and start fluids-N-saline. Hydration helps mobilize and clear pulmonary secretions
- Attach pulse oximeter and check oxygen saturation, blood for arterial blood gas (ABG) analysis is sent if oxygen saturation is low
- Quickly assess the general condition of the patient, check her pulse, blood pressure (BP), respiratory rate (RR) and temperature
- Send calls to physician and anesthetist.

POINTS TO BE NOTED IN HISTORY

1. *Suspect asthma* if patient gives previous history of attacks of breathlessness associated with cough, wheeze, tightness in chest, shortness of breath and production of sputum.
2. *Assess the severity of disease:* If the patient gives previous history of such attacks then ask about
   a. Their frequency (whether 1 or 2 times per week, or daily).
   b. Do they interfere with her sleep and how often is she awakened at night with these symptoms (1-2 times per month or more than 4 times per week).
   c. Whether she is able to carry on with her routine chores or there is limitation of her activities. All of these will help assess the severity of bronchial asthma and its pharmacological management. The NAEP (National asthma education program) has defined criteria to classify the severity of asthma (Table 8.1).[7]

Table 8.1: Classification of Asthma Severity and Control in Pregnant Patients				
*Asthma control**	*Well controlled*	*Not well controlled*	*Poorly controlled*	*Very poorly controlled*
Asthma severity** Symptom frequency/ Salbutamol use	Intermittent ≤2d/ week	Mild persistent >2d/ week, but not daily	Moderate persistent Daily symptoms	Severe persistent Throughout the day
Night time awakening	≤ Twice per month	>Twice per month	> Once per week	≥ 4/wk
Interference with normal activity	None	Minor limitation	Some limitation	Extremely limited
FEV_1 or peak flow % predicted/ personal best	>80%	>80%	60-80%	< 60%

* Assess asthma control in patients on long-term control medications to determine whether step up, step down or no change in therapy required.

** Assess severity for patients who are not on long-term control medication, to determine starting controller therapy based on severity.

3. *Enquire about the precipitating factors:*
   a. Exercise
   b. Exposure to irritants or allergens. Association between asthma and allergy is common.[3] Usual allergens are animal dander, urine and saliva, house dust mites, cockroach antigens, pollens and mold. Other irritants are tobacco smoke, strong odors, air pollutants and some food additives.
   c. Following some infection.
   d. Any drug intake which could have precipitated the attack- drugs such as aspirin and beta-blockers can act as triggers.
   This knowledge will help in prevention of further attacks by avoiding the trigger.
4. *History of asthma in previous pregnancy and its severity.* Asthma severity seems to follow the same course in subsequent pregnancies.[8]
5. *The treatment history*—Medications that the patient is taking to control the attack
   a. Beta agonist inhalers
   b. Low dose steroid inhalers.
   c. Other drugs such as theophylline, cromolyn or leukotriene receptor antagonist (LTRA).
   d. Oral steroids
   e. If the patient needed ventilatory support in any previous attack
   All this information has a bearing on the pharmacological management of asthma attack as per the **step therapy** approach to asthma severity (Table 8.2).
6. *Menstrual and obstetric history:* Ask for period of amenorrhea, early USG done for dating, presence of fetal movements, status of tetanus immunization, past obstetric history.

> **History in this case:** This patient gives history of similar episode in this pregnancy two months ago, as well as in last pregnancy for which she required to be admitted to hospital. She is presently on budesonide inhaler 4 puffs daily (medium dose) and salmetrol inhaler 2 puffs twice daily. Today, despite taking her regular dose and salbutamol inhaler her symptoms are not subsiding.

POINTS TO BE NOTED IN EXAMINATION

General Examination

- Assess the general condition of the patient, whether conscious, oriented, extent of respiratory distress.
- Look for pallor, cyanosis or jaundice, pedal edema and swelling over body. Assess the hydration of the patient.
- Check vitals
  Check peripheral pulses—rate, rhythm, volume.
  Monitor blood pressure.
  Count respiratory rate and rhythm.

Cardiovascular and Respiratory System Examination

- Auscultate the heart and check for murmur or any extra sound.
- Auscultate the lungs and confirm bronchospasm (presence of rhonchi). Check for crepitations or absent breath sounds.

Abdominal (P/A) Examination

- Check for hepatosplenomegaly
- Check the height of uterine fundus, fetal presentation, fetal heart sound (FHS).

Examination in this case:
Patient is conscious, oriented, not cyanosed, and is not able to complete sentences in one breath.
Pulse-120/min, RR-30/min (using accessory muscles of respiration), BP-130/88 mm Hg
Cardiovascular examination- No murmur
Respiratory system-Bilateral rhonchi present with occasional crepts.
P/A -Fundal height -34 weeks corresponding to period of amenorrhea, cephalic presentation and FHS 140/min.

Diagnosis

From history and examination, a diagnosis of severe acute asthmatic attack with 34 weeks pregnancy is made.

Further management will include performing certain investigations and tests to confirm the diagnosis, and simultaneously starting the treatment.

INVESTIGATIONS

- Complete hemogram
- Blood group ABO & Rh
- Blood urea
- Serum electrolytes
- Random blood sugar
- Urine routine exam.
- Pulmonary function are assessed by FEV_1 (spirometry) and PEFR (using peak flow meter).
- Fetal status to be assessed by cardiotocography (CTG) and biophysical profile.

TREATMENT

In a pregnant patient step-care therapeutic approach, as per Table 8.2, should be followed for treating asthma as it increases the number and dosage of medication according to asthma severity. Patients with poorly controlled asthma are stepped up 1 step and very poorly controlled asthma are stepped up 2 steps. After control is sustained for a few months a cautious step-down approach to therapy may be followed.

Table 8.2: Step therapy medical management of asthma during pregnancy[11]
Asthma severity and Medications*
Mild intermittent
1. No daily medications, salbutamol as needed
Mild persistent
2. Low- dose inhaled corticosteroid (alternative cromolyn, LTRA, or theophylline**)
Moderate persistent
3. Medium- dose inhaled corticosteroid (alternative: low-dose inhaled corticosteroid and LABA, LTRA, or theophylline)
4. Medium- dose inhaled corticosteroid and LABA (alternative: medium-dose inhaled corticosteroid plus LTRA, or theophylline)
Severe persistent
5. High- dose inhaled corticosteroid and LABA
6. High- dose inhaled corticosteroid and LABA and oral prednisolone

*   Starting therapy for a specific level of severity
** Theophylline (serum level 5-12 µg/mL)
    LABA-long-acting β agonist (salmeterol and formoterol)

ACUTE EXACERBATION IN PREGNANCY

The treatment for acute asthmatic exacerbation in pregnancy is the same as for the nonpregnant patient. A low threshold for hospitalization should be followed for pregnant patients. Airway inflammation has been found to be the basic underlying pathology and is seen to be present in all cases. The aim of management is to treat the inflammation in order to decrease airway responsiveness and prevent symptoms of asthma or an acute attack.

- Give **salbutamol** 5 mg in 3 ml normal saline as nebulizer via oxygen mask.
- Maintain **hydration** by giving IV fluids—1 liter normal saline 8 hourly.
- Put the patient on noninvasive BP (NIBP**) monitor** and **ECG monitor**.
- If **oxygen saturation** < 92 percent or features of life-threatening attack send **ABG**.

LIFE-THREATENING ATTACK OF ASTHMA

Signs of life-threatening asthma are confusion, coma, cyanosis, feeble respiratory effort, bradycardia, hypotension, a silent chest and a PEFR (peak expiratory flow rate) of < 33 percent predicted (approx.160 L/min). Predicted PEFR is 480 L/min.

- Measure PEFR every 15 min. Signs of improvement are a rise in PEFR above 50 percent predicted
- Repeat **salbutamol** 5 mg via nebulizer (up to 3-4 doses) every 15 min till improvement is there
- If after 3 doses of salbutamol there is not much change in severity of symptoms, oxygen saturation remains poor or there is development of side effects, one must give parenteral corticosteroids Give inj. **hydrocortisone** 200 mg IV (may be repeated 4 hourly if required)
- Consider subcutaneous **terbutaline,** 0.25 mg if patient does not respond to the above treatment
- Ensure that physician is available
- An inhaled anticholinergic, **ipratropium bromide** 500 μg may be added to a repeat dose of salbutamol via nebulizer, if the response to the above therapy is not satisfactory
- In patients who are refractory to inhaled therapies consider giving IV **aminophyline** 250 μg over 10 minutes under ECG control. Serum levels need to be monitored. Aminophylline is said to cause neonatal irritability and apnea; hence the pediatrician should be informed. It is not given if patient is already taking oral theophyllines
- Monitor fetal heart rate at regular intervals, or monitor continuously by CTG
- Monitor and record pulse, BP, respiratory rate, oxygen saturation and the drugs that have been given
- If patient still does not improve arrange for portable X-ray to rule out pneumothorax or consolidation. Tension pneumothorax must be relieved on an emergency basis by inserting a chest drain, or by putting an intravenous cannula into the second intercostal space in the midclavicular line and replacing it with a chest drain.

Patient showing signs and symptoms of life-threatening attack and a deteriorating PEFR would require ICU care and maybe intubation. ABG is sent and anesthetist is called. A $PaCO_2$ of >4 kPa or PaO_2 of <8 kPa indicates severe respiratory compromise and intubation is strongly indicated.

Patient who shows improvement will have relief in her breathing and wheeze; heart rate, respiratory rate and oxygen saturation return to near normal; chest clears up on auscultation and PEFR rise above 50 percent predicted. The patient should also perceive fetal movements. These patients will require further observation and assessment (both maternal and fetal) to decide on the need for ongoing therapy.

- Patients showing an improvement in FEV_1, or PEFR above 70 percent sustained for 60 minutes after last treatment, no distress and reassuring fetal status may be discharged and followed up in the outpatient clinic.
- Patients showing lesser improvement in FEV_1 ,or PEFR more than 50 percent but less than 70 percent predicted and persistence of mild-to-moderate symptoms need to be individualized for further management (whether continued treatment in emergency room, discharge home or hospitalization).

- Patients showing poor response of FEV_1 or PEFR less than 50 percent need hospitalization and continuation of therapy.

OBSTETRIC MANAGEMENT

Planning the timing and mode of delivery is important because of potential fetal and maternal complications. Perinatal mortality for asthmatics is twice that in controls.[9]

Maternal mortality although rare can occur in a case of status asthmaticus and rises to 40 percent when a pregnant asthmatic requires ventilatory support.[10]

The fetus is particularly prone to maternal respiratory changes. With respiratory alkalosis in the asthmatic mother, the fetus may develop hypoxemia well before the maternal perception of respiratory compromise. Hence the need for close fetal monitoring by CTG and biophysical profile. Aggressive management of acute asthma exacerbations as discussed above may prevent fetal compromise.

When to Terminate Pregnancy and how?

Once the acute exacerbation is controlled the patient can continue with pregnancy till fetal maturity is reached, provided the fetal parameters are normal. In the presented case, patient is 34 weeks pregnant and should benefit if delivery is postponed to 37 weeks. In case of fetal compromise labor can be induced with PGE2 gel, which is safe. Cesarean delivery for acute exacerbation of asthma is rarely needed. However, delivery may benefit the respiratory status of a patient with unstable asthma who has a mature fetus.

During Labor

- Asthma medications are continued during labor and delivery. Women who have received systemic steroids in the past 4 to 6 weeks are given IV steroids (100 mg hydrocortisone 8 hourly) during labor and for 24 hrs after delivery to prevent adrenal crisis.
- Pediatrician and anesthetist are kept informed.
- Patient is kept hydrated.
- Adequate analgesia is required to prevent bronchospasm and to reduce oxygen consumption. Epidural analgesia is ideal for labor. Regional anesthesia is preferred over general anesthesia for cesarean section. A nonhistamine release narcotic such as Fentanyl is preferable to Meperidine or Morphine.
- In the event of postpartum hemorrhage $PGF_{2\alpha}$ and methyl ergometrine are avoided as they cause bronchospasm, instead other oxytocin is used.

Breastfeeding

There is no contraindication to breastfeeding as only small amounts of asthma medications are secreted in breast milk.

Advice on Discharge

- Patient should continue the asthma medication - short-acting β agonist 2 to 4 puffs every 3 to 4 hours as per the need.
- She should continue with oral steroids if already started, at a dose of 40 to 60 mg in single or two divided doses for 3 to 10 days.
- Inhaled corticosteroids should be started or continued till further medical follow up.
- Next visit for medical follow-up visit is scheduled in 5 days time.
- If pregnancy is continuing fetal movements are monitored and patient is followed up weekly.
- If patient has delivered, postnatal follow up is done after six weeks and medical follow-up is done after 5 to 7 days for monitoring treatment.

KEY POINTS

- Pregnant women with asthma should continue their asthma medication during pregnancy to avoid asthma symptoms and exacerbations.
- Aim of asthma therapy during pregnancy is to maintain adequate fetal oxygen saturation by preventing hypoxic episodes in the mother.
- Step care therapeutic approach is followed for treating asthma during pregnancy.
- Serial ultrasound and fetal surveillance for fetal growth and activity are recommended in pregnant patients with moderate-to-severe asthma.
- Inhaled **salbutamol** is the recommended **rescue therapy** in acute asthmatic attack in pregnancy.
- Inhaled **corticosteroids** are the first line **controller therapy** in pregnant patients with persistent asthma and **budesonide** is the drug of choice.
- Oral corticosteroids are required for very poorly controlled asthma.
- Asthma medications should be continued during labor and delivery.
- Women who have received systemic corticosteroids in the past 4 weeks should be given intravenous corticosteroids (inj. hydrocortisone 100 mg 8 hourly) during labor and for 24 hrs after delivery to prevent adrenal crisis.

REFERENCES

1. Wendel PJ. Asthma in pregnancy. Obstet Gynecol Clin North Am 2001;28:537-51.
2. National Asthma Education and Prevention Program Expert Panel Report: Managing asthma during pregnancy: recommendations for pharmacologic treatment- 2004 update. J Allergy Clin Immunol 2005;115:34-46.
3. Dombrowski MP, Schatz M. ACOG Practice Bulletin: Asthma in pregnancy. Obstet Gynecol 2008;111:457-64.
4. Hargreave FE, Dolovich J, Newhouse MT. The assessment and treatment of asthma: A conference report. J Allergy Clin Immunol 1990;85:1098-1111.
5. National Asthma Education Program: Report of the Working Group on Asthma in Pregnancy: Executive Summary. Management of Asthma in Pregnancy. National Heart, Lung and Blood Institute. NIH Publication No. 93-3279A, March 1993.
6. Dombrowski MP, Schatz M, Wise R, Momirova V, Lindon M, Mabie W, et al.Asthma during pregnancy. National Institute of Child Health and Human Development Maternal- Fetal Medicine Units Network and the National Heart, Lung, and Blood Institute. Obstet Gynecol 2004;103:5-12.
7. US Department of Health and Human Services, Public Health Service, National Institute of Health: Guidelines for the Diagnosis and Management of Asthma. NIH Publication No. 91-3042, August 1991.
8. Gluck JC, Gluck PA. The effects of pregnancy on asthma, a prospective study. Ann Allergy 1976;37:164-8.
9. Gordon M, Nishwander KR, Berendes H: Fetal morbidity following potentially anoxigenic, obstetric conditions: Bronchial asthma. Am J Obstet Gynecol 1970;106:421-9.
10. Cunningham FG, Leveno KJ, Bloom SL, Hauth JC, Rouse DJ, Spong CY. Medical and surgical complications in pregnancy. In: Williams Obstetrics, 23rd edn, USA: McGraw Hill, 2010. pp. 996-1012.
11. Dombrowski MP, Schatz M. Asthma in pregnancy. Clin Obstet Gynecol 2010;53:301-10.

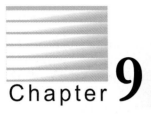

Chapter 9

Jaundice in Pregnancy

Ashok Kumar, Nargis Begum, Minu

INTRODUCTION

Jaundice is the visible yellow coloration of skin, sclera and mucosa. It is observed when serum bilirubin rises >2 mg % (normal levels 0.3 to 1.0 mg %). The liver serves multiple functions which involve the biotransformation of insoluble compounds (For example drugs, toxins, bilirubin), the metabolism and excretion of cholesterol and bilirubin, the production of plasma proteins (For example albumin, coagulation factors, alpha- and beta-globulins, transferrin, haptoglobin) and the metabolism of amino acids, carbohydrates and lipids. Liver cell injury or necrosis is measured by determining aspartate aminotransferase (AST) and alanine aminotransferase (ALT) levels, while liver synthetic function (depressed in cirrhosis or severe acute liver disease) is quantified by determining albumin level and prothrombin time. Cholestasis and biliary obstruction are evaluated by measuring alkaline phosphatase, bilirubin, 5'-nucleotidase or gamma-glutamyl transpeptidase (GGT) levels.[1]

Jaundice occurs in 1 in 1500 pregnancies. The physiological changes and normal values of liver function tests during pregnancy are shown in Table 9.1 and 9.2 respectively. In tropical countries like India, morbidity and mortality due to liver diseases in pregnancy is very high.[3] There are various causes of jaundice in pregnancy (Table 9.3). Viral hepatitis (VH) is the most common cause of jaundice in pregnancy and hence it will be discussed in this chapter. The most common causes of viral hepatitis are the five hepatotropic viruses: Hepatitis A (infectious hepatitis and short-incubation period), Hepatitis B (serum hepatitis and long-incubation hepatitis), Hepatitis C (parenterally transmitted non-A non-B hepatitis), Hepatitis D (delta agent), and Hepatitis E (enterically transmitted non-A non-B hepatitis). The etiologic spectrum of various types of hepatitis during pregnancy is shown in Table 9.4. Hepatitis E is most common type of hepatitis in pregnancy especially in third trimester. Precise serological identification of the type of hepatitis is required to define the management and prognosis during pregnancy (Table 9.5).

In the developed world, the course of viral hepatitis is not altered by the pregnancy *per se*. However in developing world, fulminant course, increased fetal and maternal mortality, preterm delivery, and abortion are common in women having viral hepatitis during pregnancy.[5] Perinatal transmission have been observed in HBV, HCV and HEV infection.

The incidence of HAV in pregnancy is 1 in 1000.[6] If the patient is infected in the third trimester, preterm labor can occur and the newborn should receive passive immunoprophylaxis within 48 hours of delivery.[7] Hepatitis A does not lead to chronic infection and rarely leads to serious complications. The overall case fatality rate is less than 1 percent.[8]

Acute HBV infection occurs in 2 per 1000 pregnant women.[9] There is increased risk of prematurity, meconium stained liquor, intrauterine growth retardation and neonatal death in severe

Table 9.1: Changes in liver function test during pregnancy[2]

- ALT/AST/GGT/Serum Bilirubin decreases 25 percent below normal values due to hemodilution
- Clotting factors VII,VIII, & X/Fibrinogen synthesis increases
- Proteins and albumin synthesis decreases by 20 percent due to estrogen influence or increased plasma volume
- Fibrinolytic activity decreases
- Alkaline phosphatase (ALP) levels is elevated two to four fold secondary to placental alkaline phosphatase levels

Table 9.2: Normal values of liver function tests in normal pregnancy

| | | *Normal value in females* | | |
| | *Nonpregnant* | *Pregnant* | | |
		1st trimester	*2nd trimester*	*3rd trimester*
AST (U/L)	7-40	10-28	11-29	11-30
ALT (U/L)	0-40	6-32	6-32	6-32
GGT (U/L)	11-50	5-37	5-43	5-41
ALP (U/L)	30-130	32-100	43-135	130-410

Table 9.3: Causes and prognosis of jaundice in pregnancy

A.	**Peculiar to pregnancy**
Acute fatty liver	Rare; variable prognosis
Toxemia	Rare; Hepatic hemorrhage may be complication
HELLP syndrome	Hemolytic anemia, elevated liver function tests, low platelet count, rare, poor prognosis
Recurrent cholestasis	Common, good prognosis, familial, reoccurs, fetal wastage
Hyperemesis	Rare cause of jaundice
B.Intercurrent	
Viral hepatitis	Main cause of jaundice :
	Hepatitis A
	Hepatitis B
	Hepatitis C
	Hepatitis E
	HSV, CMV, EBV, yellow fever
Gallstone	Rare cause of jaundice, ultrasound diagnosis
Chronic liver disease	Rare, prognosis variable
Drug induced hepatitis	Rare, common drugs : isoniazid, rifampicin, paracetamol

Table 9.4: Etiological spectrum of hepatitis in third trimester of pregnancy from Lok Nayak Hospital[4] (n=97)

Hepatitis	A	B	C	E	A+B	B+E	A+E	Non A-E	N
AVH	1	5	0	25	1	2	0	40	69
	(1.4%)	(7.2%)	(0%)	(36.2%)	(1.4%)	(2.8%)	(0%)	(57.9%)	(71%)
FHF	4	2	0	21	0	2	3	6	28
	(14.3%)	(7.14%)	(0%)	(75%)	(0%)	(7.1%)	(10.7%)	(21.4%)	(29%)
Total	5	7	0	46	1	4	3	46	97
	(5.2%)	(7.2%)	(0%)	(47.4%)	(1.03%)	(4.1%)	(3.1%)	(47.4%)	

Table 9.5: Simplified diagnostic approach of hepatitis serological tests

Serologic tests of patient's serum

HBsAg	IgM Anti-HAV	IgM Anti-HBc	Anti-HCV	IgM Anti-HEV	Diagnostic Interpretation
-	+	-	-	-	Acute hepatitis A
+	-	+	-	-	Acute hepatitis B
-	-	+	-	-	Acute hepatitis B
+	-	-	-	-	Chronic hepatitis B
+	+	+	-	-	Acute hepatitis A and B
-	+	+	-	-	Acute hepatitis A and B
-	-	-	+	-	Acute hepatitis C
-	-	-	-	+	Acute hepatitis E

fulminant cases. The interferon and ribavirin combination therapy causes birth defects in infants so usage of effective contraception is recommended during the treatment and 6 months after treatment ends.

The incidence of hepatitis C virus in pregnant women is variable:0.14 percent in UK, 1.1 percent in Australia, 1.3 percent in Taiwan, 3.2 percent in US. A study from Lok Nayak Hospital showed 1.03 percent incidence rate of hepatitis C in asymptomatic pregnant women.[10] The associated risk factors for HCV transmission are acupuncture, tattooing, dilatation and curettage. The rate of vertical transmission is increased in cases having associated HIV infection. In pregnancies with no detectable levels of HCV RNA, vertical transmission is rare.

One distinctive clinical feature of hepatitis E, compared with other forms of viral hepatitis, is its increased incidence and severity in pregnant women especially those infected in third trimester fatality rates range between 15 to 25 percent. The complications associated with HEV infection are abortion, intrauterine death, preterm labor and fulminant hepatic failure (FHF). Transmission of HEV infection from mother-to-child was found to vary from 23.3 percent to 100 percent in India and 33.3 to 50 percent in Argentina[11,12] and associated with very high perinatal morbidity and mortality. The babies born to HEV infected mother had anicteric hepatitis, hypothermia, hypoglycemia and hepatic necrosis.[13] However there are no long-term effects of hepatitis E. Transmission does not differ depending on route of delivery as long as no signs of acute maternal disease are present.

CASE SCENARIO-1

A 24-year-primigravidae reports to emergency at 28 week of gestation with history of fever for 1 week, nausea, loss of appetite, yellow discoloration of eye, urine, malaise and pain in right upper quadrant of abdomen.

Comments: The fever and systemic symptoms indicate she should be considered for the diagnosis of acute viral hepatitis.

Differential Diagnosis

- Viral hepatitis (common in all the three trimesters)
- Drug induced hepatitis (common in all the three trimesters)
- Intrahepatic cholestasis of pregnancy (common in 2nd and 3rd trimester)
- Gallstones disease(common in all the three trimesters)
- Pre-eclampsia/eclampsia (common in 3rd trimester)
- Hemolytic anemia, elevated liver function tests, low platelet count (HELLP syndrome).(common in 3rd trimester)
- Acute fatty liver of pregnancy (common in 3rd trimester)
- Hepatic rupture (common in 3rd trimester)
- Hyperemesis gravidarum (common in 1st trimester)

POINTS TO BE NOTED IN HISTORY

- Booked/Unbooked
- Relation to period of gestation
- Duration of yellowish of eyes/Nausea/Vomiting/Pruritus/Abdominal pain
- History of clay-colored stools (**indicate obstructive jaundice**)
- High-colored urine
- Systemic symptoms: fever, malaise, anorexia, weight loss, sore throat (**Flu like symptoms occur with viral hepatitis**)
- History of any abdominal swelling, hematemesis, bleeding per rectum (**to rule out Portal hypertension**)
- Sleep pattern disturbance, altered sensorium (**Hepatic encephalopathy**)
- Drug history (**intake of hepatotoxic drug**)
- Past history of blood transfusion/accidental exposure (**transmission of Hepatitis B & C infection occurs via transfusion of blood products , by needle stick injuries**)
- Past history of jaundice
- History of past pregnancy (**intrahepatic cholestasis of pregnancy recurs in 30 to 50 percent next pregnancy**) and use of birth control pills
- History of multiple partners or intravenous drug abuse (**association with transmission of HBV or HCV infection**)
- History of jaundice in family members (**association with transmission of HBV or HCV infection**)

> **History in this case:**
> History of fever for 7 days, anorexia, malaise, vomiting, dark yellowish urine, clay-coloured stools and abdominal pain. No history of any drug intake.

POINTS TO BE NOTED IN EXAMINATION

Aim is to Find Out

1. Severity of hepatitis (LFT, Prothrombin time, ultrasound of abdomen)
2. Cause/type of hepatitis (viral markers)
3. Complication of hepatitis: In terms of involvement of CNS, coagulation system, renal and respiratory system
4. Presence of preterm labor/labor depending on period of gestation
5. Evaluation for fetal well-being (look for FHS, IUGR in patients who had history of hepatitis remote from term).

General Physical Examination

- Conscious/Drowsy/Restless
- Pulse rate/Respiratory rate/Temperature/Blood Pressure
- Pallor/Icterus/Pedal Edema
- Signs of vitamin deficiency and hypoprotinemia – stomatitis, cheilosis, easy pluckability of hair
- Petechie/Bruises/Itch marks/spider angioma/nevi
- Tremors
- Urine output
- JVP

Cardiovascular and Respiratory System Examination

Abdominal (P/A) Examination

- Hepatosplenomegaly
- Ascites

- Prominent abdominal veins
- Fundal height – whether corresponding to period of gestation
- Presence of uterine contraction, fetal heart sounds

Pelvic Examination

- Vaginal discharge/bleeding/leaking: amount, color and smell
- Cervical Os: closed or open

> **Examination in this case:**
> Patient conscious, cooperative, well-oriented, afebrile.
> PR-82/m, Pallor⁻/Pedal edema⁻/Icterus⁺, BP-118/70 Hg/mm, Chest/CVS normal
> P/A- hepatomegaly, soft, tender. No ascites. A live pregnancy of 28 weeks.

INVESTIGATIONS

- Blood Group, Rh Factor
- Complete blood count: Hemoglobin, total leukocyte count (TLC) (rule out acute infection), differential leukocyte count (DLC), platelet count (rule out HELLP), peripheral smear (see for hemolysis, and type of anemia if present, for malarial parasite).
- Mean corpuscular volume (80-96 fL), Mean corpuscular hemoglobin concentration (33-37%), mean corpuscular hemoglobin (27-33 pg).
- Bleeding Time/Clotting Time/Clot Retraction time
- Coagulation Profile: Prothrombin Time (Test & Control), APTT-32-37 sec, d Dimer-0.5 mg/dL, Serum Fibrinogen-150-600 ng/dL, Fibrin degradation product-<10µg/dL
- Liver Function Test [ALT, AST, ALP, S. Biluribin (direct bilirubin & indirect bilirubin), T. Protein, S. Albumin]
- Kidney function test (serum creatinine, urea, electrolytes)
- Blood sugar random (to rule out acute fatty liver of pregnancy)
- Urine- Routine (to rule out pre-eclampsia)
- Viral Markers (HBsAg, anti-HBcIgM, HBeAg,anti-HAV IgM, anti-HCV, anti-HEV IgM)
- Ultrasound upper abdomen for hepatosplenomegaly
- Ultrasound for fetal cardiac activity

> **Investigations in this case:**
> ALT- 1790 U/L, AST- 1560 U/L, S. Bil- 8.6 mg% (D. Bil- 6.3 & I.Bil- 2.3), ALP- 350 U/L, PT- c-14s; t-16s, S. Alb-3.2 g%, mild leukopenia with a relative lymphocytosis, Viral markers—Anti-HAV IgM positive.

Diagnosis

Acute Hepatitis A

MANAGEMENT

- Hospitalization of patient (helps to monitor diet, liver function test, clinical course)
- Supportive treatment with fluid and adequate rest
- High carbohydrate and low protein diet (20 gm)
- Hygienic measures
- Vitamin K 10 mg I/M daily for 3 days
- Follow-up with LFT
- Pregnancy need not be terminated
- Steroids have no role
- Breastfeeding can be continued

PROGNOSIS

- No teratogenic effects on fetus reported
- Complete recovery with no residual disease in most cases.
- 15 percent patients have relapsing hepatitis A infection, i.e. recurring infection in 6 months.

PREVENTION

- Vertical and perinatal transmission occurs via contamination of maternal feces in mother of hepatitis A in third trimester/after delivery
- New born remains susceptible to hepatitis A from mothers who continues to excrete virus in her stool for weeks
- Neonatal immunoprophylaxis is rarely necessary as most neonatal infections are mild and herald life-long immunity
- *Prophylaxis:* ISG 0.02 ml/kg within 2 weeks of exposure to HAV infected mother and new born of mothers with HAV infection.

CASE SCENARIO-2

A 30 year G2P1L1 reports to emergency at 38 week of gestation with jaundice, HBsAg positive since 1year, vomiting, and abdominal pain along with labor pain.

Examination in this case:
Patient conscious and cooperative, afebrile, PR-82/m, pallor⁻/pedal edema⁻/icterus⁺, BP—110/78 Hg/mm, Chest/CVS- Normal. P/A- hepatomegaly, soft, tender. No ascites. A live term pregnancy.

Investigations in this case:
ALT- 1250 U/L, AST- 2458 U/L, S. Bil- 7.8 g% (D. Bil- 5.3& I.Bil- 2.5), ALP- 264 U/L, PT- c-14s; t-16s, S. Alb-3.2 g%, Viral markers- HBsAg & HBV DNA positive.

Diagnosis

Acute on chronic hepatitis B

Features of Acute Hepatitis in this Case

- Clinical feature- flu like symptoms, malaise, anorexia, nausea, arthralgia, rash
- Marked rise of serum transaminases
- 50 percent develop jaundice

Features of Chronic Hepatitis B in this Case

HBsAg positive since 1 year
Other features indicating hepatitis B infection are given in (Table 9.6).

Table 9.6: Points clinching the diagnosis of hepatitis B Infection
• First serological marker to appear- HBsAg (appears 4 week before onset of clinical symptoms) and remains detectable for 1 to 6 weeks.
• Chronic HBV carrier state diagnosed by presence of HBsAg or HBeAg 6 months after initial exposure.
• HBeAg detected during 1st month of acute infection indicates acute viremia and infectivity.
• Recovery indicated by conversion of HBeAg to anti-HBe antibody.

Table 9.7: Vertical transmission of Hepatitis B		
Maternal serum markers	*Maternal hepatitis B*	*Neonatal outcome*
HBsAg, HBeAg and IgM Anti- HBc	Acute	Acute hepatitis, recovery usually
HBsAg, HbeAg	Chronic	Chronic carrier (20-95%)
HBsAg, Anti Hbe	Chronic	Chronic carrier (0-20%)
HBsAg	Chronic	Fulminant hepatitis

Prognosis

- Incidence of transmission depends on **acute/chronic stage, period of gestation and HBeAg status** (Table 9.7).
- Acute maternal infection in first trimester resolves and risk of neonatal infections is minimal
- HBV infection during second and third trimester pose threat of vertical transmission between 10 to 90 percent respectively
- HBeAg is marker of active viral replication; if both HBsAg and HBeAg positive risk of infection to child is 70 to 90 percent
- Most infection occur at the time of delivery due to contact by maternal blood
- Mode of delivery does not affect transmission.

TREATMENT

- Hospitalization considered for clinically severe illness
- Treatment usually supportive
- Maintenance of adequate calorific diet and fluid intake
- Intravenous hydration may be required, if patient has persistent vomiting
- Vigorous or prolonged physical activity should be avoided
- Drugs metabolized by liver, must be avoided
- Vitamin K 10 mg I/M daily for 3 days
- Fetal heart sound monitoring should be done
- Investigate for HBeAg and HBeAb
- Induction of labor has no role
- If patient goes in labor spontaneously, vaginal delivery is preferable to cesarean section in view of coagulation disturbance and high-risk of intraoperative and postoperative bleeding. Arrange adequate amount of fresh frozen plasma (FFP) and blood for emergency.
- Active management of third stage of labor to prevent postpartum hemorrhage (PPH)
- If PPH occurs, FFP and blood should be transfused.

Postpartum Management

- Isolation of new born not necessary
- 0.5 mL of HBIG soon after birth preferably within 1 hr (atleast 48 hrs) and 1st dose of 0.5mL (1.0 μg) of HBV vaccine
- Repeat of HBV vaccine at one and 6 months (prevents 95% of neonatal cases of hepatitis B)
- Breastfeeding not contraindicated
- Preterm infants weighing less than 2000 g born to mothers who are HBsAg positive require an additional vaccine dose, and the first dose should not be counted due to the potentially reduced immunogenicity in these patients.
- All infants should be tested for Anti-HBsAg and HBsAg 9 to 18 months after delivery.[14]

CASE SCENARIO-3

A 22 year G2P1L1 reports to emergency at 35 week of gestation with deep jaundice, restlessness, irritative behaviour, anorexia, malaise, vomiting and abdominal pain.

History in this case:
History of fever for 7 days, restlessness since night, anorexia, malaise, vomiting, dark-yellowish urine, clay-colored stools and abdominal pain. No history of any drug intake.

Examination in this case:
Patient restless, noncooperative, violent behavior, afebrile, PR-82/m, Pallor[+]/Pedal edema[+]/Icterus[+], BP-120/80 Hg/mm, Chest/CVS- Normal. P/A- hepatomegaly, soft, tender. No ascites. A live pregnancy of 35 weeks.

Investigations in this case:
ALT- 3740 U/L, AST- 4520 U/L, S. Bil- 15.8 g% (D. Bil- 12.6 & I.Bil- 3.2), ALP- 568 U/L, PT- c-14s; t-50s, S. Alb-2.4 g%, Viral markers-Anti-HEV IgM positive.

Diagnosis

Acute liver failure due to Hepatitis E
Most common cause of acute liver failure in pregnancy is **acute viral hepatitis**
Other causes are:
• Drug induced liver disease
• Budd-Chiari syndrome
• Acute fatty liver of pregnancy

MANAGEMENT OF ACUTE LIVER FAILURE

• Must be monitored in intensive care unit (patients are generally very sick and mortality is high) (Table 9.8)
• Avoid precipitating factors and discontinue oral proteins
• Administer fluid and electrolytes as per requirement and parenteral calories initially (3000K Cal/day: 10 to 25 percent Dextrose)
• Correct hypokalemia (60 meq/day KCl) and correct acidosis (sodium bicarbonate)
• Measures that affect intestinal bacteria: Ampicillin 2 to 4 gm/day to sterilize bowel and to decrease endogenous NH_3 production
• Lactulose 30 to 45 ml 6 hourly/retention enema/high bowel wash
• Control infection (antibiotics)
• Correct coagulopathy: Vitamin K 10 mg I/M daily for 3 days
• FFP, platelets as per the condition of the patients

Table 9.8: Major complications and their pathogenesis in viral hepatitis during pregnancy	
Major complications	*Pathogenesis*
Hypoglycemia	Decrease glucose synthesis
Hypotension	Hypovolemia
Encephalopathy	Cerebral edema
Septicemia	Bacterial/fungal infection
Gastrointestinal hemorrhage	Stress ulceration
Intracerebral hemorrhage	Coagulopathy
Respiratory failure	Decrease vascular resistance, ARDS
Renal failure	Hepatorenal syndrome, Acute Tubular Necrosis, Hypovolemia

- Mannitol, if intracranial tension is increased
- Steroids have no role in improving the condition of mother
- Fetal heart sound monitoring
- Termination of pregnancy does not prevent the development of FHF or change the outcome (induction of labor has no role in patients with acute viral hepatitis, including hepatitis E , patients with AFLP/HELLP may benefit from early induction of labor).
- If patient goes in labor spontaneously, vaginal delivery is preferable to caesarean section in view of coagulation disturbance and high risk of intra-operative and post-operative bleeding.
- Active management of third stage of labor to prevent postpartum haemorrhage (PPH)
- If PPH occurs, fresh frozen plasma and blood should be given.

KEY POINTS

- Pregnancy causes physiological changes in liver functions and biochemical testing, which should be recognized before starting work up for liver disease.
- Viral hepatitis A to D does not affect pregnant women differently. However, Hepatitis E can be fulminant and fatal.
- Treatment of acute infection during pregnancy is similar to treatment in nonpregnant females and consists mainly of supportive care.
- It is recommended that all pregnant women undergo testing for HBsAg during early prenatal visit; even if they have been previously tested or vaccinated.
- Number of strategies has been employed to prevent mother-to-child transmission in HBV infection. Most effective strategy is combination of HepB Ig and Hep B vaccine to new born within 12 hours of birth followed by completion of vaccine series at 1 and 6 months of age.
- Nucleoside analogue therapy can be used for HBsAg positive women with high-serum HBV DNA concentration.
- Perinatal transmission observed in hepatitis B, hepatitis C and hepatitis E infection.
- Termination of pregnancy does not change the course or outcome in viral hepatitis. Vaginal delivery is preferred to operative delivery in view of the high-risk of bleeding.
- Breastfeeding is not contraindicated in women with hepatitis A, chronic hepatitis B, hepatitis C and hepatitis E.

REFERENCES

1. Chopra S, Griffin PH. Laboratory tests and diagnostic procedures in evaluation of liver disease. Am J Med 1985;79:221-30.
2. Smoleniec JS, James DK. Gastrointestinal crises during pregnancy. Dig Dis 1993;11:313-24.
3. Asimuakopoulos, G. Pregnancy and liver disease. Rev Med Chir Soc Med Nat Iasi 2006;110:326-33.
4. Beniwal M, Kumar A, Kar P, Jalani N, Sharma JB : Prevalence and severity of acute viral hepatitis and fulminant hepatitis during pregnancy : A prospective study from North India. Ind J Med Microbiology 2003;21:184-5
5. Khuroo MS, Teli MR, Skidmore S, So MA, Khuroo MI. Incidence and severity of viral hepatitis in pregnancy. Am J Med 1981;70:252-55.
6. Leikin E, Lysikiewicz A, Garry D, Tejani N. Intrauterine transmission of hepatitis A virus. Obstet Gynecol 1996;88:690-1.
7. American Academy of Pediatrics. Hepatitis A. In: Red Book 28th. Elk Grove, IL: American Academy of Pediatrics; 2009:329-37.
8. ACOG Practice Bulletin No. 86: Viral hepatitis in pregnancy. Obstet Gynecol 2007;110:941-56.
9. Haun L, Kwan N, Hollier LM. Viral infections in pregnancy. Minerva Ginecol 2007;59:159-74.
10. Kumar A, Sharma KA, Gupta RK, Kar P, Murthy NS. Hepatitis C virus infection during pregnancy in North India. Intl J Gynaecol Obstet 2005;88:55-6
11. Khuroo MS, Kamili S, Jameel S. Vertical transmission of hepatitis E virus. Lancet 1995;345:1025-26.
12. Kumar A, Beniwal M, Kar P, Sharma JB, Murthy NS. Hepatitis E in pregnancy. Int J Gynaecol Obstet 2004;85:240-44.
13. Center for Disease Control and Prevention. A Comprehensive Immunization Strategy to Eliminate Transmission of Hepatitis B Virus Infection in the United States: recommendations of the Advisory Commitee on Immunization Practices. 54. Center for Disease Control: December 23, 2005. RR-16.
14. Okada K, Kamiyama I, Inomata M, Imai M, Miyakawa Y. e antigen and anti-e in the serum of asymptomatic carrier mothers as indicators of positive and negative transmission of hepatitis B virus to their infants. N Engl J Med 1976;294:746-9.

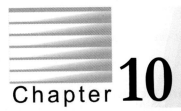

Chapter 10

Antepartum Hemorrhage

Sangeeta Gupta

INTRODUCTION

Antepartum hemorrhage (APH) is defined as bleeding from or into the genital tract occurring during pregnancy after the period of viability is reached or during labor before birth of the baby. It is one of the commonest complications of pregnancy affecting 2 to 5 percent of all pregnancies.[1] Maternal and fetal morbidity and mortality from antepartum hemorrhage are considerable and are associated with high demands on health resources.[2] The various causes are:

Placenta Previa

The placenta is located partially or completely in the lower uterine segment. Incidence is about 0.4 to 0.8 percent.[3] Maternal risks are a consequence of postpartum hemorrhage, anesthetic and surgical complications and morbidly adherent placenta. Fetal morbidity is attributed to prematurity.
The various grades of placenta previa are:
- *Total placenta previa*: Internal os is completely covered by placenta
- *Partial placenta previa*: Internal os is partially covered by placenta
- *Marginal placenta previa*: The placental edge is at the margin of the internal os
- *Low lying placenta*: The placenta is implanted in the lower uterine segment such that the placental edge does not reach the internal os but is in its close proximity

Abruptio Placentae

It is bleeding after premature separation of a normally situated placenta. The incidence varies from 0.5 to 1.8 percent.[4] Abruption is concealed in 20 to 35 percent and revealed in 65 to 80 percent cases. The maternal risks are hypovolemic shock, acute renal failure, disseminated intravascular coagulation and postpartum hemorrhage. Perinatal mortality exceeds 50 percent, with most of the perinatal deaths being stillbirths. Four grades of placental abruption have been described:[5]
- *Grade 0*: Asymptomatic patient with a small retroplacental clot
- *Grade 1*: Vaginal bleeding, uterine tetany and tenderness maybe present; no signs of maternal shock or fetal distress
- *Grade 2*: External vaginal bleeding possible; no signs of maternal shock but fetal compromise or distress is recognized
- *Grade 3*: External vaginal bleeding possible; marked uterine tetany yielding board like consistency on palpation; persistent abdominal pain, with maternal shock and fetal demise; coagulopathy maybe evident in 30 percent cases

Local Lesion

Hemorrhage due to lesion on cervix or vagina like erosion, polyp or carcinoma

Vasa Previa

Vasa previa describes fetal vessels coursing through the membranes over the internal cervical os and below the fetal presenting part, unprotected by placental tissue or the umbilical cord. This can be:
- *Vasa previa type 1*- secondary to a velamentous cord insertion in a single or bilobed placenta
- *Vasa previa type 2*- fetal vessels run between lobes of a placenta with one or more accessory lobes

The incidence varies between one in 2000 and one in 6000 pregnancies.[6-9] Unlike placenta previa, vasa previa carries no major maternal risk, but their is significant risk to the fetus. When the fetal membranes are ruptured the unprotected fetal vessels are at risk of disruption with consequent fetal hemorrhage. Vasa previa presents with fresh vaginal bleeding at the time of membrane rupture and fetal heart rate abnormalities such as decelerations, bradycardia, a sinusoidal trace or fetal demise. The mortality rate is around 60 percent.[10] Because the fetal blood volume is around 80–100 mL/kg, the loss of small amounts of blood can have major implications for the fetus, thus rapid delivery and aggressive resuscitation and blood transfusion are essential. In the antenatal period, in the absence of vaginal bleeding, vasa previa cannot be diagnosed clinically. In the intrapartum period, in the absence of vaginal bleeding, vasa previa can be diagnosed clinically by palpation of fetal vessels in the membranes at the time of vaginal examination and confirmed by direct visualization with amnioscope. Delivery is achieved by category 1 emergency cesarean section.

Indeterminate Bleeding or Marginal Bleeding

When there is no clear cause, hemorrhage is classified as unexplained, although they are often attributed to marginal bleeds or bleeds arising from the placental edge. The principal concern is their association with preterm delivery and a small increase in the risk of fetal congenital abnormality.

CASE SCENARIO-1

Mrs.XY, 26 years G2P1A0L1 presents to the casualty with 36 weeks pregnancy with vaginal bleeding.

> **Comments:** The patient is a case of **APH** at 36 weeks pregnancy

Differential Diagnosis

- Different causes of APH
  - Placenta previa
  - Abruptio placentae
  - Vasa previa
  - Indeterminate causes
- Excessive show
- Rupture uterus

POINTS TO BE NOTED IN HISTORY

- Character of bleeding:
  - Number of episodes
  - Painful or painless
  - Color of blood
- History of trauma or coitus: Trauma is likely to precipitate abruption whereas coitus may precede episode of placenta previa.
- History suggestive of pre-eclampsia: Associated with abruption
- Smoking or cocaine abuse: Associated with abruption

- Prolonged rupture of membranes (more than 24 hours)
- Following episode of sudden bout of heavy leaking (as in polyhydramnios) or manipulation like external cephalic version suggestive of abruption
- Previous abruption or placenta previa (8 to 10 fold increased risk)[11]
- Fetal movements

> **History in this case:** Patient had an episode of painless bleeding one hour back. There is history of passage of fist sized clot. The bleeding was fresh red in color and soaked her clothes. The patient is perceiving fetal movements.

Points to be noted in Examination

General Examination

- General condition
- Vital signs- pulse, blood pressure (BP), respiratory rate (RR) and temperature
- Pallor, jaundice, pedal edema

Cardiovascular and Respiratory System Examination

Abdominal Examination

Fundal height, presentation, fetal heart sound, tender uterus, consistency, uterine contractions and features suggestive of multiple pregnancy.

Word of caution: No per speculum or per vaginal examination to be done in the emergency ward or labor room

> **Examination in this case:**
> Pulse-110/min, BP- 90/70 mm Hg, pallor +, no pedal edema
> General and systemic examination unremarkable
> Abdominal examination- Fundal height 36 weeks corresponding to period of gestation, cephalic, free, FHS 136/min and regular, uterine contour well made out, uterus relaxed non-tense non-tender
> Local examination: Patient has trickle of fresh blood through introitus and her thighs are smeared with blood.

Diagnosis

The above findings are suggestive of a clinical diagnosis of low lying placenta.

Immediate Management

- Call for help immediately
- After history and rapid evaluation, resuscitate immediately.
  - Insert a thick bore intravenous cannula (gauge 16), collect blood for investigations and start intravenous fluids.
  - Intravenous (IV) fluids- Infuse normal saline or ringer's lactate initially at the rate of one liter in 15 to 20 minutes and about 2 liters in the first hour.
  - Administer oxygen by mask or nasal cannula at the rate of 6 to 8 liters/minute.
- Catheterize the bladder to monitor urinary output
- Continuous monitoring of vitals, input- output and fetal heart rate, every 15 minutes
- Arrange adequate amount of cross-matched blood and blood products.
  - Blood transfusion is given if patient has moderate-to-severe bleeding, is pale or fetal heart sound is absent.
  - Transfusion of fresh frozen plasma and other blood components may be required for correction of coagulopathy.
- In cases of Rh negative pregnancy administer anti-D.

INVESTIGATIONS

- Blood grouping and cross matching
- Hemoglobin and hematocrit
- Platelet count
- Coagulation profile: Bleeding time (BT), clotting time (CT), clot retraction time (CRT) and prothrombin time (PT). Activated thromboplastin time (APTT) and fibrinogen levels require assessment when severe abruption presents, as disseminated intravascular coagulation (DIC) is a serious complication.
- Serum electrolyte, blood urea and blood sugar
- Urine examination for albumin and sugar
- Ultrasonography (USG) - Clinical suspicion of low lying placenta should be raised in all women with vaginal bleeding after 20 weeks of gestation. A high presenting part, an abnormal lie and painless or provoked bleeding, irrespective of previous imaging results, are more suggestive of a low-lying placenta but may not be present, and *the definitive diagnosis usually relies on ultrasound imaging.*[12]
  - Ultrasonography is done to localize the placenta, to assess the gestational age, fetal cardiac activity, amount of liquor, anomalies and multiple pregnancy.
  - Transvaginal scans improve the accuracy of placental localization and are safe particularly for posteriorly situated placentas[12] or when transabdominal findings are uncertain or equivocal. There is no association of transvaginal scan with increased risk of bleeding.[13]
  - If placenta is in the upper segment, look for retroplacental clots, though absence of clots does not rule out abruption. The sensitivity of ultrasound for presence of abruption is poor (24%).[14]

> **Investigations in this case:**
> Hemogram- Hb 8 gm%, Hct 27%, platelet count- 1, 70,000/cc
> BT, CT, CRT- within normal range
> Urine routine examination-normal
> USG: Single live fetus, gestational age 36 weeks 3 days, cephalic, placenta posterior partially covering os, liquor adequate, no gross congenital anomalies

Final Diagnosis

G2P1A0L0 with 36 weeks pregnancy with single live fetus in cephalic presentation with *placenta previa.*

FURTHER MANAGEMENT

The two options of further management of placenta previa are *expectant* or *active* management. The treatment of a woman with bleeding from a placenta previa is determined by two key factors- the degree of hemorrhage and fetal maturity. In this patient active management of placenta previa is indicated as maternal condition is compromised and fetal maturity is 36 weeks.

Active Management of Placenta Previa

Immediate termination of pregnancy

Indications

- Fetal maturity 36 weeks or more
- Patient in labor
- Patient hemodynamically unstable
- Severe anemia

- Fetal distress or demise
- Malformed fetus

Mode of Delivery

Cesarean section is undertaken for all cases except Type 1 placenta previa. It is the only option in patients with profuse, life-threatening hemorrhage. Available data suggest that the distance between the leading placental edge and cervix deemed sufficient to allow vaginal delivery should be at least 20 mm.[15]

Lower segment Cesarean Section (LSCS) for Placenta Previa

- All cases of placenta previa should be managed at a tertiary care center and a consultant obstetrician should be available in delivery suite from the beginning during cesarean section of placenta previa.
- In placenta previa with previous cesarean scar, placenta accreta is very likely and a consultant should be available on floor during the cesarean section (detailed management of morbidly adherent placenta is discussed elsewhere in the book).
- There is controversy regarding the type of anesthesia during cesarean for placenta previa. General anesthesia has been preferred in the past because of fears that epidural anesthesia may exacerbate hypotension. But there is a growing body of evidence supporting the use of regional anesthesia as a safe alternative to general anesthesia in both elective and emergency cesarean delivery in cases of placenta previa.[16,17]
- The cesarean section of a case of placenta previa is associated with increased risk of hemorrhage due to atony and bleeding from the sinuses in lower uterine segment which lacks contractile properties. While undertaking the cesarean section, the location of placenta is a principal factor of interest to the obstetrician:
  - In a posteriorly placed placenta the method of delivery follows an entirely normal pattern.
  - In an anteriorly placed placenta there is greater risk of intraoperative hemorrhage. The fetus may be delivered by approaching the amniotic sac beyond the lower or lateral edge of the placenta by separating it from the uterine wall and artificially rupturing the amniotic membrane, if possible- even if this can be achieved the intraoperative blood loss may still be greater due to the increased vascularity of the anterior uterine wall. However, when there is no placenta free window, one may have to go through the placenta to deliver the baby. Early cord clamping should be done to prevent fetal exsanguination.
- The difficulties an obstetrician is likely to encounter during cesarean section for placenta previa:
  - Presence of large blood vessels in the lower uterine segment,
  - Poorly developed lower segment,
  - The placenta in the uterine incision and
  - Extraction of the baby through an inadequate incision calling for extending the incision at either ends or in T-shape.
- If there is bleeding from the placental site it may be controlled by
  - Ligating the specific bleeder if visible.
  - Taking mattress stitches through the musculature of the lower uterine segment.
  - Administration of oxytocic drugs (Oxytocin infusion 20 units, IV methergin 0.25 mg, intra-myometrial prostaglandins).
  - Pressure with hot mops for 2 to 3 minutes.
- Balloon tamponade: Bakri has reported the successful arrest of bleeding from placenta bed in 5 cases of placenta previa by using a large volume, fluid filled tamponade balloon.[18]
- Bilateral uterine artery ligation or internal iliac ligation may be required if above measures fail.
- Hysterectomy is a last resort. Total hysterectomy is necessary to control bleeding from the lower uterine segment. However, it should be opted for early in multiparous women to avert severe morbidity and mortality.

Double Set up Examination

It is the vaginal examination in operation theatre with two teams of surgeons available. It has limited indications in modern obstetrics and should be carried out when termination of pregnancy has to be done:

- If ultrasound is not available
- Discrepancy in amount of bleeding, clinical presentation and ultrasound findings
- In low lying placenta to determine the mode of delivery

It is contraindicated in:

- Active, profuse hemorrhage mandating immediate delivery
- Malpresentation
- Fetal distress
- Major degree placenta previa

Steps: Two teams of surgeon, anesthetist and pediatrician should be present in the theatre; blood should be available and cesarean tray ready. One of the obstetricians should be scrubbed and ready to operate. Intravenous line is inserted and fluid is on flow. No anesthesia is given. Patient is put in lithotomy position; bladder is catheterized and gentle per speculum examination done to rule out local lesion. Two fingers are gently introduced into the vagina and presenting part is felt through the fornices after stabilizing presenting part by abdominal hand. If bogginess is felt through fornices, there is likelihood of placenta previa. One finger is cautiously introduced into the cervix and placental edge palpated. If placenta is felt within 2 centimeters of the os, patient is taken up for LSCS. If the lower 3 cm of lower segment is free of placenta, induction of labor is done with artificial rupture of membranes (ARM) and oxytocin. If after amniotomy patient continues to bleed, LSCS should be undertaken. If brisk vaginal bleeding occurs anytime during the procedure, it should be abandoned and immediate cesarean section performed.

CASE SCENARIO-2

G3P2A0L2 with 7 months amenorrhea reports to the emergency with second episode of painless bleeding in last 7 days. The bleeding is fresh, red in color and small in amount and patient perceives normal fetal movements.

> **Examination in this case:**
> Pulse-80/min, BP- 100/70 mm Hg, no pallor or pedal edema
> Abdominal examination- Fundal height 30 weeks corresponding to the period of gestation, cephalic, free, FHS 136/min and regular, uterine contour well made out, uterus relaxed non-tense non-tender
> Local examination- No active bleeding
> **Investigations in this case:**
> Blood group- B+
> Hb 8 gm%, Hct- 27%, platelet count- 1, 70,000/cc, BT,CT,CRT- within normal range. Urine routine- normal
> USG- Single live fetus, getational age 30 weeks 3 days, cephalic, placenta reaching up to os, liquor adequate, no gross congenital anomalies.

In this case of placenta previa, patient can be managed expectantly as fetus is premature, maternal condition is stable and there is no active bleeding.

Expectant Management

Macafee[19] and Johnson[20] introduced expectant management to achieve maximum fetal maturity possible while minimizing maternal and fetal risks:

- Admit the patient in labor room.
- Sedate with 7.5 mg injection morphine intramuscularly.

- Start intravenous fluids and send samples as discussed earlier.
- Arrange blood or transfuse if hemoglobin is less than 10 gm%. Liberal use of transfusion is essential to prevent maternal morbidity due to anticipated blood loss.
- Monitor vitals (pulse rate and blood pressure), fundal height and abdominal girth and input-output and watch for vaginal bleeding.
- Administer corticosteroids for fetal lung maturity-Injection betamethasone 12mg intramuscular two doses twelve hours apart.
- If bleeding stops, patient can be shifted to the ward after 24 hours. She is given hematinics and allowed restricted activity. Correction of anemia is a vital component of expectant management.
- Administration of Anti-D in Rh negative women.
- A gentle per speculum examination is done after 5 to 7 days of stoppage of bleeding to exclude local pathology.
- When the fetus is 37 weeks, pregnancy is terminated.
- Conservative management should be abandoned prematurely, if patient has bleeding and maternal condition is unstable.

Inpatient versus Out-patient care

There is paucity of evidence to guide place of care and current trials show that either form of care is not associated with increased adverse outcome.[21,22] The decision on pattern of care will be based on history of antenatal hemorrhage during pregnancy, the grade of placenta previa, patient's social circumstances and obstetrician and patient preference.[13] All women at risk of major antepartum hemorrhage should be encouraged to remain close to the hospital of confinement for the duration of the third trimester of pregnancy.[12] If women are managed at home, they should be encouraged to ensure they have safety precautions in place, including having someone available to help them should the need arise and, particularly, having ready access to the hospital.

It should be made clear to any woman being managed at home that she should attend hospital immediately when she experiences any bleeding, contractions or pain (including vague suprapubic period-like aches).

Cervical Cerclage

The use of cervical cerclage to reduce bleeding and prolong pregnancy is not supported by sufficient evidence to recommend this practice outside of a clinical trial.[12] The two studies have shown benefit but the number of cases were small and cerclage requires further evaluation.[23,24]

Conservative Aggressive Management of Placenta Previa using Tocolysis

Tocolysis for treatment of bleeding due to placenta previa may be useful in selected cases.[25-29] There does not appear to be any significant detrimental effect on the bleeding pattern. However, beta-mimetics were used in the studies to date and, as these are known to be associated with significant adverse effects, the agent and optimum regime are still to be determined; further research is needed in this area.[12]

Screening for Placenta Previa (Placental Localization)

Routine ultrasound scanning at 20 weeks of gestation should include placental localization.[12] Further imaging would depend on type of placenta previa and symptoms:
- In cases of asymptomatic women with suspected minor previa, follow-up imaging can be left until 36 weeks of gestation.
- In cases with asymptomatic suspected major placenta previa or a question of placenta accrete, imaging should be performed at around 32 weeks of gestation to clarify the diagnosis and allow planning for third-trimester management, further imaging and delivery.
- Women who bleed should be managed individually according to their needs.

CASE SCENARIO-3

G4P1A2L1 with 34 weeks pregnancy presents with complaints of vaginal bleeding (dark colored clots) and abdominal pain.

Examination in this case:
Pulse-100/min, BP- 160/90 mm Hg, pallor and pedal edema are present
Cardiovascular and respiratory system-normal
Abdominal examination- fundal height corresponds to 36 weeks (more than period of gestation), uterus tense and tender, cephalic presentation, FHS regular
Local examination- Trickle of dark red colored bleeding
Investigations in this case:
Hb 9 gm%, platelet count- 99,000/cc, BT, CT, CRT- within normal range, PT-normal
Renal function tests- normal
USG- Single live fetus, cephalic presentation, gestational age 34-35 weeks, placenta fundo-anterior, liquor adequate
Since placenta was located in upper segment and clinical diagnosis of placental abruption was made, pelvic examination was done with following findings- cervix 2 finger loose, early effaced, membranes intact, vertex at -2 station, ARM done and blood stained liquor drained.

Management

The findings are suggestive of diagnosis of placental abruption grade 2 and the patient requires immediate delivery by cesarean section. Cesarean section is taken up after initial resuscitation of the mother and arranging adequate blood and blood products.

The management of *placental abruption* is guided by grade of abruption at presentation, the presence of concomitant pathology, condition of the mother and the fetus and the fetal gestation. Management is divided into general (already discussed) and specific measures.
Specific measures to be considered are as follows:[30]
• Immediate delivery
• Expectant management
• Management of complications like hemorrhagic shock, DIC, acute tubular necrosis and postpartum hemorrhage

Immediate Delivery

The need for immediate delivery depends on the severity of abruption and whether the fetus is live or dead.

If Fetus is Dead (Grade 3 Abruption), Vaginal Delivery is the Goal[30]

• Maternal resuscitation is emphasized as fetal death due to abruption implies that the blood loss is about 2 liters though visible vaginal bleeding may not be severe and maternal condition may apparently be well preserved. Such patients should be transfused minimum of two units of blood or as per need. About 30 percent of these cases are associated with coagulopathy and if present, should be simultaneously and actively corrected by transfusion of appropriate blood products. Rapid delivery is the key to correction of coagulopathy.
• Rapid and aggressive fluid replacement is required. However, in patients with co-existing pre-eclampsia there is risk of fluid overload and pulmonary edema and fluid replacement is best monitored by insertion of central venous catheter pressure monitoring. A good guide is to maintain central venous pressure (CVP) of 4 to 8 cm of water.
• Once resuscitation is initiated, labor is induced by artificial rupture of membranes and oxytocin infusion. There is no restriction of induction delivery time.

- The only indication of cesarean section in a dead fetus is uncontrollable bleeding or failure of conservative management. Couvelaire uterus may be the cause of failed induction but is not an indication for cesarean section.
- In severe abruption when vaginal bleeding, tonically contracted uterus and fetal hypoxia are present, it may pose a challenge to differentiate it from rupture uterus.

If the Fetus is Alive

The degree of abruption and the state of the fetus are important determinants regarding mode of delivery.
- In mild-to-moderate cases of abruption, the mode of delivery is determined by the condition of the fetus and its presentation.
- Abnormal fetal heart rate patterns are an indication for cesarean delivery.
- Patients who are allowed vaginal delivery, continuous fetal heart monitoring must be available to identify early abnormal fetal heart rate patterns. Vigilance must be maintained for development of hyperstimulation.

Expectant Management

It is considered in cases of mild placental abruption occurring before 37 weeks of gestation and mother is hemodynamically stable. The fetal condition should be monitored closely, when expectant management is opted for. The timing of delivery depends on further bleeding, the fetal condition, gestational age and neonatal services available. Induction of labor is usually advocated at 37 weeks, though no evidence exists to support it. The speculative argument is that undetected damage might have occurred to the integrity and function of placenta and in the face of uncertainty delivery at term offers more advantages. If the initial scan shows retroplacental clots, the clot may be monitored by serial scans.

KEY POINTS

- Antepartum hemorrhage effects about 2 to 5 percent of all pregnancies.
- Placenta previa complicates 0.5 percent of all pregnancies.
- Previous cesarean is one of the most important risk factor for placenta previa. The risk of occurrence is 0.65% after one cesarean section and increases to 10% after 4 or more cesarean sections.
- Conservative management of placenta previa allows safe prolongation of pregnancy, improving perinatal morbidity and mortality.
- Cesarean section of placenta previa should be performed by senior obstetrician.
- Abruptio placentae affects about 0.5 to 1.8 percent pregnancies.
- The diagnosis of Abruptio placentae is made clinically rather than by imaging.
- Management of Abruptio placentae depends on the grade. If fetus is dead, vaginal delivery should be the goal. Correction of coagulopathy is essential.

REFERENCES

1. McShane PM, Het PS, Epstien. Maternal and perinatal mortality MF resulting from placenta previa. Obstet Gynecol 1985;65:176-82.
2. Confidential Enquiry into Maternal and Child Health. Saving Mothers' Lives: Reviewing maternal deaths to make motherhood safer – 2003–2005. The Seventh Report of the Confidential Enquiries into Maternal Deaths in the UK. London: CEMACH; 2007.
3. Drife J. Bleeding in pregnancy. In: Chamberlain G, Steer PJ (eds). Turnbull's Obstetrics.3rd edn .London: Churchill Livingstone, 2006. pp. 211-28.
4. Rasmussen S, Ingrens KM, Dalaker K. The occurrence of placental abruption in Norway 1967-1991. Acta Obstet Gynecol Scand 1996;75:222-8.

5. Sher G, Statland BE. Abruptio placentaee with coagulopathy: A rational basis for management. Clin Obstet Gynecol 1985;28:15-23.
6. Catanzarite V, Maida C, Thomas W, Mendoza A, Stanco L, Piacquadio KM. Prenatal sonographic diagnosis of vasa previa: ultrasound findings and obstetric outcome in ten cases. Ultrasound Obstet Gynecol 2001;18:109-15.
7. Oleyese KO, Turner M, Lees C, Campbell S. Vasa previa: an avoidable obstetric tragedy. Obstet Gynecol Surv 1999;54:138-45.
8. Smorgick N, Tovbin Y, Ushakov F, Vaknin Z, Barzilay B, Herman A, et al. Is neonatal risk from vasa previa preventable? The 20-year experience from a single medical center. J Clin Ultrasound 2010;38:118-22.
9. Stafford IP, Neumann DE, Jarrell H. Abnormal placental structure and vasa previa: confirmation of the relationship. J Ultrasound Med 2004;23:1521-2.
10. Fung TY, Lau TK. Poor perinatal outcome associated with vasa previa: is it preventable? A report of three cases and review of the literature. Ultrasound Obstet Gynecol 1998;12:430-3.
11. Monica G, Lilja C. Placenta previa, maternal smoking and recurrence risk. Acta Obstet Gynecol Scand 1995;74:341-5.
12. Royal College of Obstetricians and Gynaecologists. Green-top Guideline No. 27: Placenta previa, placenta previa accreta and vasa previa: diagnosis and management. London: RCOG; 2011.
13. Brown RN. Antepartum haemorrhage: bleeding of placental and fetal origin. In: Studd J, Tan SL, Chervenak FA (eds). Progress in Obstetrics and Gynecology ; vol 17. London: Elsevier, 2006.pp. 203-16.
14. Glantz C, Purnell L. Clinical utility of sonography in the diagnosis and treatment of Placental abruption. J Ultrasound Med 2002; 21:837-40.
15. Bhide A, Prefumo F, Moore J, Hollis B, Thilanganathan B. Placental edge to internal os distance in the late third trimester and mode of delivery in placenta previa. Br J Obstet Gynaecol 2003;110:860-64.
16. Parekh N, Husaini SW, Russell IF. Caesarean section for placenta previa: a retrospective study of anaesthetic management. Br J Anaesth 2000;84:725-30.
17. Hong JY, Jee YS, Yoon HJ, Kim SM. Comparison of general and epidural anesthesia in elective cesarean section for placenta previa totalis: maternal hemodynamics, blood loss and neonatal outcome. Int J Obstet Anaesth 2003;12:12-6.
18. Bakri YN, Amri A, Jabbar FA. Tamponade-balloon for obstetrical bleeding. Int J Gynecol Obstet 2001;74:139-42.
19. Macafee CHG, Millar WG, Harley G. Maternal and fetal mortality in placenta previa. J Obstet Gynecol Br Emp 1962;52:313-24.
20. Johnson HW, Williamson JC, Greeley AV. The conservative management of some varieties of placenta previa.Am J Obstet Gynecol 1945;49:398-406.
21. Mouer JR. Placenta previa; Antepartum conservative management, inpatient versus outpatient. Am J Obstet Gynecol 1994;70:1683-85.
22. Wing DA, Paul RH, Millar LK. Management of the symptomatic placenta previa: a randomized, controlled trial of inpatient versus outpatient expectant management. Am J Obstet Gynecol 1996;175:806-11.
23. Cobo E, Conde-Agudelo A, Delgado J, Canaval H, Congote A. Cervical cerclage: an alternative for the management of placenta previa? Am J Obstet Gynecol 1998;179:122-5.
24. Tessarolo M, Bellino R, Ardiuno S,Leo L Weirdis T, Lanza A. Cervical cerclage for the treatment of patients with placenta previa. Clin Exp Obstet Gynecol 1996;23:184-87.
25. Cotton DB, Read JA, Paul RH, Quilligan EJ. The conservative aggressive management of placenta previa. Am J Obstet Gynecol 1980;137:687-95.
26. Silver R, Depp R, Sabbagha RE, Dooley SL, Socol ML, Tamura RK. Placenta previa: Aggressive expectant management. Am J Obstet Gynecol 1984;150:15-22.
27. Sharma A, Suri V, Gupta I. Tocolytic therapy in conservative management of symptomatic placenta previa. Int J Gynaecol Obstet 2004;84:109-13.
28. Besinger RE, Moniak CW, Paskiewicz LS, Fisher SG, Tomich PG. The effect of tocolytic use in the management of symptomatic placenta previa. Am J Obstet Gynecol 1995;172:1770-8.
29. Towers CV, Pircon RA, Heppard M. Is tocolysis safe in the the management of third-trimester bleeding? Am J Obstet Gynecol 1999;180:1572-8.
30. Konje JC, Taylor DJ. Bleeding in late pregnancy. In: James DK, Weiner CP, Steer PJ, Gonik B (eds). High-risk pregnancy: Management options. 3rd edn. Philadelphia: Elsevier, 2006. pp.1259-175.

Chapter **11**

Fetal Distress During Labor

Asmita M Rathore, Avantika Gupta

INTRODUCTION

Fetal distress as defined by the WHO's ICD-10 includes fetal stress at the time of labor or delivery.[1] It is a clinical situation where clinician feels that fetus is hypoxic or acidotic and the concern is significant enough to warrant intervention usually in the form of operative delivery. Though the term "fetal distress" has been commonly used in clinical practice for a long time, it is obscure, imprecise and nonspecific. The American College of Obstetricians and Gynecologists (ACOG) has now recommended replacement of the term fetal distress with "nonreassuring fetal status," followed by a further description of findings (e.g., repetitive variable decelerations, fetal tachycardia or bradycardia, late decelerations, or low biophysical profile).[2] Babies with fetal distress are usually delivered in good health, but in some cases fetal distress can lead to problems such as cerebral palsy, mental retardation, hypoxic ischemic encephalopathy and seizures.

CAUSES OF FETAL DISTRESS

Antepartum

1. Maternal hypotension (epidural anesthesia, supine position)
2. Post maturity
3. Placental insufficiency (pre-eclampsia, IUGR etc.)
4. Abruptio placenta
5. Chorioamnionitis

Intrapartum

1. Hypertonic contractions
2. Scar dehiscence
3. Cord around the neck
4. Cord compression in oligohydramnios
5. Cord prolapse
6. Abnormal uterine contractions
    Labor poses physiological stress to the fetus. Normally uterine contractions do not reduce the oxygen supply to the fetus as the store of oxygen in the placental bed is adequate to meet the fetal

needs during the contractions. Thus, under normal conditions, a healthy baby receives an adequate supply of oxygen during the period of uterine contractions. But uterine contractions may result in reduced oxygen supply to the fetus if there is placental insufficiency, uterine contractions are very frequent or very prolonged or there is umbilical cord compression. The fetus is usually able to compensate if the hypoxia is mild and therefore shows no abnormal response. However, severe fetal hypoxia will result in fetal distress. The pathophysiology of fetal distress is described in Figure 11.1. The main objective of fetal monitoring during labor is to identify the fetuses at risk of hypoxia. The indicators of fetal distress used in clinical practice are:

• Fetal heart rate (FHR) abnormalities
• Meconium stained liquor (MSL) and
• Cord prolapse

Though continuous electronic monitoring along with fetal scalp blood sampling (FBS) is considered to be the gold standard for diagnosing fetal distress, intermittent auscultation remains the most commonly used method of fetal monitoring in labor.

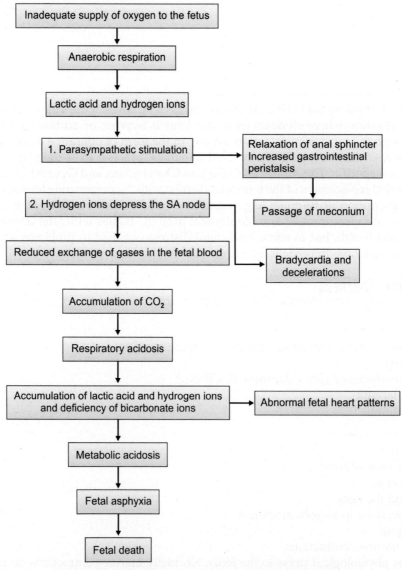

Figure 11.1: Mechanism of development of fetal distress

FHR ABNORMALITIES

FHR monitoring is the most commonly used modality to assess fetal condition during labor. The methods used are (a) intermittent auscultation using stethoscope or hand held Doppler or (b) continuous electronic fetal heart monitoring using cardiotocography (CTG) machines.

Guidelines for Intrapartum Fetal Heart Monitoring

ACOG guidelines for intrapartum surveillance state that intermittent auscultation following a uterine contraction or continuous electronic monitoring is acceptable for both low and high-risk pregnancies. Evaluating at an interval of every 30 minutes in low-risk and every 15 minutes in high-risk pregnancies in first stage of labor and every 15 minutes in second stage in low-risk and every 5 minutes in high-risk pregnancies is acceptable. FHR has to be heard for a full minute after a contraction.[3]

According to the Royal College of Obstetricians and Gynaecologists (RCOG) guidelines, all patients having normal labor should be monitored with FHR checked by auscultation for a full minute after uterine contraction and at least every 15 minutes in the first stage of labor and every 5 minutes in the second stage of labor. Criteria for initiating continuous electronic fetal monitoring include- onset of any intrapartum risk factor, evidence of FHR deceleration, baseline FHR <110 beats per minute (bpm) or >160 bpm.[4]

CASE SCENARIO-1

A 28-year-old primigravida was admitted in labor room with spontaneous onset of labor at 40 weeks gestation. On examination it was a full term pregnancy with vertex presentation. The patient was in active labor with good uterine contractions. Per vaginal (P/V) examination showed fully effaced 6 cm dilated cervix with vertex at -1 station and adequate pelvis. Patient was monitored with partogram and intermittent FHR auscultation. After half an hour a post contraction drop in FHR to 100 beats /min was detected and she was shifted to CTG monitoring. The following CTG trace was observed:-

> **Comment:**
> - Baseline-165/min – Nonreassuring
> - Beat to beat variability - Nonreassuring
> - Late decelerations lasting for <3 mins – nonreasssuring
> - Accelerations-absent – significance uncertain
> **Interpretation:** Pathological

Diagnosis

A diagnosis of nonreassuring fetal status was made.

Abnormalities of FHR Diagnosed on Intermittent Auscultation

Suspicious Pattern

FHR 100-110/min or 160-180/min or early deceleration i.e. post contraction drop recovering within 30 seconds

Pathological Pattern

a. Fetal bradycardia <100/min in between contractions
b. Irregular fetal heart and late deceleration (FHR <100/min lasting for >30 sec following contraction)
c. Persistent fetal tachycardia >180/min in between contractions, in absence of maternal tachycardia

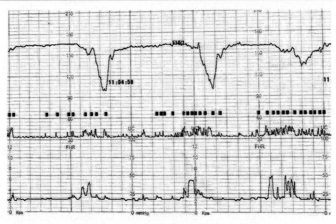

Figure 11.2: Intrapartum CTG trace

If abnormalities are detected on intermittent auscultation, continuous CTG monitoring should be instituted if possible and further decision is based on CTG findings. If facility for CTG is not available, then decision should be based on findings of intermittent auscultation and clinical review as per protocol.

Interpretation of CTG Trace (Figure 11.2)

The CTG trace is interpreted on the basis of four variables -baseline FHR, beat to beat variability, decelerations and accelerations, each of which is classified as reassuring, nonreassuring or abnormal on the basis of criteria given in Table 11.1. The CTG trace is then categorized in one of the following three categories based on these four variables:
- *Normal CTG* is when all four features fall in to reassuring category
- *Suspicious CTG* when one feature is nonreassuring and the rest are reassuring
- *Pathological CTG* when two or more features are nonreassuring or one or more features are abnormal

MANAGEMENT OF PATHOLOGICAL CTG[5]

- Firstly, check the contact and connections of the CTG probe. It is also important to rule out the effect of recent vaginal examination, recent vomiting or vasovagal episode or topping up of epidural analgesia infusion.
- Do P/V examination for explanatory signs of distress like cord prolapse or abruption.

The immediate management is intrauterine resuscitation using following measures:

	Baseline FHR/bpm	FHR Variability/bpm	Decelerations in FHR	Accelerations in FHR
		Table 11.1: CTG fetal heart rate features and classification[4]		
Reassuring	110–160	≥5	Absent	Present
Non-reassuring	100–109 or 161–180	<5 for ≥40 mins but <90 mins	Early decelerations or variable decelerations or single prolonged deceleration lasting ≤3 mins	Absence of accelerations in an otherwise normal CTG is of uncertain significance
Abnormal	<100 or >180 or sinusoidal pattern for ≥10 mins	<5 for ≥90 mins	Atypical variable decelerations or late decelerations or single prolonged deceleration lasting >3 mins	Absence of accelerations in an otherwise normal CTG is of uncertain significance

Change Maternal Position and give Oxygen

Prolonged maternal supine position can result in supine hypotension syndrome which is characterized by reduced venous return due to the pressure of the gravid uterus on inferior vena cava (IVC). This IVC compression can cause a drop in the cardiac output which leads to diminished uterine blood flow. Changing the maternal position to left lateral position may relieve this pressure on IVC. It may also help in taking the pressure off the umbilical cord in cases with oligohydramnios.

Fetal distress develops mainly due to deficiency of oxygen supply to the placenta. Oxygen is given in a hope that it would increase the oxygen supply to the fetus. However, presently there is no evidence that oxygen administration to the woman during labor is beneficial to the baby.[6]

Improve Maternal Hydration

Administration of intravenous (IV) fluids to the mother, particularly crystalloids helps in correcting hypotension by increasing intravascular volume and thereby improving uterine perfusion. Cochrane review by Hofmeyer has shown that maternal hydration appears to increase amniotic fluid volume and prevents oligohydramnios and thus cord compression during labor.[7]

Cease Abnormal Uterine Contractions

Oxytocin administration may cause tachysystole leading to fetal distress. Uterine contractions cause constriction of blood vessels and cord compression due to increased intrauterine pressure, thereby reducing the blood flow to the placenta. Normally, FHR may slow down during a contraction but recovers to normal as the uterus relaxes. Abnormal FHR in absence of contractions or persisting after contractions is suggestive of fetal distress. Excessive uterine activity can be ceased by initiation of tocolytic agents. Uterine relaxation may improve placental blood flow and therefore fetal oxygenation. RCOG recommends following regimens for tocolysis:
- Intravenous or subcutaneous terbutaline (250 µg)
- Sublingual glyceryl trinitrate (GTN) or spray (400 µg)
- Intravenous salbutamol (100 µg)
  However, β agonists may be responsible for producing adverse maternal cardiovascular effects and can also lead to hemorrhage by causing uterine relaxation.

Keep Monitoring

Continuous FHR monitoring with CTG allows the obstetrician to view the fetal heart beat in relation to the uterine contractions. If there is nonreassuring FHR or there are persistent late decelerations or it is difficult to interpret CTG, fetal scalp blood sampling for pH is indicated.

Notify and Inform

The senior consultant must be informed about the case. It must be a norm to keep the woman and her relatives appraised of the situation at all the times and involve them in clinical decision making.

Confirm Fetal Hypoxia

Routine use of CTG may lead to unnecessary interventions in the form of instrumental and operative delivery. Moreover, continuous CTG does not have any advantage in reducing fetal mortality or neurological handicap.[8] Thus CTG should be supplemented by additional tests to confirm fetal acidosis before any intervention. FBS is considered as a gold standard to identify fetal acidosis.

Fetal Scalp Blood Sampling

It should be performed in cases with abnormal FHR during labor after maternal consent if there are no contraindications to it.

Contraindications to FBS are:
- Preterm fetus <34 weeks
- Active genital Herpes infection, HIV, Australia antigen positive patient
- Cervical dilatation <3 cm
- Sepsis
- Malpresentation or placenta previa

Fetal scalp blood pH should be interpreted taking into account the previous pH measurement, the rate of progress in labor and the clinical features of the mother and the baby. The trend of serial fetal pH values would be more important than the absolute value in assessing recovery because the process of reversing fetal metabolic acidosis usually takes 20-30 minutes or longer depending on the degree of acidosis[4].

Lactate in fetal blood can be measured to evaluate fetal metabolic acidosis. A bedside handheld lactate meter is simpler as it requires less amount of blood i.e. 5 mL vs 35-50 mL required for fetal blood sampling for pH. Lactate level in blood is superior to fetal blood pH as it correlates well with cord blood hydrogen ions. The actions to be taken based upon fetal scalp pH and blood lactate levels are given in Table 11.2.

There are various tests which can be performed as an alternative to FBS:
- Intrapartum fetal stimulation tests
- Fetal ECG
- Pulse oximetry

Intrapartum Fetal Stimulation Tests

FHR acceleration in response to vibroacoustic stimulation or fetal scalp stimulation has been recommended as a substitute to FBS. Monitoring is continued if there is acceleration in response to this stimulation (reactive response) as it is associated with a reassuring sample pH and indicates an intact autonomic system and a non acidotic fetus[9]. These tests are of value when stimulation occurs when the FHR is at its baseline and the acceleration can be evoked above the baseline.

These tests can be used as a step before FBS and would reduce the need for FBS by 50 percent. However, Cochrane systemic review found that there is insufficient evidence to base recommendation for these tests in evaluation of fetal well being in labor in the presence of non-reassuring CTG trace.[10]

Method: Place the patient in lateral position and place an acoustic stimulator transabdominally close to the fetal head. Activate acoustic stimulator for 1-3 seconds. For scalp stimulation, keep a firm digital pressure on the scalp or scratch the scalp. If there is no change in fetal response, stimulation may be repeated at one to five minute intervals for a maximum of three times. It is said to be reactive if there is accelerations of [3] 15 beats/minute lasting for [3] 15 seconds and nonreactive otherwise. Fetuses that respond to either of these stimuli with fetal heart acceleration are very unlikely to have an acidotic scalp blood pH and if there is no response, 50% will show acidosis on fetal scalp blood sample.

Pulse Oximetry

A specially devised instrument called oximeter is placed over the fetal face following rupture of membranes. As it is minimally invasive and easy to use, it helps in avoiding invasive test like FBS.

Table 11.2: Management according to fetal scalp pH and blood lactate levels		
FBS result/pH	*Corresponding blood lactate*	*Subsequent action*
≥ 7.25	>4.8 mmol/L	Repeat FBS if FHR abnormalities persist
7.21 – 7.24	4.2-4.8 mmol/L	Repeat FBS within 30 minutes or consider delivery if rapid fall in pH since last sample
≤ 7.20	<4.2 mmol/L	Delivery indicated because acidosis develops after significant anaerobic metabolism

Oxygen saturation of a healthy fetus varies from 40 to 70 percent. An oxygen saturation of £30 percent for a time period of ³10 minutes correlates with a scalp pH of 7.20 or below.[11] It has an advantage over FBS as it can be used at 2 cm dilatation and has a better predictability in the presence of meconium. However, any condition which attenuates vascular pulsations may result in an inadequate signal.

ST Waveform Analysis of Fetal ECG for Intrapartum Surveillance (STAN)

Reduced oxygen supply to the fetal myocardium during labor can alter the shape of the fetal ECG, notably the elevation or depression of the ST segment. Electrodes are placed after the rupture of membranes. STAN technology uses computer analysis of ECG in combination with visual interpretation of CTG. A Swedish multicentric trial found that the use of STAN with CTG could bring about 75% reduction in the number of babies with metabolic acidosis as compared to CTG alone.[12]

Expedite Delivery

Expedite delivery if
- Adjunctive tests are not available or are contraindicated
- No response to the stimulation test
- Fetal scalp blood pH < 7.2 or lactate > 4.8 mmol/L
- There are additional signs of distress e.g. thick MSL
  According to the current guidelines (ACOG and RCOG) delivery must be achieved within 30 minutes of diagnosing fetal distress. Delivery must be planned by the fastest route, depending upon the stage of the labor. If the findings do not favor spontaneous or instrumental vaginal delivery, cesarean should be done (*Category 1 Cesarean-i.e. when there is immediate threat to life of woman or fetus*).

After Delivery

Delivery should be attended by an experienced pediatrician. Following delivery, umbilical cord blood samples from both umbilical artery and umbilical vein should be taken to check for birth asphyxia. Arterial blood is more representative of fetal metabolic condition as arterial acedemia may occur with normal venous pH. APGAR scores at 1 and 5 minute should be checked and all results should be recorded in the mother's and newborn's notes.

MECONIUM STAINED AMNIOTIC FLUID

The detection of MSL during labor is worrisome to the obstetrician; however, it is an unreliable marker of fetal distress. Meconium staining of amniotic fluid is seen frequently as the fetus matures and by itself is not an indicator of fetal distress.
- At term, the incidence of MSL is 10 to 15 percent.
- In preterm pregnancies, the incidence is <5 percent and Listeria sepsis or chorioamnionitis should be considered if meconium staining is present.
- However, in post-term (> 42 weeks) pregnancies, the incidence is 50 percent. It is considered physiological in post-term pregnancy but would be pathological if FHR monitoring is associated with nonreassuring FHR pattern.
  The current RCOG and NICE guidelines suggest that both thin and thick meconium is associated with a similar outcome.[4] Presence of a slight degree of meconium staining in the amniotic fluid without FHR abnormalities requires vigilance and does not necessarily indicate immediate delivery. MSL usually indicates the presence of fetal hypoxia or an episode of fetal hypoxia in the past. Therefore, fetal distress may be present or the fetus may be at a high-risk of distress. There is also a risk of meconium aspiration at delivery of the baby.

CASE SCENARIO-2

A primigravida with 37 weeks pregnancy came in spontaneous labor. Intermittent auscultation was being done for fetal heart monitoring. Patient was getting good contractions and had spontaneous rupture of membranes. Vaginal examination was done when thick meconium stained liquor was detected at 3 cm dilatation with 50 percent effacement. Patient was shifted to CTG monitoring which showed normal fetal heart pattern.

MANAGEMENT OF MECONIUM STAINED LIQUOR

1. Shift the patient to continuous CTG monitoring if possible or the frequency of intermittent auscultation should be increased to every 15 minutes.
2. Counsel the mother that meconium is a variation and not necessarily a complication. Explain about the 1 to 5 percent risk of meconium aspiration at the time of delivery irrespective of the mode of delivery.
3. Consider amnioinfusion.
   Amnioinfusion: It is a technique which involves infusion of crystalloids inside the amniotic cavity with the aim to dilute the meconium, thereby reducing the risk of meconium aspiration. It also helps in relieving cord compression by correcting oligohydramnios. It has a great potential to be a useful adjunct in the management of repetitive variable and prolonged decelerations in cases with oligohydramnios or MSL.
   According to Cochrane review 2010, amnioinfusion is associated with substantive improvement in perinatal outcome in settings where facilities for perinatal surveillance are limited. It is not clear whether the benefits are due to dilution of meconium or relief of oligohydramnios.[13]
   Evidence is scarce on the possibility of rare but serious maternal adverse effects of amnioinfusion such as endometritis, amniotic fluid embolism and uterine scar rupture.
   Technique of amnioinfusion – Pass Ryle's tube above the presenting part and infuse normal saline or Ringer's lactate 500 mL over 30 min at a rate of 15 mL/min then 500 mL at a rate of 3 mL/min (30 drops/min); maximum 1L of fluid can be infused.
   Containdications: Chorioamnionitis, multiple pregnancy, antepartum hemorrhage, previous cesarean section, maternal cardiac disease, cervical dilatation >7 cm.
4. Presence of MSL mandates the use of partogram to ensure normal progress of labor. There is currently no evidence to suggest that meconium aspiration syndrome would be prevented by cesarean section as neither the conditions nor the timings of aspiration can be predicted. If the FHR is within normal range with good variability and accelerations, it is said to be reassuring implying that the baby is tolerating labor well and labor can be continued with intensive monitoring.
5. At both vaginal and operative deliveries, perform thorough suctioning of the mouth and pharynx after delivery of the head and before delivery of the shoulders. A pediatrician should attend the delivery.

> **Management in this case:** In this case, the woman was in spontaneous labor, had no other associated risk factor, there was normal FHR pattern on CTG and no contraindication for amnioinfusion. So the decision for amnioinfusion and continuation of labor with strict monitoring was taken after discussion with the woman.

CORD PROLAPSE

Cord prolapse has been defined as the descent of the umbilical cord through the cervix alongside (occult) or past the presenting part (overt) in the presence of ruptured membranes.
Cord presentation is the presence of the umbilical cord between the presenting part and the cervix, with or without membrane rupture. The overall incidence of cord prolapse ranges from 0.1-0.6 percent.[14] One should feel for the cord at every vaginal examination during labor and after spontaneous rupture of membranes if risk factors are present.

Risk Factors for Cord Prolapse[15]

1. Malpresentations:
   - Breech: Overall 2.5 to 3.0 percent
     - Frank breech: 0.4 percent
     - Complete breech: 5 percent
     - Footling presentation: 10 percent
   - Shoulder (Transverse lie): 5 to 10 percent
   - Compound presentation: 10 to 20 percent
   - (Vertex presentation: 0.14%)
2. Prematurity
3. Fetal congenital anomalies like anencephaly
4. Polyhydramnios
5. Multiple pregnancies: 10 percent
6. Grandmuliparity (> 5 deliveries): 10 percent
7. Unengaged presenting part
8. Obstetric manipulations: 10 to 15 percent
   - Artificial rupture of membranes (ARM)
   - Vaginal manipulation of fetus with ruptured membranes
   - During external cephalic version
   - Internal podalic version
   - Stabilizing induction of labor
   - Insertion of uterine pressure catheter

CASE SCENARIO-3

A multigravida was being induced at 36 weeks period of gestation in view of pre-eclampsia. Per vaginal examination showed that cervix was 4 cm dilated, 70 percent effaced and the vertex was at -3 station. ARM was done for augmentation of labor. Immediately after ARM, cord was felt in the vagina and pulsations were felt in the cord. Fetal heart rate was 90 per minute.

Comment: Cord presentation missed in earlier P/V examination must have become overt cord prolapse after ARM. Cord prolapse with presence of cord pulsations is an indication for immediate delivery. Since vaginal delivery is not imminent in this patient, a category 1 cesarean should be done within 30 minutes or less.

MANAGEMENT OF CORD PROLAPSE[14,16]

- If the fetal heart is absent, deliver the baby in the manner that is safest to the mother.
- If fetus is alive, deliver immediately:
  - instrumental delivery – only if prerequisites are fulfilled
  - cesarean section if vaginal delivery is not imminent

In the mean time following measures are instituted:

1. Start oxygen by mask/nasal cannula at a rate of 4 to 6 L/min.
2. Adjust maternal position to reduce cord pressure- Trendelenberg's position (raising the foot end/Sim's position (left lateral decubitus) or genu-pectoral position (knee chest position).
3. Wearing high-level disinfected gloves insert a hand into vagina and push the presenting part up to decrease pressure on the cord and dislodge the presenting part from the pelvis.
4. Don't attempt to replace the cord back into the uterus and avoid unnecessary handling of the cord to prevent reactive vasoconstriction and fetal hypoxia.
5. Quick retrograde filling of bladder with 500 to 700 cc saline.
6. Place the other hand on abdomen in the suprapubic region to keep the presenting part out of the pelvis. Once presenting part is firmly held above pelvic brim, remove the other hand from

vagina and keep the hand on abdomen until cesarean section. If available, give terbuatline 0.25 mg subcutaneous or salbutamol 0.5 mg IV slowly over 2 minutes to reduce contractions.
7. Paired cord blood samples should be taken for pH and base excess measurement.

To conclude, though fetal distress is the commonest reason for intervention during labor, the diagnosis is imprecise. Under diagnosis can increase perinatal morbidity whereas over diagnosis can increase interventions. Thus any indicator of suspected fetal distress should be interpreted in context of the clinical situation and management individualized.

Prevention[14]

- ARM should be avoided whenever possible if presenting part is mobile. If necessary, it should be performed with arrangements in place for immediate cesarean delivery.
- Avoid unnecessary vaginal examination and obstetric intervention with ruptured membranes and a high presenting part as there is a risk of upward displacement of the presenting part and resultant cord prolapse.
- One should feel for the cord at every P/V examination during labor and after spontaneous rupture of membranes.
- Women with transverse, oblique or unstable lie should be advised admission at 38 weeks of gestation.
- Women with preterm premature rupture of membranes should also be advised admission.

KEY POINTS

- The term fetal distress should always be specified with description of findings, e.g. repetitive variable decelerations, fetal tachycardia or bradycardia, late decelerations etc.
- Low-risk patients can be monitored with intermittent auscultation.
- CTG should be interpreted using standard uniform criteria and should be supplemented by adjunctive tests to reduce false positive results.
- Expedite delivery if FHR abnormalities persist, fetal scalp blood pH is <7.2 & there are additional signs of fetal distress, e.g. meconium staining otherwise continue FHR monitoring
- Fetal scalp or vibroacoustic stimulation test can be used as an alternative to fetal scalp sampling where facilities for the latter are not available.
- Always get umbilical cord blood pH in cases of fetal distress
- Both thick and thin MSL require strict intrapartum fetal surveillance
- Amnioinfusion is beneficial in cases with MSL and repeated variable decelerations due to cord compression.
- Rule out cord prolapse at every vaginal examination during labor.
- In cases of cord prolapse, delivery must be achieved within 30 minutes of the diagnosis.

References

1. International Classification of Diseases (ICD version 2007). Pregnancy, childbirth and the puerperium: Complications of labor and delivery. World Health Organisation website [online] Available from http://www.who.int/classifications/aaps/icd/icd10online/?go60.htm+o68
2. ACOG committee opinion. Inappropriate use of the terms fetal distress and birth asphyxia. Number 197, February 1998 (replaces no. 137, April 1994). Committee on Obstetric Practice. American College of Obstetricians and Gynecologists. Int J Gynaecol Obstet 1998;61:309-10.
3. American Academy of Pediatrics and the American College of Obstetricians and Gynecologist: Intrapartum and postpartum care of the mother. In Guidelines for Perinatal care, 5th ed.Washington, DC, AAP and ACOG, 2002.
4. National Collaborating Centre for Women's and Children's health(NICE) (2007). Intrapartum care of healthy women and their babies during childbirth. [online] NICE website. Available from http://www.nice.org.uk/nicemedia/pdf/Intrapartum Care September 2007 mainguideline.pdf

5. NICE/RCOG. Electronic fetal monitoring algorithm derived from guidelines; Useful algorithmic summary of the 2001 NICE/RCOG guidelines-still current advice. RCOG website [online] Available from http://www.nice.org.uk/nicemedia/pdf/efmguidelinenice.pdf

6. Fawole B, Hofmeyr GJ. Maternal oxygen administration for fetal distress. Cochrane Database Syst Rev 2003;(4):CD000136.

7. Hofmeyr GJ, Gülmezoglu AM. Maternal hydration for increasing amniotic fluid volume in oligohydramnios and normal amniotic fluid volume. Cochrane Database Syst Rev 2002;(1):CD000134.

8. Alfirevic Z, Devane D, Gyte GM. Continuous cardiotocography (CTG) as a form of electronic fetal monitoring (EFM) for fetal assessment during labor. Cochrane Database Syst Rev 2006;3:CD006066.

9. Clark SL, Gimovsky ML, Miller FC. Fetal heart rate response to scalp blood sampling. Am J Obstet Gynecol 1982;144:706.

10. East CE, Smyth R, Leader LR, Henshall NE, Colditz PB, Tan KH. Vibroacoustic stimulation for fetal assessment in labour in the presence of a nonreassuring fetal heart rate trace. Cochrane Database Syst Rev 2005;(2):CD004664.

11. Schmidt S, Koslowski S, Sierra F. Clinical usefulness of pulse oximetry in the fetus with nonreassuring heart rate pattern. J Perinat Med 2000;28:298-305.

12. Amer-Wahlin J, Hellsten C, Noren H. Cardiotocography only versus cardiotocography plus ST analysis of fetal echocardiogram for intrapartum fetal monitoring. A Swedish randomised controlled trial. Lancet 2001;358:534-38.

13. Hofmeyr GJ. Amnioinfusion for meconium-stained liquor in labour. Cochrane Database Syst Rev. 2002;(1):CD000014.

14. Royal College of Obstetricians and Gynaecologists 2008. Umbilical cord prolapse. Green-Top Guideline NO. 50, RCOG 2008. Available at http://www.rcog.org.uk/womens-health/clinical-guidance/umbilical-cord-prolapse-green-top-50

15. Klatt TE. Breech, other malpresentations and umbilical cord complications. In: Danforth's Obstetrics & Gynaecology, 10th edition. Philadelphia, USA: Lippincott Williams & Wilkins, 2008. pp. 413.

16. Managing Complications in Pregnancy & Childbirth: A Guide for midwives & doctors. Department of Reproductive Health & Research, WHO 2003.

Chapter 12

Shoulder Dystocia

Poonam Sachdeva, Muntaha, Vandana K Benwal

INTRODUCTION

Shoulder dystocia is defined as "a difficulty in delivery of the shoulder that requires additional obstetric maneuvers to release the shoulder after gentle downward traction has failed".[1,2,3]

The mean head to body delivery time during a normal delivery is 24 seconds. When this delivery time exceeds 60 seconds, it is called shoulder dystocia. Overall, the incidence of shoulder dystocia varies between 0.6 to 1.4 percent.

Though there is a relationship between shoulder dystocia and fetal size, it is not a good predictor, as majority of infants with birth weight >4500 grams do not develop shoulder dystocia and 48 percent of shoulder dystocias occur in infants with birth weight less than 4000 gms.[3] Neonates having shoulder dystocia have significantly disproportionate shoulder to head ratio and chest to head ratio as compared to those with equally macrosomic newborns delivered without dystocia.

Shoulder dystocia may be either unilateral or bilateral. Commonly, the posterior shoulder is in the sacral bay but the anterior shoulder remains above the symphysis pubis (unilateral). Rarely, both the shoulders remain above the symphysis pubis (bilateral).[3,4]

Fetal Hazards[4,5]

Shoulder dystocia is associated with significant fetal morbidity and even mortality.
- Fetal asphyxia
- Fetal injuries which occur in 25 percent.
- Injury to brachial plexus is most common and occurs in 66 percent. Most of them recover but less than 10 percent may result in permanent brachial plexus dysfunction.
- Fracture humerus may occur in 17 percent.
- Fracture clavicle may occur in 38 percent
- Claw hand deformity may occur due to injury to C-7 to T-1.
- Erb's palsy may occur due to injury to C 5-6 & sometimes C-7 spinal nerves.
- Sternocleidomastoid hematoma may form.
  Over a period of one year, 80 percent of these injuries recover.

Maternal Hazards

- Increased operative delivery and morbidity
- Postpartum hemorrhage due to uterine atony
- Postpartum hemorrhage due to vaginal lacerations

Table 12.1: Predisposing factors for shoulder dystocia	
Pre-labor	*Intrapartum*
Previous shoulder dystocia	Prolonged 1st stage of labor
Macrosomia (But 50% occur in normal-sized babies)	Secondary arrest
Obesity(BMI > 30kg/m²)	Prolonged 2nd stage of labor
Diabetes Mellitus	Mid-pelvic instrumental delivery (more with ventuse than forceps)
Anencephaly	Oxytocin augmentation
Multiparity	
Post-maturity	

CASE SCENARIO

A 30-years-old woman G3 P2 L2 with 38 weeks pregnancy is admitted to the labor room with labor pains. She is obese with gestational diabetes and is on diabetic diet. Estimated fetal weight is about 3.5 kg. She has leaking per vaginum for the last 24 hours.

Comment: The attending obstetrician should recognize that there exists a risk for shoulder dystocia during delivery as the patient has several high-risk factors like big baby, obesity, diabetes and multiparity.

Predisposing Factors[4] (Table 12.1)

Though predisposing factors for shoulder dystocia have been identified, risk assessment for prediction of shoulder dystocia is insufficient to prevent large majority of cases. Conventional risk factors predict only 16 percent of shoulder dystocia that results in infant's morbidity and majority of cases occur in women with no risk factors. *Shoulder dystocia is thus an unpredictable and an unpreventable event.*

Prevention[6]

Prediction is not possible accurately, so care is to be taken to reduce the time interval between delivery of the fetal head and body.

History in this case: Patient had leaking per vaginum for the last 24 hours. So labor augmentation was done with oxytocin. Second stage of labor was prolonged with cervix being fully dilated for more than one hour. Hence it was decided to apply ventuse cup. The aforesaid facts in the history should alert the obstetrician to the possibility of shoulder dystocia.

Diagnosis

A dagnosis of shoulder dystocia is made as there is
1. Definite recoil of the head back against the perineum called as 'Turtle sign'.
2. Difficulty with delivery of the face and the chin
3. Failure of restitution of the fetal head
4. Failure of the shoulder to descend

MANAGEMENT[2,3,4,7]

There are some Do's and Don'ts for the management:

Don'ts

a. Do not be panicky
b. Do not give traction over the baby's head
c. Do not apply fundal pressure

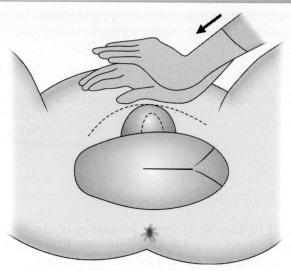

Figure 12.1: Moderate suprapubic pressure

Do's

a. Call for extra-help
b. Clear the infant's mouth and nose
c. Call anesthetist and the pediatrician
d. Drain the bladder if full
e. Perform a wide mediolateral episiotomy if not made earlier
f. Get the ultrasonography (USG) machine at the bedside to note the side of the back

Step I

Moderate suprapubic pressure should be applied by an assistant while downward traction is applied to the fetal head for 30 seconds (Figure 12.1). Intermittent pulling should be avoided.

Mechanism: This will reduce bisacromial diameter (2 cm) and rotates the anterior shoulder towards the oblique diameter.

If this method fails then proceed to the next step.

Step II

McRobert's maneuver: Maternal thighs should be abducted and sharply flexed onto patient's abdomen (Figure 12.2).

Mechanism: This results in rotation of the symphysis pubis upwards and decreases the angle of pelvic inclination. Though this does not increase pelvic dimensions, pelvic rotation cephalad frees the impacted shoulder.

This maneuver is the single most effective intervention with reported success rates as high as 90% and has low rate of complications.

Step III

Wood's corkscrew maneuver: In this, posterior shoulder is rotated to the anterior position (180°) by a screwing movement. This is done by inserting two fingers in the posterior vagina. Simultaneous suprapubic pressure is applied (Figure 12.3).

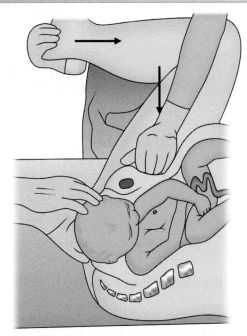

Figure 12.2: McRobert's maneuver

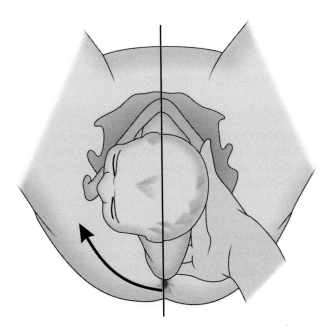

Figure 12.3: Wood's maneuver

Mechanism: This pushes the bisacromial diameter to an oblique diameter and helps easy entry of the bisacromial diameter into the pelvic inlet. In this, the fetal shoulders are the screw and the maternal pelvis is the threads. If this fails proceed to the next step.

Step IV

Rubin's maneuver: He recommended two maneuvers. First the fetal shoulders are rocked from side-to-side by applying force to maternal abdomen. If this is not successful, the pelvic hand reaches the

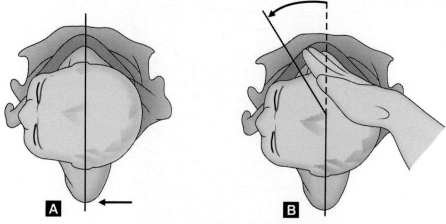

Figure 12.4: Rubin's maneuver

most easily accessible fetal shoulder which is then pushed towards the anterior surface of the chest (Figure 12.4).

Mechanism: This maneuver most often results in abduction of both shoulders, which in turn produces a small shoulder-to-shoulder diameter and displacement of the anterior shoulder from behind the symphysis pubis.

Step V

Extraction of posterior arm: It consists of carefully sweeping the posterior arm of the fetus across the chest, followed by delivery of the arm. The shoulder girdle is then rotated into one of the oblique diameters of the pelvis with the subsequent delivery of the anterior shoulder.

Step VI

Hibbard maneuver: In this maneuver pressure is applied to the fetal jaw and neck in the direction of the maternal rectum, with strong fundal pressure applied by an assistant as the anterior shoulder is freed. However, strong fundal pressure applied at the wrong time may result in even further impaction of the anterior shoulder.

Step VII

Zavanelli maneuver: In this maneuver the fetal head is flexed and the fetus is replaced within the pelvis. Thereafter baby is delivered by an emergency caesarean section. The first step is returning of the head to the occipitoanterior or occipitoposterior position if the head had rotated from either position. The operator flexes the head and slowly pushes it back into the vagina following which cesarean delivery is performed. Terbutaline 250 µg subcutaneous is given to produce uterine relaxation.

Step VIII

Fracture of the clavicle: Deliberate fracture of the clavicle by pressing the anterior clavicle against the ramus of the pubis can be performed to free the shoulder impaction. However, it is difficult to fracture the clavicle of a large neonate. The fracture will heal rapidly and is not as serious as a brachial nerve injury, asphyxia or death

Step IX

Cleidotomy: Consists of cutting the clavicle with a scissors or other sharp instrument and is usually used for a dead fetus or in anencephaly.

Flow chart 12.1: Summary of sequences of steps

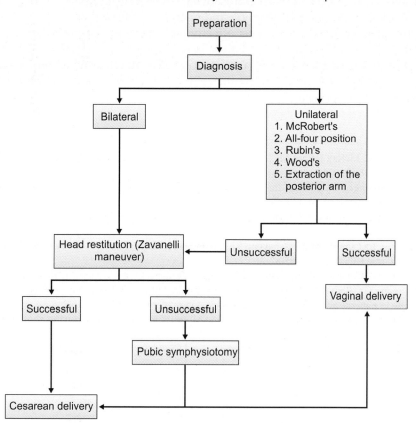

Step X

Symphysiotomy: Hartfield[8] suggested this maneuver but maternal morbidity was significantly high due to urinary tract injury.

The American College of Obstetricians and Gynecologists (ACOG) has concluded that there is no evidence that any one maneuver is superior to another in releasing an impacted shoulder or reducing the chances of injury. Performance of the McRobert's maneuver however was deemed a reasonable initial approach.

> **Management in this case:**
> The baby's head was delivered by ventuse but the shoulders could not be delivered for more than 60 sec. A diagnosis of shoulder dystocia was made. Suprabupic pressure was used but failed to deliver the shoulder. Subsequently McRobert's technique was tried and with some difficulty the shoulder was delivered. The baby was fine after some resuscitative efforts. (Flow chart 12.1)

KEY POINTS

- The mean head to body delivery time in normal birth is 24 seconds. When this delivery time exceeds 60 seconds, it is called shoulder dystocia.
- Shoulder dystocia may occur if the patient has high-risk factors like macrosomia, obesity, diabetes and multiparity.
- Neonates developing shoulder dystocia have significantly disproportionate shoulder to head ratio and chest to head ratio.

- Shoulder dystocia is associated with significant fetal morbidity and even mortality and increased maternal morbidity due to uterine atony and operative intervention.
- McRobert maneuver is the single most effective intervention with reported success rates as high as 90%.
- According to ACOG no maneuver is superior to another in releasing an impacted shoulder or reducing the chances of injury. Performance of the McRobert's maneuver however is deemed a reasonable initial approach.

REFERENCES

1. Beall MH, Spong C, McKay J, Ross MG. Objective definition of shoulder dystocia: a prospective evaluation. Am J Obstet Gynecol 1998;179:934-7.
2. Fernando A. Prolonged Pregnancy. In: Fernando A, Shirish ND, Bhide AG (eds). Practical guide to high-risk pregnancy and delivery. 3rd Ed. Elsevier, 2008.pp. 287-89.
3. Royal College of Obstetricians and Gynaecologists. Green-top guideline No.42: Shoulder dystocia. London; RCOG press, 2005.
4. Abnormal labor. In: Cunningham FG, Leveno KJ, Bloom SL, Hauth JC, Rouse D, Spong C (eds).Williams Obstetrics. 23nd Ed. Mc Graw Hill, 2010.pp. 481-87.
5. Baskett TF, Allen AC. Perinatal implications of shoulder dystocia. Obstet Gynecol 1995;86:14-7.
6. Beall MH, Spong CY, Ross MG. A randomized controlled trial of prophylactic maneuvers to reduce head-to-body delivery time in patients at risk for shoulder dystocia. Obstet Gynecol 2003;102:31-5.
7. Bruner JP, Drummond SB, Meenan AL, Gaskin IM. All-fours maneuver for reducing shoulder dystocia during labor. J Reprod Med 1998;43:439-43.
8. Hartfield VJ. Symphysiotomy for shoulder dystocia. Am J Obstet Gynecol 1986;155:228.

Chapter 13

Obstructed Labor and Rupture Uterus

Swaraj Batra, Binni Makkar, Shweta Tahlan

INTRODUCTION

Obstructed labor is one of the preventable causes of maternal and perinatal morbidity and mortality. Maternal mortality due to this condition ranges between 1 to 13 percent and perinatal mortality from 74 to 92 percent.[1] It is found to be directly or indirectly responsible for about half of all maternal deaths affecting mainly primigravida and grand multipara. Maternal deaths occur as a result of ruptured uterus as well as genital sepsis in women who undergo cesarean section done for obstructed labor.[1] Reports from India, Nigeria ,Ghana ,Ethiopia and Bangladesh indicate that up to 75 percent of cases of uterine rupture are seen with unscarred uterus and obstructed labor is one of the top five causes of maternal mortality.[2,3,4,5,6] Incidence of obstructed labor and rupture uterus in Lok Nayak hospital is about 1.6 percent and 0.1 percent respectively.

Definition

When in spite of good uterine contractions, the progressive descent of presenting part is arrested due to mechanical obstruction, labor is said to be obstructed.[1]

Causes

Obstructed labor occurs due to a mismatch between the presenting part of the fetus and the maternal pelvis (Table 13.1).

Table 13.1: Causes of Absolute Disproportion			
Maternal condition		*Fetal condition*	*Malpresentation*
Bony deformities	*Soft tissue abnormalities*		
Severe kyphosis	Cervical fibroids	Macrosomia	Persistent occipito posterior
Severe scoliosis	Ovarian tumor	Hydrocephalus	Mentoposterior
Poliomyelitis	Pelvic kidney	Iniencephaly	Shoulder
Rickets	Excessive fat	Conjoint twins	Brow
Osteomalacia	Vaginal atresia	Fetal ascites or tumors	Impacted/aftercoming head of breech
Maternal dwarfism	Vaginal septum	Impacted shoulders	Compound presentation
Pelvic fracture.		Locked twins	

In obstructed labor, there is increase in intensity, duration and frequency of uterine contractions. Relaxation phase progressively decreases. Ultimately, a state of tonic contraction develops. Lower segment elongates and becomes thinner to accommodate the fetus driven by upper segment. A circular groove encircling the uterus is formed between active uterine segment and distended lower segment called pathological retraction ring (Bandl's ring).

In primigravida, further retraction ceases in response to obstruction and state of uterine exhaustion is seen. In multiparae, retraction of upper segment continues with progressive dilatation and thinning of lower segment with progressive rise of Bandl's ring ultimately leading to uterine rupture.

CASE SCENARIO-1

A 24-year-old primigravida with 9 months amenorrhea presented to casualty with complain of labor pains for 2 days associated with leaking per vaginum for 24 hours.

Comments: Patient has nonprogress of labor and obstructed labor should be ruled out as the cause of nonprogress.

POINTS TO BE NOTED IN HISTORY

- History of prolonged and difficult labor
- History of *Dai* handling
- History of fever and leaking and their duration in view of onset of sepsis in later stages.
- History of severe pain in abdomen

History in this case:
History of prolonged labor with labor pains for 2 days and leaking for 24 hours

POINTS TO BE NOTED IN EXAMINATION

General Examination

- General condition-whether exhausted, dehydrated
- Temperature, pulse, respiratory rate (RR) and blood pressure (BP).
  In obstructed labor, in early stages, the general physical examination is usually normal. Patient may appear dehydrated and exhausted in later stages. She may have tachycardia and hypotension. Pallor may be demonstrable. There may be metabolic acidosis due to accumulation of lactic acid produced by contracting uterine and skeletal muscles.

Cardiovascular and Respiratory System Examination

- If should be examined for any abnormality

Abdominal Examination

- Uterus may be tonically contracted over the fetus and there may be difficulty in palpating fetal parts.
- Liquor may have drained out completely
- Note fetal size
- Look for signs of obstructed labor:
  - Stretching of lower uterine segment
  - Bandl's ring (in later stages) which runs obliquely over the uterus causing sharp demarcation of upper and lower uterine segment

- Bladder may be drawn up into the abdomen and with continuing pressure of the presenting part against the pubis, the bladder neck gets compressed. The bladder may become edematous and there may be blood-stained urine
- The bowel may be distended in later stages.
- Fetal distress or absent fetal heart sound (FHS) in later cases
- There may be features of chorioamnionitis and the uterus may be tender to touch.

Local and Vaginal (P/V) Examination

- Vulval edema may be there
- Vagina may be hot and dry
- Cervix- whether loose hanging or well applied over the presenting part
- Station of the head and its position or malpresentation should be noted
- A large caput and irreversible moulding may be there in late stages
- Liquor- whether foul smelling, meconium/blood stained. In late stages, liquor may be completely drained out and labor may be dry
- Type of pelvis and feto/cephalopelvic disproportion (CPD) should be noted.

> **Examination in this case**
> General examination- -Patient was dehydrated and febrile to touch, appeared mildly pale.
> Pulse-110/min, BP-110/70 mm Hg, Temp-101°F, RR-24/min
> Abdominal examination- Uterus was term size, hard, slightly tender with cephalic presentation 3/5th palpable above pelvic brim. The lower uterine segment appeared stretched out and Bandl's ring was seen midway between umbilicus and symphysis pubis.FHS was absent.
> Left occipitoposterior position with large caput coming to 0 station and irreversible moulding was present. Vagina was dry and hot with no liquor draining. On bimanual examination head was not engaged, there was CPD.
> Urine ketones were ++

Diagnosis

Obstructed labor

INVESTIGATIONS

Hemogram, blood sugar, blood urea, serum electrolytes and arterial blood gases (ABG) should be checked. Urine should be examined for ketones

MANAGEMENT

Initial Management in such Cases

- Patient should be initially stabilized and dehydration should be corrected by rapid infusion of Ringer's solution, at least 1 liter is given in running drip. For such patients at least 2 liters of fluids are needed to correct dehydration
- Blood should be cross matched and kept arranged and investigations sent
- Parenteral broad spectrum antibiotics should be administered to avoid sepsis
- Tetanus immunization status should be checked and active immunization is given if required
- Maintain an observation chart to record urine output, pulse, BP and temperature
- Bladder should be catheterized before any operative procedure
- Nasogastric tube may be used to empty the stomach before general anesthesia is given.

Mode of Delivery

The choice of the mode of delivery depends on the stage of labor, level of the presenting part and the associated maternal and fetal complications.

- If the case is detected early with good fetal condition, **cesarean section** gives good results. After incising the abdomen, preferably through a midline subumbilical incision, the peritoneal cavity is entered high up, to avoid injury to the bladder. An assistant can help to disimpact the fetal head per vaginum. Fetus can also be delivered by pulling the feet through the uterine incision. Care must be taken to avoid lateral tears if head is jammed in the pelvis as this can compromise the blood supply to the already bruised myometrium and attempts at securing hemostasis could endanger the ureters. If there is lateral extension or tear, the uterus should be exteriorized and one hand should be placed posterior to the broad ligament to visualize and suture the torn area, remaining close to the uterus. Methergine/oxytocin/prostaglandins can be given to prevent postpartum hemorrhage
- For cases presenting late with a dead fetus, cesarean section is a safe option. **Destructive operations** may also be considered in such cases especially in regions with poorly developed health services, although these procedures have no place in modern obstetrics. When facilities for cesarean section are absent or unsafe, these procedures may allow safe delivery of mother, in addition to avoiding a uterine scar that may rupture if she is unable to obtain suitable antenatal care in subsequent pregnancy.
- **Symphysiotomy** seems to have no place in modern obstetrics as a cesarean section is a better option. It is a good alternative when facilities for cesarean are not available. Specific indications for symphysiotomy include engaged head arrested by mid-pelvic or outlet contraction, arrested abnormal presentation like brow or face, especially when the disproportion does not permit the safe application of forceps.

Management in this case:
- The patient was resuscitated with rapid infusion of 1 liter of Ringer's solution.
- Simultaneously, blood was sent for complete blood count and cross match.
- Intravenous (IV) broad spectrum antibiotics were started.
- An emergency cesarean section was done after catheterization under anesthesia. A still born baby (birth weight- 3.5 kg) was delivered. Per operatively lower segment was thinned out and bladder was advanced with slightly hematuric urine.
- Postoperatively- bladder was kept catheterized for 2 weeks. IV antibiotics were continued for the same period. Speculum examination was done before removing the catheter to confirm healthy status of anterior vagina. Patient remained afebrile and was discharged after stitch removal with advise on contraception, spacing and antenatal care in next preg.

CASE SCENARIO-2

A 30-year-old G3P2L2 with POG of 37 weeks presented with complains of labor pains for 2 days associated with leaking per vaginum for 12 hours. Patient also gave history of *Dai* handling. Her last two pregnancies were full term vaginal deliveries at home with uneventful postpartum period.

Comments: Patient has presented with prolonged labor. She is a multigravida and is more at risk of rupture uterus if there is obstructed labor

History in this case:
Third gravid
History of prolonged leaking and *Dai* handling

Examination in this case:
Patient was dehydrated and had tachycardia. BP-100/80 mm Hg. There was moderate pallor.
Abdominal examination –
- Uterus was term size with fetus lying in transverse lie
- Strong contractions present
- The lower segment was stretched out.
- FHS was not localized.
Per vaginal (P/V) examination –
- Cervix 5 cm dilated
- Fetal hand lying at the introitus., shoulder felt at brim
- No liquor draining
- Pelvis gynecoid

Diagnosis

Term pregnancy with transverse lie with hand prolapse, in obstructed labor with intrauterine fetal demise

Management in this case:
- The patient was managed by initial stabilization (as discussed previously) followed by emergency cesarean section.
- Postoperatively patient was managed in similar manner as the previous case.
- Destructive operations like decapitation or internal podalic version were not considered as lower segment was stretched. Such procedures may be considered in these cases (if there are no signs of imminent rupture) especially in countries like India where health facilities are not very well developed. These procedures may allow safe delivery of mother, in addition to avoiding a uterine scar which may rupture if she is unable to obtain obstetric care in future pregnancies.

COMPLICATIONS OF OBSTRUCTED LABOR

Immediate Complications

- With prolonged obstruction, there are increased chances of *sepsis*, both intrapartum and postpartum
- Postpartum uterine exhaustion and sepsis can lead to *hemorrhage* and *shock*
- In late stages *rupture uterus* may be seen in parous women.

Late Complications

Various organ systems may get involved as a result of injuries from prolonged obstructed labor
- The most common of all injuries is the *obstetric fistula formation*. Base of the bladder is nipped in between the presenting part and symphysis pubis and undergoes pressure necrosis. The devitalized tissue becomes infected and later may slough off resulting in development of genito-urinary fistula in 2nd week after delivery
- In addition to vesicovaginal fistula, other injuries can occur like total urethral loss, stress incontinence, hydroureteronephrosis, renal failure, rectovaginal fistula
- *Scarring of genital tract* may also be seen
- There may be pituitary and hypothalamic dysfunction that frequently leads to amenorrhea-*Sheehan's syndrome*
- *Pelvic inflammatory disease* also increases with obstructed labor
- There is a high rate of *secondary infertility* in these patients owing to combined effects of amenorrhea (Sheehan's syndrome), pelvic inflammatory disease and genital tract scarring

- Some women may develop *foot drop* resulting from excessive compression of sacral plexus by the fetal head
- It could also result in perineal nerve damage and nerve damage to bladder resulting in complex *bladder dysfunction.*

PREVENTION OF OBSTRUCTED LABOR

1. There should be provision of more primary care centers and better access to comprehensive antenatal and emergency health services with skills to provide basic emergency obstetric care and availability of skilled attendants at delivery can decrease the incidence of this condition.[7]
2. As the risk of obstructed labor is closely related to physical size, particularly the pelvic size of the mother, micronutrient supplementation for the chronically malnourished population appears to be an attractive intervention to reduce maternal and fetal mortality. These interventions must be targeted at younger age groups.
3. External cephalic version for breech presentation and transverse lie can be initiated. The use of early induction of labor to confer the benefits of delivering smaller babies is debatable.[8]
4. It is wise to look for the presence of risk factors during early labor to facilitate early referral to a center with adequate facilities for performing emergency procedures.
5. There should be routine use of partogram for timely diagnosis of this condition. The classic pattern attributable to CPD especially in a primigravida, is secondary arrest of dilation. In parous women, there could be arrest of descent, usually in the second stage of labor in spite of good pains.

RUPTURE UTERUS

Uterine rupture is a life-threatening condition for both mother and fetus. The profile of causes and mortality varies between developed and developing countries. However, the limitation of health services in the latter and a rising cesarean section rate in the former means uterine rupture is increasing in most of the regions of the world. The hospital based incidence of uterine rupture varies from 1 in 100 to 500 deliveries in developing countries to 1 in 3000 to 5000 in hospitals with well developed health services.[9] Maternal death from uterine rupture is rare but severe maternal morbidity associated with hemorrhage and emergency obstetric hysterectomy is common. In developing countries maternal mortality from uterine rupture may be from 5 to 15 percent and fetal loss can exceed 80 percent.[10] Uterine rupture is one of the most serious accidents seen during pregnancy.

1. *Rupture during pregnancy:* It is quite rare and may be seen in cases of weakening of uterus caused by previous dilatation and curettage (D& C) or grand multiparae due to neglected labor.
2. *Rupture during labor:* It is of two types
   a. *Traumatic:* It is due to
      - Intrauterine manipulations such as version, destructive operations, forceps extraction performed by unskilled personnel
      - Accidents.
   b. *Spontaneous:* It may occur due to
      - Obstructed labor
      - Uterine defects such as malposition (e.g. pendulous belly)/weakening of uterine wall by cesarean section/myomectomy.
   c. *Misuse of oxytocic drugs* is the cause in occasional cases.

Multiparity is recognized as a powerful predisposing cause. This is explained partly by weakening of uterine wall and strong uterine contractions trying to overcome obstruction due to malpresentation or CPD.

Morbid Anatomy

Rupture is said to be **complete** if all the coats including peritoneum are torn and **incomplete** if peritoneum is intact.

Predisposing Factors

1. *Overstretching of lower uterine segment:* This is the underlying cause of uterine rupture in cases of obstructed labor. In this situation, normal changes in uterus become greatly exaggerated; retraction in upper segment proceeds to an extreme degree while stretching becomes extreme in passive portion longitudinally and circumferentially which is made to accommodate the greater part of fetal body. In consequence, the retraction ring rises higher progressively and is then a pathological phenomenon (Bandl's ring). Finally the lower segment ruptures due to continuous stretching, hypoxia, myometrial edema and necrosis. Fetus suffers from prolonged hypoxia and dies.
2. *Intrauterine manipulation:* In these cases, rupture starts in the cervix or lower uterine segment, runs up the body and usually follows the lateral uterine wall, opening up the broad ligament resulting into broad ligament hematoma. The tears may extend deeply into the vault as well. Majority of these are incomplete ruptures.
3. *Abnormalities of uterus:* These include scar in the uterus from previous cesarean section or myomectomy. Rupture of uterine scar after lower segment cesarean section (LSCS) is very rare, i.e. 0.4 percent.
4. *Previous cesarean scar:* In 4 percent of women becoming pregnant after classical cesarean, scar gives way during labor or pregnancy. Rupture in these cases is usually longitudinal and situated in the anterior uterine wall near the midline. All cases of previous cesarean section should be booked for delivery in a place with facility for cesarean section.

CASE SCENARIO-3

A 23-year-old G2P1L1 with period of gestation of 38 weeks with previous LSCS presented with complaints of labor pains for 4 hours. Her last delivery was by a LSCS done for fetal distress 3 years back in a private hospital. Per operatively there were no complications and her postoperative period was uneventful.

On examination: Her vitals were stable.

Abdominal examination—Uterus was term size with cephalic presentation. There was no scar tenderness and FHR was 140/min; estimated fetal weight was 2.8 kg.

P/V—cervix was 3 cm dilated and 80 percent effaced with vertex at -2 station with left occipito transverse position. Membranes were present and pelvis was adequate.

The patient was planned for vaginal birth after cesarean (VBAC) as previous section was done for non recurrent cause 3 years back with uneventful postoperative period. She was not postdated, baby was average size, there was no scar tenderness and there was no CPD. The patient was shifted to labor room and continuous fetal heart monitoring was done along with strict watch on features of scar dehiscence.

> **Comments:** All women undergoing labor after previous cesarean section should be carefully assessed for possibility of VBAC and monitored for signs of scar rupture.

POINTS TO BE NOTED IN HISTORY

- History of prolonged and difficult labor
- History of previous scar in the uterus—note the type of surgery done on the uterus—lower segment section/classical section/myomectomy, when was the procedure performed, by whom and for what indication. Details of postoperative period, interval between pregnancies, period of gestation of present pregnancy as postdated pregnancy may be a contraindication to VBAC.
- In patients with imminent rupture due to obstructed labor, patient may complain of constant pain in lower abdomen while contractions become progressively stronger and tetanic and she has features of obstructed labor.

- Patient may give history of very strong contractions followed by sudden cessation along with features of shock.

POINTS TO BE NOTED IN EXAMINATION

- Tachycardia and scar tenderness may indicate scar dehiscence
- Fetal heart rate abnormalities such as variable and late decelerations are common and among most reliable early signs of imminent rupture
- Vaginal bleeding may be seen varying from minimal to heavy bleeding. In some cases, there may be bleeding into broad ligament resulting into broad ligament hematoma
- Bladder signs and symptoms are also important. In early stage of lower uterine segment rupture, there may be bladder tenesmus and hematuria. This is particularly so in cases of rupture of previous lower segment scar
- Sudden rupture is usually attended by severe shock and acute abdominal pain. There is sudden feeling of something giving away. There is pallor, tachycardia, low BP and shifting dullness in the abdomen due to intraperitoneal bleed.
- Cessation of uterine contraction occurs if there is complete rupture leading to expulsion of fetus in peritoneal cavity. In such cases, two abdominal swelling can be differentiated- one representing the fetal parts and other the retracted uterus. FHS is absent and presenting part if felt earlier by per vaginum examination may recede.
- In case of scar rupture in patients with previous cesarean section, rupture, may remain unnoticed initially for sometime due to gradual oozing from the previous scar site. In the initial stage, there may be fetal heart decelerations before FHS disappears.

> **Further course of events in this case:**
> After 2 hours patient started complaining of constant severe pain in lower abdomen. CTG started showing decelerations and in no time the fetal heart disappeared.
> On examination patient had tachycardia with BP of 90/70 mm Hg.
> Abdominal examination - Uterine contour was ill defined and fetal parts were found to be superficially palpable. Fetal heart sound was not localized.

Diagnosis

Rupture uterus.

MANAGEMENT

- Immediate laparotomy is indicated in such patients.
- Investigations should be sent before taking the patient for laparotomy:
  - Complete blood count
  - Blood urea
  - Blood sugar
  - Arterial blood gases
  - Bleeding time (BT), clotting time (CT), clot retraction time (CRT) should be checked and corrected if deranged before surgery.
- If the patient is in shock, she should be initially resuscitated by rapid infusion of 2 to 3 liters of crystalloid solution. Simultaneously blood sample is sent for cross match followed by transfusion of packed cells.
- After abdomen is opened, fetus and placenta removed, decision must be taken whether to remove the uterus or do the repair by suturing the rent.
- In case of rupture of lower segment scar, the edges of the rent are usually neat and are usually treatable by excising the previous scar and resuturing the edges. If the patient has completed her family, tubal ligation should also be done along with the repair after consent.

- In most other cases of uterine rupture, margins are ragged and irregular and suturing may not be feasible and therefore subtotal hysterectomy may be indicated. If there is no overt sepsis, with no involvement of cervix or paracolpos, subtotal hysterectomy is the procedure of choice. This can be done more rapidly and carries less risk of damage to bladder. However, repair should be attempted if patient has no living issue.
- Total abdominal hysterectomy is needed if cervix and paracolpos are involved or if there is sepsis associated with rupture.
- In all cases of obstructed labor, it is essential to check the integrity of bladder and indwelling catheter should be kept for 2 weeks. Also the patient must have blood culture and cervical swab taken for culture and sensitivity.
- At the time of discharge the patient should be explained and it should be clearly mentioned on the discharge slip that in future pregnancy mode of delivery should be by cesarean section at 34 to 36 weeks of period of gestation and pregnancy should be avoided preferably for at least 2 years by using appropriate spacing methods.

Management in this case:

The patient was taken up for immediate laparotomy.

Simultaneously blood sample was sent for complete hemogram, coagulation profile and cross match.

Per operatively, there was rupture of previous uterine scar and there was 800 cc of hemoperitoneum with dead fetus partially lying in the peritoneal cavity.

The fetus was delivered and uterine rent was repaired after freshening the margins of previous scar.

Per operatively two units of packed cell transfusion was also given.

Postoperative period was uneventful. Patient was discharged with the advice to avoid further pregnancy for at least 2 years and to have cesarean section at 36 weeks of gestation during next pregnancy.

KEY POINTS

- Obstructed labor is the one when inspite of good uterine contractions, the progressive descent of presenting part is arrested due to mechanical obstruction.
- Obstructed labor is found to be directly or indirectly responsible for about half of maternal deaths affecting mainly primigravida and grand multipara. It can easily be prevented by various ways like provision of comprehensive antenatal care, routine use of partogram and early referral of high-risk cases.
- Management includes initial stabilization followed by emergency cesarean section in most of the cases.
- Postoperatively, bladder should be kept kept catheterized for two weeks in order to prevent formation of genitourinary fistulae.
- All cases of previous cesarean section should be booked for delivery in a place with facility for cesarean section.
- Fetal heart rate abnormalities such as variable and late decelerations are common and among most reliable early signs of imminent rupture.
- Immediate laparotomy is indicated in cases of uterine rupture after initial resuscitation.

REFERENCES

1. Adhikari S, Dasgupta M, Sanghamita M. Management of obstructed labour: a retrospective study. J Obstet Gynaecol Ind 2005;55:48-51.
2. Bartlett LA, Mawji S, Whitehead S, et al. Afghan Maternal Mortality Study Team. Where giving birth is a forecast of death: maternal mortality in four districts of Afghanistan, 1999-2002. Lancet 2005;365:864-70.
3. Dumont A, de Bernis L, Bouvier-Colle MH, Bréart G; MOMA study group. Cesarean section rate for maternal indication in sub-Saharan Africa: A systematic review. 2001 Lancet 20;358:1328-33.
4. Ebeigbe PN, Enabudoso E, Ande AB. Ruptured uterus in a Nigerian community: a study of sociodemographic and obstetric risk factors. Acta Obstet Gynecol Scand 2005;84:1172-4.

5. Rahman MH, Akhter HH, Khan Chowdhury ME, Yusuf HR, Rochat RW. Obstetric deaths in Bangladesh, 1996-1997. Int J Gynaecol Obstet 2002;77:161-9.

6. Tonks A. Pregnancy's toll in the developing world. BMJ 1994;308:353-4.

7. Hofmeyr GJ. Obstructed labor: using better technologies to reduce mortality. Int J Gynaecol Obstet 2004;85:S62-72.

8. Bullough C, Meda N, Makowiecka K, Ronsmans C, Achadi EL, Hussein J. Current strategies for the reduction of maternal mortality. BJOG 2005;112:1180-8.

9. Aboyeji AP, Ijaiya MD, Yahaya UR. Ruptured uterus: a study of 100 consecutive cases in Ilorin, Nigeria. J Obstet Gynaecol Res 2001;27:341-8.

10. Betrán AP, Wojdyla D, Posner SF, Gülmezoglu AM. National estimates for maternal mortality: an analysis based on the WHO systematic review of maternal mortality and morbidity. BMC Public Health 2005;5:131.

Chapter **14**

Atonic Postpartum Hemorrhage

Chandan Dubey

INTRODUCTION

Postpartum hemorrhage (PPH) is a leading cause of maternal morbidity and mortality worldwide. It results in the death of 140,000 women annually,[1] with the evidence of substandard care in most cases.

Primary PPH is defined as blood loss in excess of 500 mL after a vaginal delivery and over 1000 mL after a cesarean delivery within 24 hours of delivery.

More than 1000 mL loss is major PPH.

Other definitions used are, blood loss resulting in:
- A hematocrit drop of greater than 10 percent.
- Need for blood transfusion.
- Hemodynamic instability.[2]

Secondary PPH occurs after 24 hours and up to 12 weeks after delivery.

The incidence of PPH is between 4 to 6 percent when blood loss is estimated subjectively and increases to 10 percent when objective estimates are used.[3]

Out of the four causes of primary PPH, which include uterine atony, trauma to the genital tract, retained placental tissue and coagulopathy, the most common is uterine atony. It is estimated to cause over 80 percent cases of PPH.

Risk Factors for Atonic PPH

Atonic PPH often occurs in the absence of risk factors but should be anticipated in the presence of known risk factors which are:
- Labor related causes
- Induction/oxytocin
- Precipitate labor/prolonged labor
- Chorioamnionitis
- Uterine over distension
- Multiple pregnancy
- Polyhydramnios
- Fetal macrosomia
- Halogenated inhalational anesthetics

- Grandmultiparity
- Obesity

CASE SCENARIO-1

A 36-year-old lady had a normal vaginal delivery of her 5th baby. Baby weight was 4 kg. Active management of third stage was done by oxytocin infusion (10 units in 500 mL ringer lactate), controlled cord traction and uterine massage.
Her predelivery hemoglobin was 11 gm%
Pulse- 80/min and BP- 120/80 mmHg.
Resident conducting the delivery noticed a gush of bleeding after delivery of the placenta.
- **Placenta looked complete on examination**
- **Uterus appeared flabby on palpation.**
- **Estimated blood loss was 600 mL.**

> **Comment:** Grandmultiparity and fetal macrosomia are risk factors for atonic PPH in this lady. Labor room staff should be alert and ready for this emergency. The findings are suggestive of atonic PPH.

Differential Diagnosis

Traumatic PPH, retained placental tissue, coagulopathy.

Approach to Diagnosis of PPH

Diagnosis should prompt evaluation of:
- Clinical circumstances surrounding the delivery.
- General assessment of the patient.
- Evaluation of vital signs.
- Detailed physical examination.
   Clinical indicators of maternal hemodynamic status: These include maternal pulse, blood pressure (BP), peripheral pulses, cool extremities, hypothermia, pallor and change in sensorium.

Estimation of Blood Loss

- Visual estimation of blood loss tends to be imprecise, regardless of clinician's experience and is mostly underestimated by 30 to 50 percent.[4]
- The clinical status of the patient may lag behind the blood loss leading to underestimation of diagnosis in early stages. (Table 14.1)
- Significant changes may occur only when maternal blood loss is up to 30 percent.

Objective Assessment of Blood Loss

- Conical calibrated drapes for blood collection which have been shown to reduce error in estimation to less than 15 percent.[5]

Table 14.1: Benedetti's classification of hemorrhage[4]			
Hemorrhage class	Acute Blood Loss (mL)	Percent Loss	Symptoms
1	900	15	None, palpitations, dizziness, mild tachycardia
2	1200-1500	20-25	Mild tachycardia, tachypnea, diaphoresis, weakness
3	1800-2100	30-35	Overt hypotension, tachycardia (120-160/min), tachypnea, restlessness, pallor, oliguria, cold and clammy extremities
4	2400	40	Hypovolemic shock

- Weighing of blood soaked swabs, mops and drapes whose dry weight is known and is subtracted. (1gm= 1mL blood)
- Accounting for blood in placenta which is about 150 mL.[4]
- Replacing the amniotic fluid soaked drapes after delivery of baby to eliminate error due to the amniotic fluid.

MANAGEMENT

- Initial management should be prompt. Bimanual compression and massage by mobilizing and pushing the uterus cephalad should be the initial intervention in treating uterine atony. Uterine elevation stretches and compresses the uterine arteries and the myometrium is stimulated to contract.
- Bladder should be catheterized in case of persistent bleeding as a full bladder may impair contraction of uterus.

Management in this case:
- The attending nurse was asked to give 0.2 mg ergometrine intravenous (IV)
- Oxytocin infusion was increased to 20 units in 500 mL ringer lactate (RL)
- The bladder was catheterized.
- Bimanual compression of the uterus was done (Figure 14.1).
- Examination of the vulva, vagina and cervix did not reveal any trauma.
- Bleeding persisted.
- Pulse-120/min, BP- 96/70 mmHg

PPH PROTOCOL

Management of PPH involves simultaneous activation of five major steps:[6]
- Communication
- Resuscitation: A B C-**airway, breathing, circulation**
- Investigation
- Monitoring and Recording
- Treatment of the cause of hemorrhage

Communication

- *Call HELP:* Senior resident, junior resident, intern and nurse.
- Inform consultant on call, anesthetist, OT staff, and blood bank.

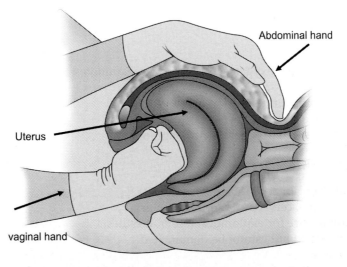

Figure 14.1: Bimanual compression and massage of uterus

Resuscitation

- Lay the patient flat; give oxygen by mask (10 to 15L/min).
- Check her pulse, BP and oxygen saturation (every 5 min/continuous monitor)
- Feel for uterine tone and rub up a contraction.
- Obtain IV access with two 16 gauge cannula.
- Urgent requisition for blood should be sent.
- Rapid infusion of crystalloids while waiting for blood to arrive, up to 2 liters, followed by 1.5 liters colloids.
- 20 to 40 U oxytocin in 500 mL RL is started and 0.2 mg ergometrine is given if not contraindicated (as in hypertension and cardiovascular disease).
- Check whether placenta is complete.
- Catheterize the bladder.
- Do per vaginal examination
- Remove clots
- Bimanual compression and massage
- Medical management—Move up along uterotonics
  - Oxytocin and ergometrine.
  - PGF 2α—Carboprost 250 mg intramuscular (IM)/intramyometrial every 15 min up to 8 doses)
  - PGE 1—Misoprostol 800-1000 µg per rectal(PR)
- In general, if there has been little/no response to methergine, do not give the second dose but move onto prostaglandin medications.
- Second medication is often hemabate, i.e. carboprost- 15-methyl PGF 2α one amp (0.25mg) IM or intra-myometrial but some centers prefer misoprostol (800-1,000 ug PR).
- If carboprost has had little/no effect move on to non-pharmacologic methods after the 2nd dose. If there is some effect, up to 8 doses may be given at 15 to 20 minute intervals.

Investigations

- Hemogram with platelet count
- Coagulation profile—prothrombin time (PT), activated partial thromboplastin time (APTT), fibrinogen.
- Bedside bleeding time (BT), clotting time (CT), clot retraction time (CRT).
- Blood for grouping and cross matching—at least 4 to 6 units packed red blood cells (PRBC) and fresh frozen plasma (FFP).
- Urea and serum electrolytes
- Arterial blood gases (ABG).

Monitoring and Recording

- Pulse, BP, respiratory rate, oxygen saturation every 5 minutes or continuously.
- Hourly urine output
- Fluid intake –amount and type
- Drugs – name, dosage and route
- CVP line may be considered if there is no coagulopathy.

Treatment of the Cause of Hemorrhage

If bleeding does not stop:
- Examine vulva, vagina, cervix and uterus for injury.
- Shift to operation theatre for exploration under anesthesia if:
  - Trauma is suspected but cannot be demarcated.
  - Bleeding persists

- – Vital signs deteriorate more than explained by manifest blood loss
- – Retained placenta
- For uterine atony, which is the cause in 85 percent cases, the following treatment options are available if uterotonic medications fail
  - – Balloon tamponade (level 1 evidence, grade A recommendation)[6]
  - – Laparotomy
    - - B-Lynch, Hayman's, square compression sutures
    - - Stepwise devascularization
    - - Internal iliac ligation
    - - Hysterectomy
  - – Pelvic arterial embolization

Balloon Tamponade

- According to a systematic review[7], balloon tamponade, B Lynch compression sutures, pelvic devascularization and pelvic arterial embolization have similar and comparable success rates of 84 to 90 percent in management of PPH.
- Several hydrostatic balloons have been used for this purpose like the Bakri balloon, Rusch balloon, Sengstaken-Blakemore esophageal catheter, Foley balloon and condom catheter.
- Balloon catheters are based on simple technology, easy to use and can be used as a *tamponade test*.
  - – *Positive test:* PPH stops after balloon inflation. No further intervention is needed as it is therapeutic.
  - – *Negative test:* PPH continues after balloon inflation indicating the need for laparotomy.
- The need for further intervention is known in a few minutes. These advantages make it the preferred first line treatment in atonic PPH.

Steps for Inserting Condom Balloon

- Foley's catheter is inserted in bladder prior to the procedure.
- Cervix and vagina are cleaned with betadine.
- Under aseptic precautions a size 16 Foley's catheter is inserted within the condom and tied near the mouth of the condom by a silk thread. Inner end of the catheter remains within the condom. Anterior and posterior lips of cervix are grasped with 2 sponge holding forceps
- Then the condom is introduced within the uterine cavity
- Foley bulb is inflated with 30 mL saline
- Outer end of the catheter is connected with a saline set, the saline is kept 60 to 70 cm above the abdomen and the condom is inflated.
- Between 200 to 500 mL saline is required to inflate the balloon
- The balloon is filled till it appears at cervix, bleeding is reduced considerably and further inflation stops
- Maximum inflation volume is up to 1000 cc.
- Outer end of the catheter is folded and tied with thread
- A vaginal pack is inserted to keep the balloon in place
- Can be kept *in-situ* for up to 48 hrs
- Gradual deflation is done

Further management in this case: The above patient continued to bleed despite bimanual compression and massage, oxytocin infusion, ergometrine, 2 doses of carboprost and misoprostol 1000 µg per rectal.
- Trauma was ruled out by thorough examination.
- Decision for balloon tamponade was taken and condom catheter was inserted.
- PPH was controlled and no further treatment was needed.

Contd...

Contd...

> **Postoperative management of this patient:**
> - Patient was shifted to postoperative ward where oxytocin infusion was given for 12 hours and broad spectrum intravenous antibiotics were given for 24 hours.
> - Her vital signs, fundal height, bleeding per vaginum and urine output were monitored till removal of the balloon 24 hours later.
> - This was done by gradual deflation with a needle inserted in the Foley tube. This prevents sudden decompression which may result in hemorrhage. It also allows time for other measures to be taken if bleeding resumes on deflation.

Blood Transfusion

- Decision for blood transfusion is based on the following factors:
  - Estimated blood loss
  - Continuing bleeding
  - Clinical condition (anemia, pre-eclampsia)
  - Response to crystalloid/colloid
  - Last recorded hemoglobin
- FFP should be started after 2 units PRBCs
- PRBC: FFP: Platelets are given in the ratio 6:4:1/ 4:4:1
- Cryoprecipitate is given if fibrinogen level is <100 mg/dL
- Rh negative uncrossmatched blood can be given in situations where delay is not acceptable.

Aim of Transfusion is to Achieve

- Hemoglobin >8g/dl
- Platelet count >75 x 10^9/l
- Prothrombin time <1.5 x mean control
- Activated prothrombin time <1.5 x mean control
- Fibrinogen >1.0 g/l.

Recombinant Activated Factor VII

- Dangerous but potentially lifesaving.
- Can have dramatic effects on DIC; less clear effects on mortality; off-label use appears to have higher risk of thrombosis.
- There are no randomized controlled trials and the reported small series are often biased; optimal dosing for obstetrical patients is not known.
- Patient must have received clotting factors (FFP, cryoprecipitate and platelets) prior to its use.
- Usually used after 10 to 12 units of packed red blood cell transfusion and still not enough. It should not to be used at the 4 to 6 unit stage.
- It does not stop surgical bleeding. It is used for DIC and generalized oozing.

CASE SCENARIO-2

A primigravida had a cesarean section done for fetal distress. There was excessive bleeding after delivery of the placenta. Placenta was complete.
Oxytocin infusion, ergometrine and carboprost failed to control the bleeding.
Uterus was atonic. B-Lynch brace suture was applied and bleeding was controlled.

> **Comment:** Uterine compression sutures like the B-Lynch brace suture are ideal for controlling atonic hemorrhage during cesarean section. They are quick, easy, effective and preferred as a first line management during cesarean in cases where fertility preservation is an issue.

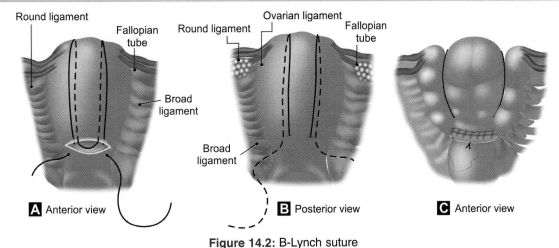

Figure 14.2: B-Lynch suture

Steps of B-Lynch Suture Application (Figure 14.2)

- To check potential efficacy of B-Lynch suture, the surgeon applies pressure to the exteriorized uterus with one hand posterior and the other anterior just below the inferiorly displaced bladder. If bleeding is controlled, then B-Lynch suture is likely to be effective
- The first suture is placed 3 cm below the transverse cesarean incision on the right taking care to dissect the bladder well away prior to this step
- The suture is then passed through the uterine cavity to a point 3 cm above the incision and about 4 cm from the lateral border of the uterus, at which point it is passed through the anterior uterine wall.
- The suture is then carried vertically over the fundus of the uterus, while the assistant maintains compression of the uterus.
- The suture is then passed through the posterior uterine wall at the level of cesarean incision and uterosacral ligament.
- The suture inside the cavity is carried horizontally to the corresponding position on the left side of the uterus and passed back through the posterior uterine wall on the left.
- The suture which is now outside the uterine cavity posteriorly is carried over the fundus and down the left side of the uterus anteriorly, again approximately 4 cm from the lateral side of the uterus. The suture is then passed through the uterine wall into the cavity at a point symmetrical to that previously done on the opposite side
- Next the suture is passed through the uterine wall below the cesarean incision at a point corresponding to the initial entry point of the opposite side.
- The two ends of the suture are tied after closing the uterine incision.
- At this time the assistant should maintain compression on the uterus so that the suture places maximum possible compression on the uterus.

B-Lynch suture requires a hysterotomy incision hence many modifications have been made which can be placed after a vaginal delivery, like horizontal or vertical square compression sutures and Hayman suture.

Hayman Suture

Involves placement of 4 sutures, 2 on each side at approximately the same place as B-Lynch suture. The suture is passed through the entire thickness of the uterus from anterior to posterior at a point where a lower segment transverse incision would have been made. Four such sutures are passed and tied over the fundus while compression is maintained by the assistant.

Stepwise Uterine Devascularization

AbdRabbo[8] first described uterine devascularization for control of intractable PPH.
- The first 2 steps involve ligation of ascending branch of uterine artery at the level of hysterotomy incision. The stitch is taken with number 1 chromic catgut or vicryl from anterior to posterior through an avascular area of the broad ligament and brought anteriorly through the myometrium taking 2 cm thickness of the myometrium without entering the cavity and then tied.
- Step 3 and 4 involve ligation of uterine artery lower down bilaterally, 3 to 5 cm below the lower segment, after mobilization and dissection of bladder well down, similar to the manner described above.
- Steps 5 and 6 involve ligation of utero-ovarian anastamosis[9] at the cornu bilaterally.

Hypogastric Artery Ligation

Hypogastric artery ligation bilaterally has been the mainstay of controlling intractable pelvic hemorrhage for a long time though a subsequent hysterectomy is required in around 40 percent cases. Even then the decreased pelvic vascularity makes the hysterectomy easier.
- It involves identification of common iliac artery and its bifurcation. The posterior peritoneum is opened just distal to this point identifying the ureter and retracting it in the medial fold. The internal iliac (hypogastric) artery and vein and external iliac artery and vein are identified.
- The hypogastric artery is isolated by blunt dissection and a right angled clamp is passed from lateral to medial side preventing injury to the underlying vein. An absorbable suture is passed under the artery 3 cm distal to the bifurcation to avoid posterior division of hypogastric artery and it is tied.
- The same procedure is carried out on the opposite side.
- Dorsalis pedis pulse is checked on both sides to rule out accidental ligation of external iliac artery.

Peripartum Hysterectomy

Hysterectomy may be required in some patients to control massive PPH even if the woman desires to retain fertility. In patients, where fertility is not an issue the obstetrician may resort to hysterectomy sooner in the course of events if the situation demands. This may be required to prevent co morbidities associated with massive hemorrhage like DIC, hypoxia, hypothermia, acidosis, shock and sometimes mortality.
- A supracervical hysterectomy may be appropriate in most cases as it is quicker, unless the cervical region is involved in hemorrhage as in placenta previa or morbid adherent placenta.
- The steps are similar to a routine hysterectomy with a few important points to be kept in mind.
- The pedicles are increased in size due to peripartum tissue edema and hypertrophy and care should be taken not to include too much tissue in the clamp. The pedicles may be taken in 2 portions.
- The pedicles should be doubly clamped and doubly ligated ensuring hemostasis.

Pelvic Arterial Embolization

Transcatheter arterial embolization is an effective second line therapeutic option if medical management fails. It has the advantage of being minimally invasive, safe and effective technique for rapid management of severe PPH with preservation of uterus. It has become a standard of care even though its effects on future fertility remain controversial.

KEY POINTS
- Uterine atony is responsible for upto 85 percent cases of primary PPH.
- Visual assessment of blood loss is imprecise and results in underestimation by 30 percent to 50 percent.Objective assessment can reduce this error to 15 percent.
- Formal protocols for managing PPH should be in place in all labor units.

- Incorrect estimation of blood loss may delay diagnosis and also result in inadequate resuscitation with fluids and blood, increasing the risk of morbidity and mortality.
- Balloon tamponade is a safe, minimally invasive, quick and effective option if medical management of atonic PPH fails. It is an appropriate first line treatment before resorting to more invasive procedures like compression sutures, devascularization or hysterectomy, for which a laparotomy will be needed.
- Decision for hysterectomy should be taken without delay if necessary in order to avert severe morbidity and mortality.

References

1. AbouZahr C. Global burden of maternal death and disability. Br Med Bull 2003;67:1-11.
2. ACOG Practice Bulletin. Clinical management guidelines for obstetrician-gynecologists number 76, October 2006: Postpartum hemorrhage. Obstet Gynecol 2006;108:1039-47.
3. Carroli G, Cuesta C, Abalos E, et al. Epidemiology of postpartum haemorrhage: a systematic review. Best Pract Res Clin Obstet Gynaecol 2008;22:999-1012.
4. B-Lynch C. A Textbook of Post Partum Hemorrhage: A Comprehensive Guide to Evaluation, Management, and Surgical Intervention. New Delhi: Jaypee Brothers Medical Publishers; 2006.
5. Toledo P, McCarthy RJ, Hewlett BJ, et al. The accuracy of blood loss estimation after simulated vaginal delivery. Anesth Analg 2007;105:1736-40.
6. Royal College of Obstetricians and Gynecologists. Prevention and Management of Post partum Hemorrhage. Green-top Guideline No. 52, May 2009, minor revisions November 2009.
7. Doumouchtsis SK, Papageorghiou AT, Arulkumaran S. Systematic review of conservative management of postpartum hemorrhage: what to do when medical management fails. Obstet Gynecol Surv 2007;62:540-7.
8. AbdRabbo SA. Step wise uterine devascularization: a novel technique for management of uncontrollable postpartum hemorrhage with preservation of the uterus. Am J Obstet Gynecol 1994;171:694-700.
9. Sentilhes L, Trichot C, Resch B, et al. Fertility and pregnancy outcomes following uterine devascularization for severe postpartum hemorrhage. Hum Reprod 2008;23:1087-92.

Chapter 15

Morbidly Adherent Placenta and Retained Placenta

Usha Manaktala, Avantika Gupta

INTRODUCTION

It is well known that placenta accreta complicates 5 percent of pregnancies with placenta previa. The incidence of morbidly adherent placenta is rising as the frequency of cesarean sections increases. This condition is also seen in the context of previous myomectomies and previous uterine curettage or evacuations associated with infection. Clark et al observed an increased incidence of placenta previa from 0.26 percent in women with a normal uterus to 0.65 percent after 1 and up to 10 percent after 4 or more cesarean sections.[1]

Adherent Placenta may be of Three Types

- Placenta accreta—Chorionic villi on the myometrial surface,
- Placenta increta—Villus infiltration into myometrium, and
- Placenta percreta—Villus infiltration through entire myometrium to breach the serosa and beyond.

Placenta percreta is associated with a maternal mortality as high as 10 percent and significant maternal morbidity, including massive hemorrhage, disseminated intravascular coagulation, hysterectomy, bladder and ureteric trauma, fistula formation, postoperative sepsis, acute respiratory distress syndrome and acute tubular necrosis.[2]

There is therefore need for reliable antenatal diagnosis, since such a condition when encountered unexpectedly at delivery will invariably lead to massive blood loss and multiple complications. Management aims to ensure a safe delivery of the fetus, along with measures for prevention and effective management of postpartum hemorrhage (PPH).

Risk Factors for Placenta Accreta

- Placenta previa
- Previous uterine surgery
- Prior cesarean section (Table 15.1)
- Prior myomectomy
- Asherman's syndrome
- Submucosal fibroid
- Age > 35 years
- Multiparity > 6 pregnancies

Table 15.1: Risk of placenta accreta in women with previous cesarean section[3]	
No. of prior CS	*Risk of placenta accreta (%)*
0	3.3
1	11
2	40
3	61
4+	67

- Endometrial ablation
- Manual removal of placenta
- Puerperal sepsis

CASE SCENARIO-1

A 29-year-old G3P1L1A1 with previous lower segment cesarean section (LSCS) 2 years back and 1 previous evacuation done for missed abortion was referred to our department at 35 weeks of gestation for placenta previa. At 32 weeks, a routine growth scan revealed anterior placenta covering the os, with a strong suggestion of placenta accreta due to thinning of myometrium overlying the placenta. There was no history of antepartum hemorrhage.

Comments: Diagnosis of placenta accreta must be considered since there is placenta previa along with scarred uterus and a history of evacuation.

RADIOLOGICAL FINDINGS IN PLACENTA ACCRETA[4]

Various radiological techniques have been used for the diagnosis of placenta accreta (Table 15.2).

Greyscale Ultrasonography (USG)

- Obliteration of the clear space, defined as the obliteration of any part of the echolucent area located between the uterus and the placenta.
- Visualization of placental lacunae, defined as multiple linear, irregular vascular spaces within the placenta (Swiss-cheese appearance).
- Interruption of the posterior bladder wall-uterine intersurfaces such that the usual continuous echolucent line appears instead as a series of dashes.
- Thinning of myometrium overlying the placenta.

Color Doppler

- Vascular lakes with turbulent flow (peak systolic velocity >15 cm/sec)
- Diffuse or focal lacunar flow
- Hypervascularity of serosa-bladder interface
- Markedly dilated vessels over peripheral subplacental zone

Table 15.2: Diagnostic performance of different radiological modalities to diagnose placenta accreta[4,5]			
	Sensitivity	*Specificity*	*PPV*
Grey scale USG	95%	76%	82%
Color Doppler	92%	68%	76%
3D power Doppler	100%	85%	88%
MRI	88%	100%	

3D Power Doppler

- Numerous coherent vessels involving the whole uterine serosa-bladder junction
- Hypervascularity
- Inseparable cotyledonal and intervillous circulation, chaotic branching, detour vessels

Magnetic Resonance Imaging (MRI)

- Uterine bulging
- Heterogenous signal intensity within the placenta
- Dark intraplacental bands on T2 weighted imaging

Transvaginal scan is better than transabdominal scan to visualize lower uterine segment. The visualization of placental lacunae had the highest sensitivity (78.6%), followed by obliteration of clear space (57%) and the interruption of the posterior bladder-uterine wall intersurface (21.4%).[6] The degree of invasion as visualized on MRI, will alter the treatment plan. MRI is a better modality when the placenta is located posteriorly or at the fundus or when the patient is very obese.

MANAGEMENT OF PLACENTA ACCRETA AND PERCRETA (FIGURE 15.1)

Antenatal Management

- Patient should be managed as an in-patient.
- Prevention and correction of anemia
- Risk of preterm delivery should be explained to the patient.
- Corticosteroid cover is given for fetal lung maturity

Perioperative Planning

- Timing of cesarean: 36 to 37 weeks[4]
- Book the elective cesarean section at appropriate gestation to avoid labor and emergency cesarean
- Counsel the woman and her family about:
  - The suspected diagnosis
  - Need for operative delivery
  - Massive hemorrhage and morbidity associated with it
  - Need for multiple blood transfusions
  - Possibility of interventional radiological procedures
  - Postoperative morbidity
  - Need for ICU care
  - Possible hysterectomy
  - Pros and cons of conservative management if fertility is to be preserved

Multidisciplinary Team

Royal College of Obstetricians and Gynaecologists (RCOG) recommends a multidisciplinary team approach for the management of placenta accreta.[4] The team should consist of:

- Consultant obstetrician – to perform the procedure.
- Consultant anesthetist should directly attend the case. Anesthetic technique needs to be carefully chosen. There is insufficient evidence to support one technique over other.
- Interventional radiologist – Uterine artery embolization through balloon catheter may be needed to control massive hemorrhage. Prophylactic transfemoral placement of balloon in internal iliac arteries for the prevention of massive hemorrhage requires further evaluation.
- Urologist – If bladder invasion is suspected, prior cystoscopy and placement of ureteric stents helps to identify the ureters during surgery.
- Hematologist – Massive blood transfusion is anticipated. Adequate blood and blood products must be cross matched. Where available, cell salvage should be considered.
- Neonatologist should be informed.

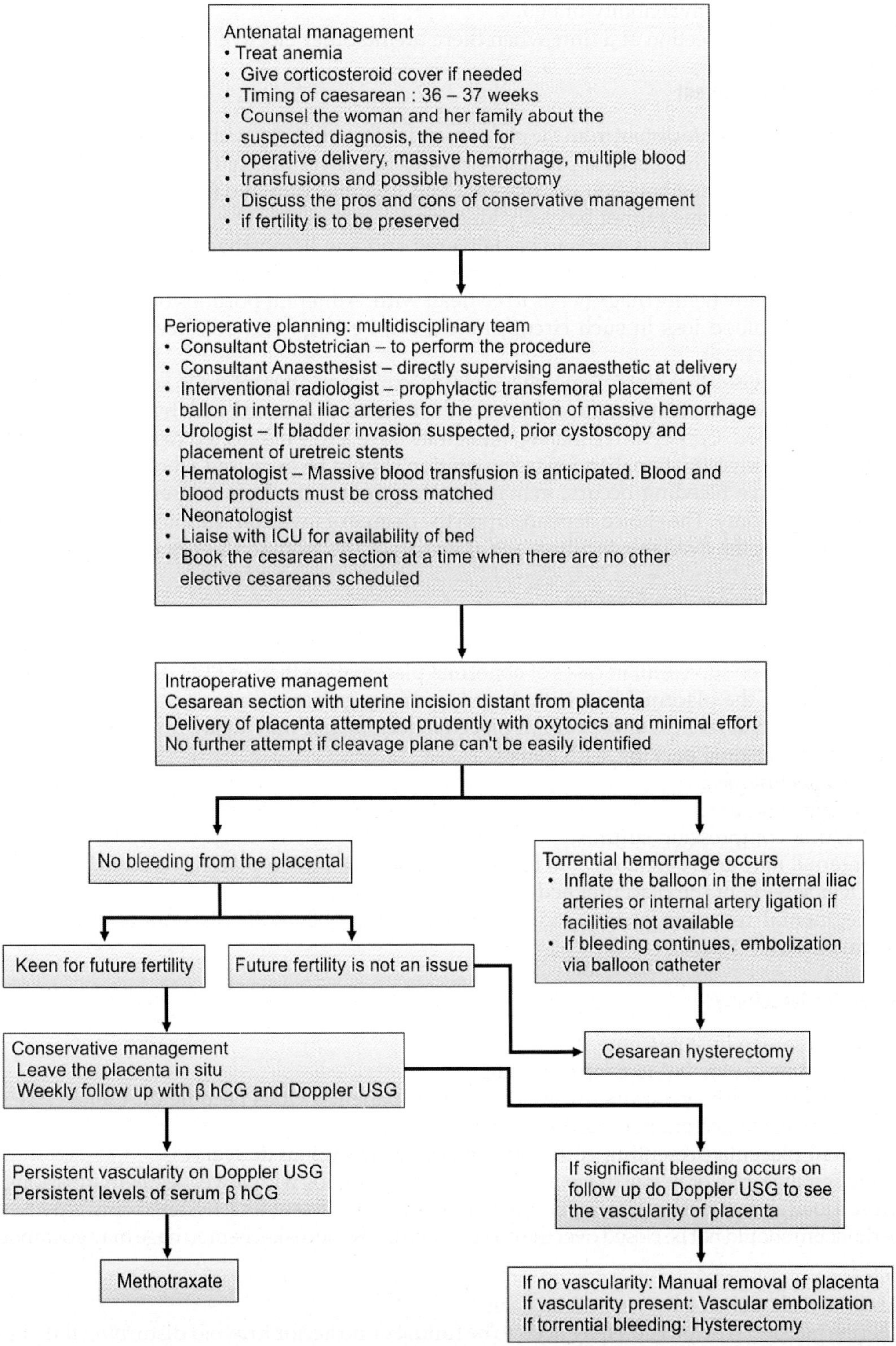

Antenatal management
- Treat anemia
- Give corticosteroid cover if needed
- Timing of caesarean : 36 – 37 weeks
- Counsel the woman and her family about the
- suspected diagnosis, the need for
- operative delivery, massive hemorrhage, multiple blood
- transfusions and possible hysterectomy
- Discuss the pros and cons of conservative management
- if fertility is to be preserved

Perioperative planning: multidisciplinary team
- Consultant Obstetrician – to perform the procedure
- Consultant Anaesthesist – directly supervising anaesthetic at delivery
- Interventional radiologist – prophylactic transfemoral placement of balloon in internal iliac arteries for the prevention of massive hemorrhage
- Urologist – If bladder invasion suspected, prior cystoscopy and placement of uretreic stents
- Hematologist – Massive blood transfusion is anticipated. Blood and blood products must be cross matched
- Neonatologist
- Liaise with ICU for availability of bed
- Book the cesarean section at a time when there are no other elective cesareans scheduled

Intraoperative management
Cesarean section with uterine incision distant from placenta
Delivery of placenta attempted prudently with oxytocics and minimal effort
No further attempt if cleavage plane can't be easily identified

No bleeding from the placental

Torrential hemorrhage occurs
- Inflate the balloon in the internal iliac arteries or internal artery ligation if facilities not available
- If bleeding continues, embolization via balloon catheter

Keen for future fertility

Future fertility is not an issue

Conservative management
Leave the placenta in situ
Weekly follow up with β hCG and Doppler USG

Cesarean hysterectomy

Persistent vascularity on Doppler USG
Persistent levels of serum β hCG

If significant bleeding occurs on follow up do Doppler USG to see the vascularity of placenta

Methotraxate

If no vascularity: Manual removal of placenta
If vascularity present: Vascular embolization
If torrential bleeding: Hysterectomy

Figure 15.1: Management of placenta accreta

- Nurse in charge should be informed to arrange for the operation theatre.
- Liaise with ICU for availability of bed.
- Book the cesarean section at a time when there are no other elective cesareans scheduled.

Intraoperative Management

- Open the uterus at a site distant from the placenta and deliver the baby without disturbing the placenta
- Attempt to deliver the placenta prudently (under the cover of oxytocics) with minimal effort only if there is a plane between the placenta and myometrium. No further attempt should be made if cleavage plane cannot be easily identified.
- If the placenta separates, it needs to be delivered and any hemorrhage that occurs needs to be dealt in the normal way. If placenta separates partially, the separated portion(s) need to be delivered and any hemorrhage needs to be dealt with. Adherent portions of placenta can be left in place, but blood loss in such circumstances can be large and massive hemorrhage needs timely management.
- The ACOG advises that since hemorrhage may occur when attempting to separate the placenta, it may be prudent to complete the delivery of the infant and proceed with hysterectomy with the placenta attached. Conservative management may have a role in selected cases but its use should be considered investigational and extreme caution should be exercised when it is attempted.[7]

If intraoperative bleeding occurs, management options vary from conservative approach to obstetric hysterectomy. The choice depends upon the degree of invasion, various clinical parameters, surgical expertise, the available facilities and the wish of the woman to preserve fertility.

Management of Intraoperative Bleeding

- Uterine artery embolization: Successful in 72 percent cases of placenta accreta.[8] Arterial embolization is less likely to be successful in cases of abnormal placentation than in PPH due to other causes.
- Hemostasis of the placental bed with Argon beam coagulator.
- Balloon tamponade: Less successful in placenta accreta and may delay timely hysterectomy.
- Uterine and vaginal packing with gauze.
- Surgical techniques:
  - B- Lynch suture.
  - Vertical compression sutures.
  - Internal iliac artery ligation – 40 to 60 percent failure rate in placenta accreta.[9]
  - Over sewing of the placental bed
  - Segmental resection of invaded myometrium together with placenta and suturing the myometrial defect.

Cesarean Hysterectomy

Proceed to cesarean hysterectomy if:
- The above measures fail to control bleeding.
- Torrential hemorrhage occurs during cesarean or patient's vitals become unstable.
- Known placenta accreta managed emergently.
- Adherent placenta presenting at the time of cesarean/vaginal delivery.

There is a high-risk of hemorrhage in subtotal hysterectomies with lower segment invasions, and therefore a total abdominal hysterectomy should be performed. If a subtotal hysterectomy is performed, the peritoneum should not be closed over the cervical stump, as concealed hemorrhage may go unnoticed.

Procedure
- Abdomen is opened by a vertical incision
- Uterine incision: The incision may need to be fundal or posterior to avoid disturbing the placenta during delivery of baby.
- The placenta is not removed and the umbilical cord is tied close to the placenta and uterus is closed in single layer.

- If placenta percreta/increta involves important vascular sites, the decision is taken for occlusion of the vascular supply by bilateral internal iliac artery ligation/ selective arterial embolization/ balloon occlusive devices.
- Blood vessels should be ligated individually as blood vessels in placenta percreta lack muscular media, are friable and do not contract well.
- Pedicles should be taken preferably at some distance from highly vascular placenta which has replaced the myometrium to prevent tearing of friable tissue.
- There should not be any traction applied to the lower uterine segment as it may lead to inadvertent tearing of peritoneum with heavy bleeding.
- If bladder is involved, intentional cystostomy is done. Affected region is resected with uterus en bloc. Bladder is closed with delayed absorbable suture. Resection and reimplantation of the ureters may also be required.

Uterine Conservation: Leaving the Placenta

If there is no bleeding and preoperative diagnosis is well confirmed, conservative management may be followed. Although it reduces the risk of hysterectomy from 85 percent to 15 percent,[10] there are certain risks associated with conservative management. There is no consensus as to whether the placenta should be removed in the postpartum period or left to resorb or to be expelled spontaneously. Interval removal of placenta can be associated with massive hemorrhage which may require laparotomy and even hysterectomy.

Prerequisites
- Only planned elective cases of placenta accreta.
- Preservation of fertility is of prime importance.
- There is no predisposing factor for sepsis.
- Minimal intraoperative blood loss.
- Patient is willing for strict follow-up which may extend up to months.

Key components
- Cut the cord at the placental insertion and leave the placenta *in situ*.
- Close the uterine incision.
- Oxytocics: 3 hours to 3 days.[10]
- Prophylactic broad spectrum antibiotics for 10 to 14 days.[10]
- Weekly follow up:
  - Clinical: Look for any hemorrhage, abdominal pain and clinical signs of any infection
  - Laboratory: Total leukocyte counts, CRP, high vaginal swab if vaginal discharge
  - Serum β hCG
  - USG to see placental size and vascularity

Further Management based on Doppler USG Findings
- *If persistent vascularity is present on Doppler USG and levels of serum β hCG are* persistently high, methotraxate can be tried.
  Role of Methotraxate: Controversial
  - It affects proliferating tissue and therefore a significant effect on degenerative tissue would seem unlikely
  - Exposes woman to potential side effects (gastrointestinal side effects, hepatic toxicity, myelosuppression, renal failure) and it also precludes breastfeeding.
  - Resolution is usually complete by 3 to 4 months regardless of methotrexate use.[11]
  - Monitoring with β hCG doesn't correlate with the volume of remaining tissue as β hCG takes longer to return to normal even when remaining trophoblast is usually reabsorbed
  Dose of methotraxate (based on case reports):
  - 6 doses of 50 mg intravenous (IV)-slow administration, alternating with 6 mg folinic acid OR
  - 1 mg/kg/week intramuscular (IM) methotraxate for 6 weeks [12]

Monitoring is then done by weekly measurement of serum β hCG and Doppler USG. If still there is persistent vascularity, vascular embolization is required.

- *If there is no vascularity on Doppler USG, manual removal of placenta may be tried.* Hemorrhage may occur during manual removal which may require vascular embolization or even hysterectomy.
- *Anytime during follow-up, if there is significant bleeding, manual removal of placenta after vascular embolization is attempted. And if bleeding is torrential, hysterectomy needs to be performed.*

RETAINED PLACENTA

The WHO states that if the placenta is not expelled within 30 minutes after delivery of the baby, the woman should be diagnosed as having retained placenta. In the absence of hemorrhage, the woman should be observed for a further 30 minutes following the initial 30 minutes, before manual removal of the placenta is attempted.[13] It affects 0.6 to 3.3 percent of normal deliveries. Following a retained placenta in one pregnancy, there is a recurrence rate of 6.25 percent.[14]

Some placentas are simply trapped behind a closed cervix (trapped placenta), some are adherent to the uterine wall but easily separated manually (retained placenta) while others are pathologically invading the myometrium (placenta accreta) (Table 15.3).

Following delivery of the baby, the retroplacental myometrium is initially relaxed. It is only when it contracts that the placenta shears away from the placental bed and is detached and expelled. Retained placenta occurs when the retroplacental myometrium fails to contract. An ultrasound examination will reveal whether the placenta is detached or not.

Risk Factors for Retained Placenta

- Gestational age < 36 weeks
- Pre-eclampsia
- Augmented labor
- High-pregnancy number
- Maternal age > 30 years
- Previous abortion

CASE SCENARIO-2

A 28-year-old P3L3 had premature rupture of membranes at 35 weeks. Labor was augmented after 24 hours and she had a vaginal delivery. After 30 minutes of delivery no signs of placental separation were observed. She was given 10 U oxytocin IM immediately after the delivery of the baby. The fundal height was not reduced but uterus was contracted and there was no postpartum hemorrhage. On vaginal examination, cervix was fully dilated and placental edge was not felt.

Table 15.3: Defferences between a trapped placenta and adherent/retained placenta		
	Trapped placenta	*Adherent/retained placenta*
Per abdomen	Fundus feel small and well contracted	Fundal height will not get reduced
Per vaginum	Edge of the placenta felt through tight cervical os	No placental edge is felt
USG	Myometrium is thickened all around the uterus and a clear demarcation is seen between the myometrium and the placenta	Myometrium is thickened in all areas except where the placenta is attached where it will be very thin or even invisible
Management	Glyceryl trinitrate 50 to 500 µg IV given as tocolysis to relax the os and release the placenta by controlled cord traction	Umbilical oxytocin injection Manual removal of placenta

Comment: This patient has risk factors for retained placenta—Preterm labor and augmentation of labor. Examination reveals that the fundal height is not reduced and placental edge is not felt on per vaginum examination.

Diagnosis

Retained placenta

MANAGEMENT OF RETAINED PLACENTA (FIGURE 15.2)

1. WHO states that if placenta is not expelled spontaneously within 30 minutes after delivery of the baby, the woman should be diagnosed as having retained placenta. However, the delay to diagnose this condition is left to the judgement of clinician, as there is no evidence for or against this definition.
2. In absence of hemorrhage, woman should be observed for a further 30 minutes following the initial 30 minutes, as 40 percent of retained placentae will be delivered spontaneously during this time with an average blood loss of 300 mL.[15]
   During this time, **oxytocics along with controlled cord traction** are tried.
   Choice of oxytocic [13]
   - *Oxytocin:* Oxytocin lasts in the circulation for only 10 minutes. Continuous infusion of 5 to 10 IU/hr increases the overall tone of the myometrium and stimulates strong phasic contractions.
   - *Ergometrine:* Since it produces a long continuous contraction for up to 90 minutes, it is not preferred. Prophylactic use of IV ergometrine is associated with increased rate of retained placenta as a result of myometrial spasm distal to fundally placed placenta.
   - *Prostaglandin analogues:* Produce increase in both background tone and contraction strength for up to 90 minutes. Therefore, their use is also not recommended.

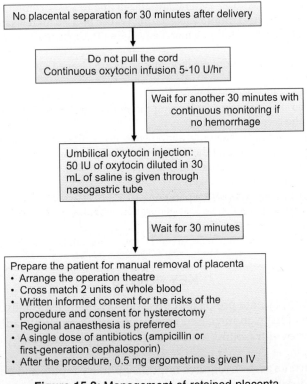

Figure 15.2: Management of retained placenta

3. Following this, if placenta is still not separated, an intraumbilical injection of oxytocin is attempted via nasogastric tube using **"Pipingas technique"**[16]
   - Cord is cut at the end to achieve a clean end for insertion of nasogastric tube
   - A nasogastric tube of size 10 is then passed along the vein until resistance is felt and *then withdrawn by 5 cm to allow for any divisions of the vein prior to its insertion* into the placenta
   - Push 50 IU oxytocin in 30 mL saline through nasogastric tube. (Trials with higher dose of oxytocin, i.e 100 IU found higher success rates, but is not yet recommended).

   Alternatively, if no nasogastric tube is available, 30 mL oxytocin is injected directly into the cord and then the cord should be massaged to encourage the drug up the cord into the placental bed. According to Cochrane review, umbilical vein injection of saline solution plus oxytocin appears to be effective in the management of retained placenta and reduces the need for manual removal of placenta by over 75 percent.[17]

4. If this is also unsuccessful after 30 minutes, **manual removal of placenta** is done (see Box).
5. If placenta is found to be adherent to the uterus at a small area after the procedure:[18]
   - Strong oxytocics, e.g. 0.5 mg ergometrine should be used to cause contraction strong enough to obstruct the blood flow through the radial arteries to the placental fragments
   - Prophylactic broad spectrum antibiotics are given to prevent endometritis
   - Closely observe for 48 hours for secondary hemorrhage
   - No sharp curettage should be tried.
6. If further hemorrhage occurs, then further gentle attempts at uterine evacuation may be necessary or even hysterectomy may be required.

Manual Removal of Placenta

- Arrange the operation theatre for manual removal of placenta.
- Cross match 2 units of whole blood as there is a risk of hemorrhage during the procedure.
- Written informed consent should be taken about the failure of the procedure, the risk of hemorrhage, blood transfusion, perforation, endometritis and the consent for hysterectomy in case of failure of the procedure or massive uncontrolled hemorrhage.
- Regional anesthesia is preferred over general anesthesia due to lesser complications.
- If the uterus is contracted, glyceryl trinitrate (50-500 mg IV) can be used for relaxation if regional anesthesia is used. Isoflurane/halothane is used in general anesthesia to cause uterine relaxation.
- *Procedure:*[18]
  - The woman is placed in lithotomy position and parts are cleaned and draped.
  - Bladder is catheterized.
  - Surgeon should wear long sterile gloves.
  - One hand is placed inside the vagina forming the fingers into a cone and if the cervix is closed, try to forcibly dilate the cervix.
  - The other hand is placed on the maternal abdomen to steady the uterus and provide counter pressure.
  - Follow the umbilical cord through the vagina up to its insertion into the placenta. Once the rough velvety interface between the uterus and placenta is identified, the plane is gently dissected using side-to-side slicing motion of the fingers.
  - Remove the placenta after complete separation.
- A single dose of antibiotics (ampicillin or first-generation cephalosporin) should be offered after manual removal of the placenta.[13]
- After the procedure, 0.5 mg ergometrine is given IV for strong uterine contraction.

KEY POINTS

- Women with anterior placenta previa and previous cesarean, especially with a short cesarean to conception interval have an increased chance of having morbidly adherent placenta.
- Antenatal diagnosis by ultrasound with color flow Doppler is usually sufficient to make the diagnosis.
- Management of placenta accreta requires multidisciplinary inputs and perioperative measures for elective planned delivery.

- Cesarean hysterectomy is the safest option for the patient with placenta accreta.
- Conservative management for adherent placenta should be reserved for the patients in whom antenatal diagnosis of placenta accreta has been made, future fertility is desired and there are facilities for strict follow-up.
- For retained placenta, injection of 50 IU oxytocin in 30 mL saline down the umbilical cord by Piping as technique is the first line option.
- If this is unsuccessful after 30 minutes, manual removal should be carried out under antibiotic cover.

REFERENCES

1. Clark SL, Koonings RP, Phelan JP. Placenta previa/and prior cesarean section. Obstet Gynecol 1985;66:89-92.
2. Bennett MJ, Sen RC. Conservative management of placenta previa percreta: report of two cases and discussion of current management options. Aust N Z Obstet Gynaecol 2003;43:249-51.
3. Silver RM, Landon MB, Rouse DJ, et al; National Institute of Child Health and Human Development Maternal-Fetal Medicine Units Network. Maternal morbidity associated with multiple repeat cesarean deliveries. Obstet Gynecol 2006;107:1226-32.
4. Placenta praevia, and vas praevia: diagnosis and management. Greentop guideline no. 27. Available at http://www.rcog.org.uk/files/rcog-corp/GTG27PlacentaPraeviaJanuary2011.pdf
5. Warshak CR, Eskander R, Hull AD, et al. Accuracy of ultrasonography and magnetic resonance imaging in the diagnosis of placenta. Obstet Gynecol 2006;108:573-81.
6. Comstock CH, Love JJ Jr, Bronsteen RA, et al. Sonographic detection of placenta in the second and third trimesters of pregnancy. Am J Obstet Gynecol 2004;190:1135-40.
7. American College of Obstetricians and Gynaecologists: Placenta. ACOG Committee Opinion No. 206. Washington, American College of Obstetricians and Gynecologists, 2002.
8. Descargues G, Douvrin F, Degré S, Lemoine JP, Marpeau L, Clavier E. Abnormal placentation and selective embolization of the uterine arteries. Eur J Obstet Gynecol Reprod Biol 2001;99:47-52.
9. Evans S, McShane P. The efficacy of internal iliac artery ligation in obstetric hemorrhage. Surg Gynecol Obstet 1985;160:250-3.
10. Doumouchtsis SK, Arulkumaran S. The morbidly adherent placenta: an overview of management options. Acta Obstet Gynecol Scand 2010;89:1126-33.
11. Armstrong C, Harding S, Dickinson J. Clinical aspects and conservative management of placenta. The Obstetrician & Gynaecologist 2004;6:132-37.
12. Panoskaltsis TA, Ascarelli A, de Souza N, Sims CD, Edmonds KD. Placenta increta: evaluation of radiological investigations and therapeutic options of conservative management. BJOG 2000;107:802-6.
13. Managing complications in pregnancy and childbirth: a guide for midwives and doctors. Geneva, World Health Organization, 2007.
14. Andrews DW. The retained placenta. In: Studd J (Ed). Progress in Obstetrics and Gynaecology. New Delhi: Churchill Livingstone 2005;16:103-22.
15. Carroli G, Belizan JM, Grant A, Gonzalez L, Campodonico L, Bergel E. Intraumbilical vein injection and retained placenta: evidence from a collaborative large randomised controlled trial. Grupo Argentino de Estudio de Placenta Retenida. Br J Obstet Gynaecol 1998;105:179-85.
16. Pipingas A, Hofmeyer GJ, Sesel KR. Umbilical vessel oxytocin administration for retained placenta: *in vitro* study of various infusion techniques. Am J Obstet Gynecol 1993;168:793-95.
17. Nardin JM, Weeks A, Carroli G. Umbilical vein injection for management of retained placenta. Cochrane Database Syst Rev 2011;5:CD001337.
18. Weeks AD. The retained placenta. In: Studd J(ed). Progress in Obstetrics and Gynaecology 16. New Delhi: Churchill Livingstone, 2005. pp. 133-54.

Chapter 16

Inversion Uterus

Poonam Sachdeva, Vidhi Choudhary

INTRODUCTION

Uterine inversion is defined as 'the turning inside out of the fundus of the uterus either into the uterine cavity or into the vagina' (Figure 16.1). It is a rare clinical condition that can occur in both puerperal and nonpuerperal uterus. Puerperal uterine inversions are far more common than nonpuerperal uterine inversions (86% versus 14%).[1] Estimates of frequency of puerperal inversions have ranged between one per 8,537 deliveries to one per 200,000 deliveries.[1,2,3]

Most of the puerperal uterine inversions are acute as compared to only 8.6 percent nonpuerperal uterine inversions. Approximately 2 percent of nonpuerperal inversions are associated with tumor, of which 20 percent are malignant. This emphasizes the need of biopsy prior to definitive treatment.

Classification

Various classification schemes describe uterine inversion

Classification on Basis of Type of Uterus[3]

- Puerperal or obstetric
- Nonpuerperal or gynecologic inversion -
  - submucous leiomyoma with fundal attachment
  - endometrial carcinoma and sarcoma.

Classification on the Basis of Duration of Inversion

- *Acute:* Diagnosed within 24 hrs of delivery
- *Subacute:* Diagnosed after 24 hrs but within 4 weeks after delivery
- *Chronic:* Diagnosed after 4 weeks of delivery.

Classification on the Basis of Severity of Acute Inversion[4,7]

- *Stage 1:* First (incomplete); the inverted fundus extends to, but not beyond, the cervical ring. The fundus remains within the uterine cavity.
- *Stage 2:* Second (incomplete); the inverted fundus extends through the cervical ring but remains within the vagina

- *Stage 3:* Third (complete); the inverted fundus extends down to the introitus.
- *Stage 4:* Fourth (total); the vagina is also involved, with complete inversion of the uterus and vagina through the vulva.

Risk Factors for Uterine Inversion

- Idiopathic—In up to 50 percent of cases, no risk factors are identified and there is no mismanagement of the third stage.
- Mismanagement of the third stage of labor (premature traction on umbilical cord and fundal pressure before separation of placenta) is the most common cause.[1]
- Other causes are:
  - Uterine atony
  - Precipitate labor
  - Fundal implantation of a morbidly adherent placenta
  - Manual removal of the placenta
  - A short umbilical cord
  - Chronic endometritis
  - Fetal macrosomia
  - Trials of vaginal birth after cesarean delivery (VBAC)
  - Myometrial weakness or uterine sacculation
  - Acute tocolysis with nitroglycerin or other potent tocolytic drugs
  - Cesarean delivery
  - Placenta previa and Placenta accreta, increta, or percreta
  - Connective tissue disorders (Marfan's syndrome, Ehlers-Danlos syndrome).

CASE SCENARIO

A 25-yr-old woman P2L2 delivered at home 6 hours back presented to the emergency in conscious state with complaints of excessive vaginal bleeding, abdominal pain and mass protruding per vaginum. Delivery was conducted by untrained birth attendant at patient's residence with failed attempt to remove placenta.

> **Comments:** Diagnosis of acute puerperal uterine inversion should be considered as she presented within 24 hrs of delivery, with vaginal bleeding, history of failure to remove placenta and complaint of a mass protruding through vagina.

Differential Diagnosis

- Uterovaginal prolapse
- Fibroid polyp
- Attached placenta over submucous fibroid
- Retained placenta without inversion

POINTS TO BE NOTED IN HISTORY

- Symptoms
  - Postpartum hemorrhage—Most common symptom
  - Severe abdominal pain
  - Sudden cardiovascular collapse
- Duration of labor (all three stages)—Prolonged labor leading to uterine atony may be a risk factor
- Personnel conducting delivery—Delivery by untrained birth attendant causing raised intraabdominal pressure may precipitate inversion.

- Factors causing abnormal placental adhesions like previous LSCS, prior curettage or chorioamnionitis can cause inversion if placenta is unduly pulled prior to separation.
- History of placental delivery
  - deliberate attempts to pull placenta prior to its separation
  - whether the placenta delivered complete or partial
  - delivery by trained or untrained personnel.
- Estimated blood loss—Shock may be out of proportion to observed blood loss as element of neurogenic shock is present in these patients.
- Obstetrical history—Risk is more in primigravidas with tendency to recur in subsequent pregnancies.

> **History in this case:** Delivery was conducted by untrained birth attendant and duration of labor was about 7 hrs with third stage lasting for 2 hrs, with failed attempt to remove placenta. There was history of excessive blood loss and pain abdomen.
> Risk factors in this case:
> - P2L2 delivered at home
> - Delivered by untrained birth attendant
> - Failed attempt to remove placenta

POINTS TO BE NOTED IN EXAMINATION

General Examination

- General condition—Fair/poor
- Vitals—Temperature, pulse, respiratory rate (RR) and blood pressure (BP).
- Pallor, hydration
- Urinary output

Cardiovascular and Respiratory System Examination

Abdominal Examination

- Abdominal tenderness
- Absence of uterine fundus on abdominal palpation\cup like depression at fundus

Pelvic Examination

- Lump in the vagina
- Polypoidal red mass in the vagina with placenta attached/submucosal polyp attached (nonpuerperal)
  - In Stage 1, dimple may be felt in the mid-line.
  - In Stages 2, 3 and 4 fundus is usually not palpable abdominally.

> **Examination in this case:**
> Patient was conscious but in poor general condition, grossly pale and dehydrated
> Pulse-120/min, BP-90/60 mm Hg, Temp-101°F, RR-24/min
> Chest-clear, CVS- tachycardia, no additional sounds
> P/A - Uterus was not palpable
> Local examination- Polypoidal, shaggy red mass with placenta attached seen protruding outside vagina.
> P/V- cervical ring was felt with inverted uterus, fundus was not felt.

Diagnosis

Inversion uterus

MANAGEMENT

The key to a successful outcome is **teamwork, resuscitation and repositioning of the uterus.**[4-8]

Initial Management and Resuscitation

- Alert obstetric emergency team
- Gain intravenous (IV) access and send all investigations
- Cross-match 4 units of blood
- Catheterize the bladder
- Treat shock by giving volume expanding fluids and oxygen.

Investigations

- Blood group and cross-match
- Complete blood count
- Coagulation profile
- Kidney function test
- Liver function test
- Ultrasound
- *USG features (Figure 16.1):* Ultrasound may be required if there is any doubt in diagnosis. Ultrasound findings in uterine inversion are:[9]
  - Uterus not seen in normal position
  - Echogenic mass is found in birth canal
  - Longitudinal scan shows U-shaped depressed longitudinal groove from uterine fundus to center of inverted part
  - Transverse scan shows hypoechoic mass in vagina with central H-shaped hypoechoic cavity due to bulge of anterior and posterior wall into groove.

Further Management

- Continuous monitoring of patient's vital signs
- Once the diagnosis is established and resuscitative measures are started, determine whether the placenta is attached to the uterus. No attempts should be made to remove the placenta as this can lead to a severe PPH.

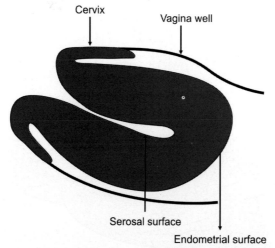

Figure 16.1: USG features

- For further manipulations general anaesthesia is used.[6,7,8]
- Transient tocolysis with terbutaline (subcutaneous injection of 0.25 mgs or infusion) or ritodrine 5 mg I/V may be required to relax the cervical ring.
- The inverted uterus should be thoroughly cleansed using antiseptic solution.
- Apply compression to the inverted uterus with a moist, warm sterile towel until ready for the procedure.

REPOSITIONING THE UTERUS: NONSURGICAL METHOD

Aim is to reposit the uterus inside without removing the placenta. It is important that the part of the uterus that came out last should be reposited first.

Manual Correction

1. *Johnson maneuver:* The inverted uterus is grasped in the palm of the hand with fingers placed posteriorly and pushed through the cervix towards the umbilicus to its normal position, using the other hand to support the uterus (Figure 16.2). Manual removal of placenta is attempted after correction. It is important that the part of the uterus that came out last (the part closest to the cervix) is reposited first. The principle behind this is that 'the uterus has to be lifted into the abdominal cavity above the level of the umbilicus before repositioning can occur. It is thought that the stretch of uterine ligaments will rectify the uterine inversion. The chances of success are quoted as 43 to 88 percent.
2. *Fenton & Singh modification:* Pressure is applied all around the periphery of mass.

Hydrostatic Correction

If correction is not achieved manually, hydrostatic method is tried.
1. *O'Sullivan's method:*[10]
   - The woman should be placed in deep Trendelenburg position (head end should be 500 cm below the level of the perineum).
   - A high-level disinfected douche system with large nozzle and long tubing (2 meters) and a warm water reservoir (3 to 5 L) should be prepared. Warm normal saline and an ordinary IV administration set can be used.

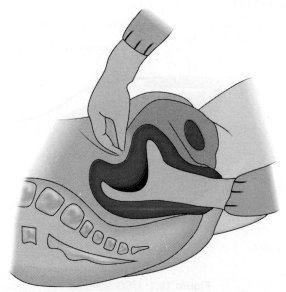

Figure 16.2: Manual replacement of the inverted uterus

- Posterior fornix should be identified (easily done in partial inversion when the inverted uterus is still in the vagina. In other cases, the posterior fornix is recognized by where the rugose vagina becomes the smooth vagina.)
- Nozzle of the douche is to be placed in the posterior fornix and with the other hand the labia is sealed over the nozzle.
- Assistant is asked to start the douche with full pressure (raise the water reservoir to at least 2 meters). The posterior fornix of the vagina will be distended by water so that it gradually stretches.
- The circumference of the orifice increases and relieves cervical constriction and results in correction of the inversion.

2. *Ogueh method:*[11]
   Proposes use of silicone cup. It is important not to seal the cup over the inverted fundus: instead, the cup should be positioned in the direction of the posterior fornix to allow vaginal distension. *Complications associated with hydrostatic methods are* infection, failure of the procedure and, theoretically, saline embolism.

Postprocedure Care

1. *Uterotonics:* After correction of inversion, uterotonics are given to maintain contraction of the uterus. Oxytocin infusion 20 units in 500 mL normal saline or Ringer's lactate is given at a rate of 60 drops per minute. If the uterus does not contract after oxytocin, ergometrine 0.2 mg or prostaglandins are given.
2. *Anibiotics:* A single dose of prophylactic antibiotics is given before correcting the inversion:
   a. For acute inversion in clean labor room:
      - Ampicillin 2 g IV plus metronidazole 500 mg I/V; OR
      - Cefazolin 1 g IV plus metronidazole 500 mg I/V.
   b. If there are signs of infection (as in this case) or the woman currently has fever, a combination of antibiotics is given until she is fever-free for 48 hours –
      - Ampicillin 2 g IV every 6 hours; plus
      - Gentamicin 1. 5 mg/kg body weight IV every 24 hours; plus
      - Metronidazole 500 mg IV every 8 hours
3. *Analgesia:* Appropriate analgesic drugs are given

> **Management in this case:**
> - After initial resuscitation, Johnson's maneuver was successful in this case.
> - Postprocedure—uterotonics were given. Uterus remained at its normal position and well contracted. Blood loss was average (100 mL).
> - Prophylactic antibiotics (ampicillin, gentamicin, metrogyl) were started prior to the procedure as patient had poor health status with history of *Dai* handling. Antibiotics were continued for 48 hrs.
> - She was transfused with 2 units of packed cells.
> - Postprocedure Hb- 9.6 gm%, TLC -9000 per cmm.
> - She was discharged on oral hematinics on day 5 in stable condition.

REPOSITIONING THE UTERUS: SURGICAL METHODS

Combined Abdominal-vaginal Correction

Abdominal-vaginal correction under general anesthesia[6,7] may be required if the above measures fail. Abdomen is opened with midline vertical incision below the umbilicus to the pubic symphysis. A bladder retractor is placed over the pubic bone and self-retaining abdominal retractors are placed.
   a. *Huntington's procedure:*[12] The constricting cervical ring is dilated digitally. A tenaculum/Allis is placed through the cervical ring and the inverted fundus is grasped. Gentle continuous traction is applied to the fundus while an assistant attempts manual correction vaginally.

b. *Haultain's procedure:*[13] If traction fails, the constricting cervical ring is incised posteriorly (where the incision is least likely to injure the bladder or uterine vessels) and digital dilatation is repeated followed by tenaculum and traction steps to reduce the inversion. The incised ring is repaired after manually removing the placenta.

c. *Ocejo:*[14] In this method the cervical ring is cut anteriorly. This method is preferred when adhesions are present in POD.

If there are signs of infection, the subcutaneous tissue is packed with gauze and loose 0 catgut (or polyglycolic) sutures are placed. Skin closure is delayed till after the infection has cleared; if there are no signs of infection the skin is closed with vertical mattress sutures of 3-0 nylon (or silk) and a sterile dressing is applied.

Others Techniques Described in the Literature

a. Vijayaraghvan et al. [15] reported a case where acute inversion of the uterus was managed under laparoscopic guidance.

b. Antonelli et al. [16] reported a case where laparotomy was performed and a silastic cup used from above for the correction of complete acute inversion of the uterus. The stated advantages of using a silastic cup were that it was gentler on the tissues and afforded easy placement and maneuvering through the constriction ring.

Abdominal Hysterectomy

This may be required in cases with intractable hemorrhage not responding to nonsurgical and conservative surgical methods.

PREVENTION OF INVERSION UTERUS

- Active management of third stage of labor.
- Avoid excessive traction on umbilical cord.
- Avoid fundal pressure.
- Avoid vigorous manual removal of placenta.

PROGNOSIS

The condition carries a good prognosis if managed correctly. Woman should be reassured that fertility and reproductive outcome are not compromised following surgical correction.

CONCLUSION

The management of acute uterine inversion should be incorporated into skills and drills training. As it is a rare condition, the precise incidence is unknown. Active management, prompt diagnosis and treatment can prevent morbidity associated with the condition.

KEY POINTS

- Acute uterine inversion is a rare and unpredictable obstetric emergency.
- Active management of third stage is a preventive measure.
- Mortality and morbidity are reduced by prompt recognition and management.
- Shock and uterine replacement must be addressed simultaneously.
- There is a need for skills and drills training because of the rarity of acute inversion.

REFERENCES

1. Baskett TF. Acute uterine inversion- a review of 40 cases. J Obstetric Gynaecol Can 2002;24:953-6.
2. Das P. Inversion of the uterus. J Obstet Gynaecol Br Empire 1940;47:525-48.
3. Donald I: Practical Obstetric Problems, 4th ed, London, Lloyd-Luke, 1974, p 731.
4. Bhalla R. Acute inversion of the uterus. The Obstetrician & Gynecologist 2009;11:13-18.
5. Grady JP. Malposition of the Uterus. Medscape education Jun 12, 2008. Available in http://emedicine.medscape.com/article/272497-overview.
6. World Health Organization 2000: Correcting uterine inversion. Available in www.who.int/reproductive-health/impact/procedures.
7. Beringer RM, Patteril M. Puerperal uterine inversion and shock. Br J Anaesth 2004;92:439-41.
8. Abouleish E, Ali V, Joumaa B, Lopez M, Gupta D. Anaesthetic management Of acute puerperal uterine inversion. Br J Anaesth 1995;75:486-7.
9. Rana KA, Patel P. Complete uterine inversion- an unusual yet crucial sonographic diagnosis. J Ultrasound Med 2009;28:1719-22.
10. Ward HR. O'Sullivan's hydrostatic reduction of an inverted uterus: sonar sequences recorded. Ultrasound Obstet Gynecol 1998;12:283-6.
11. Ogueh O, Ayida G. Acute inversion- a new technique of hydrostatic replacement. Br J Obstret Gynaecol 1997;104:951-2.
12. Huntington JL, Boston M.D. Acute inversion of uterus. Med Surg J 1921;184:376-80.
13. Haultain FWN. Br Med J 1901; ii, 974.
14. Kojima K, Suginami H, Egawa H et al. Recurrent inversion of the puerperal uterus managed with the Ocejo operation. Nippon Sanka, Fujinka Gakkai Zasshi 1995;47:1375-7.
15. Vijayaraghvan R, Sujatha Y. Acute postpartum uterine inversion with hemorrhagic shock- laparoscopic reduction: a new method of management. BJOG 2006;113:1100-02.
16. Antonelli E, Irion O, Tolck P, Morales M. Subacute uterine inversion: description of a novel replacement technique using the obstetric ventouse. BJOG 2006;113:846-7.

Chapter 17

Perineal Tear During Delivery

Latika Sahu

INTRODUCTION

There are over 500,000 natural childbirths per year and a large number of women suffer perineal tears during delivery. Approximately 50 to 60 percent of those women will need to be sutured. About 2 percent, i.e. over 10,000 women a year experience perineal tears that require anal suturing.[1] The Royal College of Obstetricians and Gynaecologists (RCOG) estimate that over 85 percent of women who have a vaginal birth will suffer some degree of perineal trauma and of these 60 to 70 percent will need suturing.[2]

Perineal trauma affects women's physical, psychological and social well-being and can disrupt breastfeeding, family life and sexual relations. It is vital for women's future well-being that perineal injuries are correctly identified and repaired timely.

Classification of Perineal Tears

The RCOG has recommended the following classification of perineal trauma for best practice.[3]
- *First degree tear:* Laceration is limited to the fourchette and superficial perineal skin or vaginal mucosa.
- *Second Degree:* Involving perineal muscles but not the anal sphincter.
- *Third Degree:* Involving the anal sphincter complex, i.e. both external anal sphincter (EAS) and internal anal sphincter (IAS).
  - *3a:* < 50% of EAS torn
  - *3b:* > 50% of EAS torn
  - *3c:* IAS torn
- *Fourth Degree:* Involving the anal sphincter complex (EAS and IAS) and the rectal mucosa.

Causes of Perineal Tears

- Rapid stretching of the perineum-as in precipitate labor
- Overstretching of the perineum – as in prolonged second stage, in big baby (>4kg), deflexed head, occipitoposterior/face presentation, shoulder dystocia, contracted pelvis
- Inelastic/rigid perineum- as in some nulliparas, scarred perineum, female genital mutilation.

CASE SCENARIO-1

A 25-year-old primipara delivered a male baby of weight 4.2 kg at home (conducted by *Dai*) and came to emergency 2 hours after delivery with complaints of fecal incontinence and excessive bleeding per vaginum since delivery.

Comments: Diagnosis of third/fourth degree perineal tear should be considered as she is complaining of fecal incontinence and excessive bleeding per vaginum.

Differential Diagnosis

- Other causes of excessive vaginal bleeding.
- Tears in other parts of genital tract.

POINTS TO BE NOTED IN HISTORY

- Duration of labor
- Parity
- Weight of the baby
- History of instrumental/manipulative deliveries
- History of delay in timing of/inadequate episiotomy, uncontrolled/neglected delivery
- Bleeding –amount
- Incontinence of feces
- Past obstetrical and gynecological history—history of perineal tears in previous delivery. Any prior surgery done on perineum producing scarring.

History in this case: She is a primipara, delivered a 4.2 kg baby at home, conducted by *Dai* and has presented with bleeding per vaginum and fecal incontinence following delivery.

POINTS TO BE NOTED IN EXAMINATION

General Examination

a. General condition
b. Pulse, blood pressure, pallor, jaundice, respiratory rate.
c. Urine output.

Cardiovascular and Respiratory System Examination

Abdominal Examination

Uterine size, whether contracted and retracted or not any other mass or abnormality present.

Pelvic Examination

On Inspection

- Amount and site of bleeding.
- Degree of perineal tear.
- Presence of fecal soiling.

Per Speculum Examination

- Bleeding from other sites—Cervix or vagina.
- Tears other than perineal area—Vaginal tear, cervical tear etc.

- Amount of damage of anal sphincter.
- Involvement of rectal mucosa.
- Presence of necrotic tissue/slough -indicate longer duration of tear.

Per Vaginal Examination

- Confirmation of per speculum findings.
- Uterine size, contracted or not.
- Levator anitone.
- Condition of the torn tissue-to decide immediate (within 24 hr) or delayed repair (after 24 hr).

Examination in this case: General condition and vitals are stable. There is a fourth degree perineal tear with bleeding and fresh edges, soiling with feces is present.

Diagnosis

Fourth degree perineal tear.

INVESTIGATIONS

- Hemoglobin, hematocrit.
- Blood group and Rh typing
- Blood sugar, urea, serum electrolytes
- Urine routine and microscopy

TREATMENT

The patient should be examined by an experienced obstetrician and shifted to operation theatre for exploration and repair of the tear under regional/general anesthesia.

- Consent—the patient should be informed about full extent of the injury sustained, structures involved and the procedure of repair.
- Examine the vagina, cervix, perineum and rectum. Place a gloved finger in the anus and lift to see the tear of anal sphincter, and rectal mucosa. Remove any fecal material, if present. Change gloves.
- Repair the rectal mucosa using interrupted 3-0/4-0 sutures 0.5 cm apart.
- Cover the muscularis layer by bringing together the fascial layer with interrupted sutures.
- Identify and grasp the torn ends of the anal sphincter complex with allis forceps and mobilize muscles to ensure that their ends can overlap each other by 0.5 – 1.0 cm. They should be sutured with 3-0 PDS/2-0 vicryl sutures by using a "figure of 8" or overlap method.[4]
- Examine the anus to ensure the correct repair of the rectum and sphincter. Then change gloves to repair the vaginal mucosa and perineal muscles.
- Repair the skin using interrupted 2-0 sutures. A cochrane review found that a continuous subcuticular stitch produced more comfortable results.[5]
- Blood transfusion (if blood loss is more) and vaginal pack may be required (if hemostasis cannot be achieved).
- Intravenous antibiotics (Cefuroxime 1.5 g and Metronidazole 500 mg) should be administered at the time of the repair.[1]

Postoperative Care

- Nil per oral for first 24 to 48 hours, then start clear fluids followed by semisolid and normal diet by 5th day
- Antibiotics—Cefuroxime and metronidazole orally for 1 week

- Avoid enema and rectal examination for 2 weeks
- Stool softener/laxatives- Lactulose 10 ml tid and Fybogel 1 sachet bd for 2 weeks
- Physiotherapy and pelvic floor exercises for 6-12 weeks
- NSAIDs, ibuprofen — for pain
- Seitz baths—sitting in a warm bath that only covers hips and buttocks
- Ice pads—Ice wrapped in a cloth applied to the area to dull the pain
- Clean the perineum and keep it dry after urination
- Use a cushion when sitting or lying down
- Not to use tampons until complete wound is healed
- Infrared light therapy—It penetrates cells in the perineal area and heats them, causing the cells to release their toxins in the sweat and therefore assists in the healing process, which can help to ease pain
- Women should be discharged from hospital after normal bowel function
- All women should be seen by a senior obstetrician at 6 weeks follow-up.

Complications

Complications may occur as a result of the tear or the repair done for it.
1. Incontinence of stool and/or flatus - Many women are able to control defecation by the use of other perineal muscles.
2. Rectovaginal fistula Requires reconstructive surgery three months/more postpartum.
3. Failure of repair requiring secondary repair
2. Hematoma—open and drain it. Close the wound if there are no signs of infection and bleeding.
5. Fear, difficulty and discomfort in passing stools in the immediate postnatal period.
6. Wound infection (8%)—Open and drain the wound. Remove infected sutures, debride the wound and give antibiotics
7. Granulation tissue formation.
8. Fecal urgency (26%)
9. Pain—Perineal pain and dyspareunia (9%)

Mode of Delivery in Future Pregnancies

There is level IV evidence that all women who have sustained an obstetric anal sphincter injury in a previous pregnancy and who are symptomatic or have abnormal end anal ultrasonography and/ or manometry should have the option of elective cesarean section.[6]

Management of 1st and 2nd Degree Perineal Tears

Suturing of vaginal mucosa, perineal muscle and skin are repaired as described above. Postoperatively analgesics and antibiotics are given.

Management of Neglected Cases

If closure in a third/fourth degree perineal tear is delayed for > 12 hours, infection is inevitable. Delayed primary closure is indicated. Close the rectal mucosa and approximate the anal sphincter with 2 or 3 sutures; close the muscle, vaginal mucosa and the perineal skin 6 days later.

Necrotizing fasciitis requires wide surgical debridement. Perform secondary closure in 2 to 4 weeks, depending on resolution of infection. Give antibiotics until necrotic tissue is cleared and the woman is fever-free for 48 hours.

Central Perineal Rupture

This is a rare accident in precipitate labor. The head is driven down and the tissue gives way in the central portion, midway between the rectum and the commissure. The head then descends through this rent, and sometimes through the rectum.

When the rectum is involved, divide the narrow bridge between the laceration and the commissure, thus making it a complete tear before suturing. If, the rectum is not involved, only suture the central tear in the perineum.

PREVENTION OF PERINEAL TEAR DURING DELIVERY

Proper management of labor especially 2nd stage of labor can reduce the incidence of perineal tears. As per cochrane review, the incidence of severe perineal trauma can be decreased by minimizing the use of episiotomy and operative vaginal delivery. [Evidence level A][7]

Antenatal Interventions

Antenatal Perineal Massage

It reduces the likelihood of perineal trauma. Massages should be performed daily from 34 weeks of pregnancy. To perform a perineal massage place one or two fingers about an inch and a half into the vagina and apply downward pressure for 2 minutes, and then applying pressure to the either side of the vaginal opening for 2 minutes each. Lubricating jelly, like K-Y Jelly, sweet almond oil, Vitamin E/ Wheatgerm oil can be used for lubrication. This softens the skin and may help it to stretch more easily during labor.[8]

Hyaluronidase Injection in the Perineum

Perineal injection of hyaluronidase has been reported to prevent perineal trauma.[9]

Exercise and Nutrition

- Good nutrition— rich in vitamin E, C and bioflavonoid (1,000 mg.) are important for tissue health and elasticity.
- Kegel exercises —ask the women to contract and hold the muscles of pelvic floor that are used to stop the flow of urine and practice contracting, holding, and slowly releasing these muscles to strengthen them.

Intrapartum Interventions to Reduce Perineal Trauma (NICE Guidelines 2007)[10]

1. Perineal massage should **not** be performed in the second stage of labour.
2. Either the 'hands on' (guarding the perineum and flexing the baby's head) or the 'hands poised' (with hands off the perineum and baby's head but in readiness) technique can be used to facilitate spontaneous birth.
3. Lidocaine spray should not be used to reduce pain in the second stage of labour.
4. A routine episiotomy should not be carried out during spontaneous vaginal birth.
5. Where an episiotomy is performed, the recommended technique is a right mediolateral episiotomy (the angle to the vertical axis should be 45 to 60 degrees).
6. An episiotomy should be performed if there is a clinical need such as instrumental birth or suspected fetal compromise.
7. Tested effective analgesia should be provided prior to carrying out an episiotomy, except in an emergency like acute fetal compromise.
8. To enable a woman who has had previous third- or fourth-degree trauma make an informed choice, discussion with her about the future mode of birth should encompass:
   - Current urgency/incontinence symptoms
   - The degree of previous trauma
   - Risk of recurrence
   - The success of the repair undertaken

- The psychological effect of the previous trauma
- Management of her labor.

Episiotomy should not be offered routinely to them.

PROGNOSIS

Prognosis of perineal tear (I-IV degree) if repaired immediately is good, with 60 to 80 percent asymptomatic at 12 months. Most women who remain symptomatic describe incontinence of flatus or fecal urgency.

KEY POINTS

- Diagnosis of fourth degree perineal tear should be considered when a woman presents with fecal incontinence and excessive bleeding per vaginum
- If the edges of the tear are fresh immediate repair should be done
- Repair should be done in operation theatre under anesthesia
- Repair is done in layers
- Postoperative care is very important
- Proper management of 2nd stage of labor can prevent perineal tear
- Good nutrition, antenatal perineal massage and exercise reduce the chance of perineal tear
- Prognosis of perineal tear repair is good.

REFERENCES

1. Buppasiri P, Lumbiganon P, Thinkhamrop J, Thinkhamrop B. Antibiotic prophylaxis for third- and fourth-degree perineal tear during vaginal birth. Cochrane Database Syst Rev 2010;(11):CD005125.
2. Royal College of Obstetricians and Gynecologists. The Management of Third- and Fourth-Degree Perineal Tears. Green-top Guideline No.29. London: RCOG; 2007 [www.rcog.org.uk/womens-health/clinical-guidance/management-third-and-fourth-degree-perineal-tears-greentop-29].
3. Sultan AH. Editorial: Obstetric perineal injury and anal incontinence. Clin Risk 1999;5:193-6.
4. Fernando R, Sultan AH, Kettle C, Thakar R, Radley S. Methods of repair for obstetric anal sphincter injury. Cochrane Database Syst Rev 2006;(3):CD002866.
5. Kettle C, Hills RK, Ismail KM. Continuous versus interrupted sutures for repair of episiotomy or second degree tears. Cochrane Database Syst Rev 2007;(4):CD000947.
6. Sultan AH, Thakar R. Lower genital tract and anal sphincter trauma. Best Pract Res Clin Obstet Gynecol 2002;16:99-115.
7. Carroli G, Belizan J. Episiotomy for vaginal birth. Cochrane Database Syst Rev 2003;(1):CD000081.
8. Beckmann M, Garrett A. Antenatal perineal massage for reducing perineal trauma. Cochrane Database Syst Rev 2006;(1):CD005123.
9. Scarabotto LB, Riesco ML. Use of hyaluronidase to prevent perineal trauma during spontaneous delivery a pilot study. J Midwifery Womens Health 2008;53:353-61.
10. National Collaborating Centre for Women's and Children's Health (UK).Intrapartum Care: Care of healthy women and their babies during childbirth. London: RCOG Press; 2007 Sep.

Chapter 18

Vulval and Paravaginal Hematomas

Latika Sahu

INTRODUCTION

Puerperal genital hematomas can be a cause of serious morbidity and even maternal death.[1] The pregnant uterus, vagina, and vulva have rich vascular supplies that are at risk of trauma during the birth process leading to hematoma formation.

Incidence of puerperal genital hematoma is 1 in 300 to 1 in 1000 deliveries.[2] Nulliparity, episiotomy and forceps delivery are the most commonly associated risk factors.[3] Hematomas may develop following injury to a blood vessel without laceration of the superficial tissue. These may occur with spontaneous or operative delivery.

Genital hemotomas can be vulval, paravaginal, broad ligament and retroperitoneal in location. Patients with vulval/paravaginal hematomas usually present with intense pain and localized, tender swelling. Broad ligament hematomas may be palpated as masses adjacent to the uterus.[4] All may result in significant blood loss that mandates resuscitation. Symptoms usually develop within a few hours of delivery. The speed of diagnosis will depend on the extent of the bleeding, its associated consequences and the level of awareness of the medical staff.

A woman with a large hematoma may be found collapsed within a few hours of delivery, whereas a woman with a small hematoma in an episiotomy may present with persisting pain over a few days. Excessive perineal pain is a hallmark symptom of puerperal hematomas and its presence should prompt a gentle pelvic examination. Continued vaginal bleeding may occur if a hematoma ruptures into the vagina.

Vulval Hematomas

In vulval hematomas bleeding is limited to the vulval tissues superficial to the anterior urogenital diaphragm. Branches of pudendal arteries- inferior rectal, transverse perineal and posterior labial arteries can be involved in vulval and vulvovaginal hematomas. Venous injury can also occur. Rapidly developing vulval hematoma causes excruciating pain.

Injury can be direct (from a pudendal needle/episiotomy) or indirect (from stretching of the vagina as the fetus passes through). Up to 87 percent of hematomas are associated with sutured perineal tears or episiotomies. Good surgical technique with attention to hemostasis in the repair of lacerations/episiotomies should limit the occurrence of this complication.[5]

Paravaginal Hematoma

The paravaginal space is bounded inferiorly by the pelvic diaphragm and superiorly by the cardinal ligament. Since it is contiguous with the paravesical, parametrial and pararectal spaces, blood arising in one connective tissue space may readily spread to any other. A paravaginal hematoma is typically confined to the upper supralevator or lower infralevator compartment, although massive hemorrhage can break through the levator barrier.

Paravaginal hematoma is usually due to rupture of paravaginal veins or damage to the descending cervical artery by the oncoming presenting part. Infralevator hematoma can be visible outside but supralevator hematoma is not visible externally and can only be diagnosed by digital examination of the pelvis.[6]

CASE SCENARIO-1

Mrs. X had a forceps delivery at 9 PM, after second stage of labor lasting 3 hr 15 min. Episiotomy and extension on the right vaginal wall were sutured. At 1 AM, patient complained of severe pain in the perineum, had tachycardia of 120/min. There was no response to analgesics.

> **Comments:** Diagnosis of vulval hematoma should be considered since she developed severe pain in the perineum 4 hours after forceps delivery.

Differential Diagnosis

- Other types of genital hematoma
- Other causes of tachycardia.

Points to be noted in History

a. Maternal factors predisposing to development of vulval hematoma:
  - Episiotomy
  - Nulliparous
  - Age > 29 years
  - Baby weight >4000g
  - Pre-eclampsia
  - Prolonged second stage of labor
  - Instrumental delivery
  - Multifetal pregnancy
  - Genital tract varicosities
  - Clotting disorders
b. Symptoms of hematoma:
  - History of excessive vaginal bleeding during delivery and after
  - Pain in vulval region
  - Abdominal pain
  - Difficulty in sitting
  - Inability to pass urine.

> **History in this case:** Primipara with second stage of labor lasting 3 hr 15 min; there was a forceps delivery followed by pain and swelling in the perineum.

POINTS TO BE NOTED IN EXAMINATION

General Examination

- General condition
- Pulse, blood pressure(BP), respiratory rate (RR)

- Pallor
- Urine output.

Cardiovascular and Respiratory System Examination
Any murmur or adventitious sound

Abdominal (P/A) Examination

- Uterine size, whether contracted or not.
- Tenderness over the uterus and other areas of abdomen.
- Presence of mass and tenderness above inguinal ligament

Pelvic Examination

Inspection of Vulva

Presence of swelling, size of swelling, site of swelling in relation to episiotomy. Bleeding from the swelling and from the vagina.

Per Speculum (P/S) Examination

Confirmation of findings on inspection, look for extent of swelling, whether margins can be defined or not. It may not be possible to carry out due to local pain. Look for presence of any other laceration

Per Vaginum (P/V) Examination

Check for size of uterus, any fullness in the fornices and confirm the site and size of swelling. A vulval hematoma is usually tense, tender and fluctuant with discoloration of overlying skin and there may be bleeding on pressing the swelling.

Per Rectal (P/R) Examination

Any swelling anterior to the rectum, extent of swelling. Note whether extending into ischiorectal fossa.

> **Examination in this case:**
> General- Pallor++, Pulse 120/min, BP 100/70 mmHg, RR 18/min
> Systemic examination—Unremarkable.
> P/A—Uterus 20 week size, well contracted, no tenderness, no other mass felt and no free fluid.
> Local examination—Vulval swelling at the region of episiotomy, size 8×9 cm, tense and tender with all the margin felt, no other laceration in vagina or cervix.
> P/V—Uterus of 20 week size, mobile, all fonices free.
> P/R - No supravaginal hematoma.

Diagnosis
Vulval hematoma.

INVESTIGATIONS

- A full blood count and coagulation screen to determine baseline values and repeated as necessary.
- Blood should be sent for crossmatching.

TREATMENT

It involves resuscitation, exploration under anesthesia and hematoma drainage
- Resuscitation with fluid replacement and blood transfusion.
- *Exploration under anesthesia:* The site in relation to episiotomy and size of hematoma are noted.

- *Hematoma drainage:* This patient had hematoma at the episiotomy site. In such cases following steps should be followed:
  - open the episiotomy sutures,
  - evacuate the clots,
  - search for any active bleeder(s) and ligate it,
  - close the dead space and
  - repair episiotomy in layers with proper hemostasis.
- Postoperative care—Foley catheter, antibiotics (e.g. cefazolin+metronidazole), analgesics.

Angiographic embolization (gaining access via femoral artery) can be used primarily or when hemostasis is not obtained by surgical methods. Internal pudendal artery with its vaginal branch and the uterine artery are embolized. The process can be done only if experienced interventional radiologist and facility for angiography is available.

CASE SCENARIO-2

Mrs. X, 29-year-old multiparous lady was brought to the causality in a state of shock 3 hour after home delivery. She complained of severe pain inside the vagina that was not associated with excessive vaginal bleeding.

> **Comments:** Diagnosis of paravaginal hematoma was considered since she was complaining of pain inside the vagina with features of shock within a few hours of delivery.

Differential Diagnosis

Other causes of postpartum shock including intraperitoneal hemorrhage and rupture uterus.

POINTS TO BE NOTED IN HISTORY

- Factors predisposing to obstetric lacerations
- Symptoms suggestive of paravaginal hematoma.

Infralevator hematoma can cause massive swelling and ecchymosis of the labia, perineum and lower vagina on the affected side, and suggillation may extend over the buttock. Anorectal tenesmus may result from extension into the ischiorectal fossa, while urinary retention may occur due to ventral spread into the paravesical space.

Supralevator hematoma cause swelling inside the vagina and features of shock.

> **History in this case:** Shock was out of proportion to the revealed blood loss, pain was inside the vagina on right side.

> **Examination in this case:**
> General—Pallor+++ Pulse 150/min, BP 80/40 mmHg, RR 30/min
> Systemic examination—Unremarkable.
> P/A—Uterus 20 week size, well contracted, no tenderness, no other mass and no free fluid.
> Local examination—No vulval swelling
> P/S—a paravaginal swelling on the right side of vagina.
> P/V—confirmed a tense, tender swelling size 8×9 cm, the entire margin felt, uterus 20 week size, mobile, and all fonices free.
> P/R examination—swelling lying anterior to rectum.

Diagnosis

Right paravaginal hematoma

INVESTIGATIONS

- Complete blood count
- Coagulation profile.
- Imaging: Ultrasound, computerized tomography (CT) and magnetic resonance imaging (MRI) scans are useful in diagnosing hematomas above the pelvic diaphragm and to assess any extension into the pelvis. MRI is particularly useful in providing information on the location, size and extent of a hematoma and in monitoring progress or resolution.[8]

MANAGEMENT

- Management aims to prevent further blood loss, minimize tissue damage, ease pain and reduce the risk of infection.
- Resuscitative measures should be initiated immediately.
- Aggressive fluid replacement and assessment of coagulation status is essential if there is heavy bleeding or signs of hypovolemia.
- Blood should be available for transfusion.
- A urinary catheter is placed to monitor fluid balance and to avoid possible urinary retention due to pain, edema or the pressure of a vaginal pack.

Immediate Treatment

a. *Management of shock:*
   - Airway, oxygen by mask, intravenous fluids
   - Patient is kept nil per oral as she may vomit and aspirate
   - Keep the patient warm
   - Maintain circulation to vital organs by elevating the legs.
b. *Surgical evacuation of the hematoma:*
   The incision should be made via the vagina. If figure of eight sutures do not achieve hemostasis, either a drain or a vaginal pack can be used.

Small, Static Hematomas (< 5 cm)

Small, static hematomas (<5 cm) can be managed conservatively. Conservative management of larger hematomas is associated with longer hospital stay, an increased need for antibiotics and blood transfusion and subsequent operative intervention.[3]

Large (> 5 cm) and Acutely Expanding Hematomas

Large (> 5 cm) and acutely expanding hematomas are managed with surgical evacuation. Incision is given at the point of maximum distention under adequate anesthesia followed by evacuation of blood clots and ligation of bleeding points. The cavity is then obliterated with mattress suture. If no bleeding vessel is identified then vagina (not the hematoma cavity) is packed for 12 to 24 hour to tamponade bleeding vessels. Drains if inserted are usually brought out through a separate site distant from the repair.[7]

Persistent Bleeding

Hematomas can recur after surgical management. Continued monitoring for signs of blood loss is essential. In case of recurrence one should re-explore the hematoma cavity. Ligation of the internal iliac artery, or hysterectomy, may be necessary. Pelvic arterial embolization can be used for the treatment of persistent bleeding, but it has limited availability.[9]

SUBPERITONEAL HEMATOMAS

Incidence-1 in 3,500 to 20,000. These are due to damage to the uterine artery. The hematoma can dissect retroperitoneally or develop within the broad ligament. Patient complains of lower abdominal pain and hemorrhage. A high index of suspicion is required to diagnose and manage these hematomas promptly before the signs of cardiovascular collapse develop. Ultrasound, CT scanning, or MRI may be used to assess the size and progress of these hematomas.

Surgical Exploration

- Look for ruptured uterus
- Ligate descending cervical artery, uterine artery and internal illiac artery
- Do hysterectomy if necessary
- Selective arterial embolization is an excellent alternative to laparotomy. The success rate is over 90 percent.[10] Complications of pelvic arterial embolization are few (<9%) and include: low grade fever, pelvic infection, ischemic buttock pain, temporary foot drop, groin hematoma and vessel perforation.
- Broad spectrum antibiotic cover should be given.
- Regular review is required to ensure that bleeding has settled and hematoma has resolved.

KEY POINTS

- The most important factor in correct diagnosis is clinical awareness.
- Excessive perineal pain is a hallmark symptom- its presence should prompt examination.
- Aggressive fluid resuscitation and blood transfusion may be required.
- Coagulation status should be monitored.
- Treatment should be carried out in an operating theatre.
- A urinary catheter should be used to prevent urinary retention and monitor fluid balance.
- Hematomas of< 5cm size at any site can be managed conservatively.
- There is no evidence to support best management in vulval/paravaginal hematoma. It can be primary repair or packing, with or without insertion of a drain.
- Vigilance should be maintained after primary repair/packing.

REFERENCES

1. Morgans D, Chan N, Clark CA. Vulval perineal hematomas in the immediate postpartum period and their management. Aust N Z J Obstet Gynaecol 1999;39:223-7.
2. Cunningham FG. Genital tract lacerations and puerperal hematomas. In: Gilstrap LC III,Cunningham FG,Van Dorsten JP (eds). Operative Obstetrics. 2nd edn. New York:Mc Graw Hill,2002.pp.223.
3. Propst AM, Thorp JM Jr. Traumatic vulvar hematomas: conservative versus surgical management. South Med J 1998;91:144-6.
4. Gabbe SG, Niebyl JR, Simpson JL, (eds). Obstetrics: Normal and problem pregnancies. 3rd edn. New York: Churchill Livingstone, 1996.pp. 523-4.
5. Ridgway LE. Puerperal emergency. Vaginal and vulvar hematomas. Obstet Gynecol Clin North Am 1995;22:275-82.
6. Creasy RK. Management of Labor and Delivery. Massachusetts: Blackwell Science, 1997.
7. Zahn CM, Hankins GD, Yeomans ER. Vulvovaginal hematomas complicating delivery. Rationale for drainage of the hematoma cavity. J Reprod Med 1996;41:569-74.
8. Nagayama M, Watanabe Y, Okumura A, Amoh Y, Nakashita S, Dodo Y. Fast MR imaging in obstetrics. Radiographics 2002;22:563-82.
9. Mousa HA, Alfirevic Z. Major postpartum hemorrhage: survey of maternity units in the U.K. Acta Obstet Gynecol Scand 2002;81:727-30.
10. Bloom AI, Verstandig A, Gielchinsky Y, Nadiari M, Elchalal U. Arterial embolization for persistent primary postpartum hemorrhage: before or after hysterectomy? BJOG 2004;111:880-4.

Chapter 19

Postpartum Collapse

Reva Tripathi, Vertika Verma

INTRODUCTION

Postpartum collapse, as the name suggests, is hemodynamic instability of a patient who has recently delivered. Postpartum collapse is a frightening obstetric complication not only because of the gravity of the situation but mostly due to its sudden occurrence. In the majority of patients revealed hemorrhage is the cause. In others where there is no external blood loss and yet patient is collapsed, either blood is being lost internally or other shock producing factors are operative.

Causes

The causes for postpartum collapse are summarized (Figure 19.1).
Hemorrhagic shock has been dealt with elsewhere and this chapter will focus on nonhemorrhagic situations.

CASE SCENARIO

A 30-yr-old female, G2P1L1, with 37 weeks pregnancy delivered vaginally 30 minutes back without any complications. She suddenly becomes dyspneic and starts gasping, her pulse is hypovolemic with rate of 122/min, systolic blood pressure (BP) is 80 mm Hg by palpatory method and her peripheries are cold.

Comments: This patient has had a postpartum collapse and resuscitation along with a quick diagnosis of the cause of collapse is essential for optimal management.

APPROACH TO DIAGNOSIS

Firstly vaginal bleeding should be checked for and the fundus of the uterus palpated as hemorrhage is the commonest postpartum problem and this will also eliminate the possibility of uterine inversion. Once vaginal bleeding appears to be average and the uterus is well contracted, one must think of postpartum collapse due to nonhemorrhagic causes.

Relevant history must be taken from the immediate caregiver while doing a quick examination of the patient keeping all the differential diagnoses in mind. Care must be taken to elicit any history which could be contributory. Quick details of antenatal or intrapartum events must be taken, e.g.

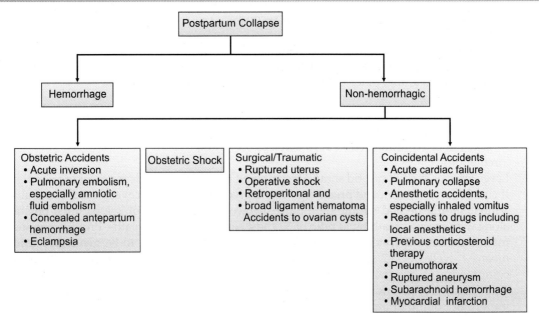

Figure 19.1: Causes of postpartum collapse

hypertension, difficult or prolonged labor, instrumental delivery and simultaneously the patient is observed for chest pain, cyanosis and signs of hypoxia which are likely to suggest a very grave situation.

Generally, there are signs of shock such as anxiety, confused look, sweating, cold clammy skin, dyspnea, rapid breathing >30/min, tachycardia >110/min, weak thready pulse, systolic BP <90 mm Hg and scanty urine output <30 mL/hr.

INVESTIGATIONS

Blood samples need to be immediately sent for:
- Blood grouping and cross-matching
- Hemogram
- Arterial blood gas analysis (ABG)
- Serum electrolytes
- Prothrombin time
- Kidney function tests
- Blood sugar estimation
- Bleeding time (BT), clotting time (CT) and clot retraction time(CRT) are bedside tests that can be immediately performed and will give some broad information about status of coagulation parameters of the patient.

MANAGEMENT

General Measures
- Mobilize staff for help and use multiparameter monitors on the patient if available.
- Initiate ABCD of basic life support.
- A- Airway assessing and opening.
  - Airway should be assessed whether open or closed. If closed, open the airway using 'head tilt chin lift' method. Any foreign body or vomitus in mouth should be suctioned or wiped out.

- B-Breathing- 'Look- Listen- Feel' for 5 to 10 seconds.
  - Look—For chest to rise and fall.
  - Listen—For air escaping during exhalation.
  - Feel—For the air flow against your cheek.
  - If patient is breathing, place patient in recovery position (left lateral)
  - If not breathing-
    - Anesthetist should be called for help.
    - Start giving rescue breaths using pocket mask or bag mask.
    - Oxygen to be administered at rate of 6 to 8 L/min.
- C- Circulation
  - Large arteries such as carotid should be palpated for 5 to 10 seconds for checking circulation.
  - If circulation is present and breathing absent, give 1 rescue breath every 4 to 5 sec. If absent, patient should be laid supine on a hard surface and chest compressions must be started along with rescue breathing at ratio of 30 chest compressions: 2 breaths. Provide one second for exhalation in between two breaths. 100 chest compressions to be given in 1 minute, means 1 cycle of 30:2 should be completed in approximately 18 seconds. Site of chest compression in pregnant patient is higher than nonpregnant women in view of raised diaphragm and position of heart that is slightly above the center of sternum, this is an important point that must be kept in mind at the time of performing resuscitation.
  - Intravenous (IV) access should be secured. It is preferable to have 2 IV lines using largest cannula available and feasible (preferably no.14). Crystalloid infusion must be given at rate of 2 liters in first hour or 3 mL of blood loss in case of revealed hemorrhage. Blood transfusion must be considered in hypovolemic shock and blood component therapy when there is deranged coagulation profile. Vasopressors may be required to maintain circulation
  - Patient should continue on continous noninvasive monitoring.
  - Bladder should be catheterized to monitor urine output.
- D- Defibrillation
  - Use automated external defibrillators if the situation warrants. Any electronic monitors should be detached before giving shock to the patient.
- At the earliest opportunity, patient should be shifted to intensive care unit for assisted ventilation and follow-up treatment.
- If feasible, an urgent chest X-ray should be done either with the help of portable X-ray machine or can be done while transferring the patient from labor room to intensive care unit as it can help in identifying the underlying cause. If a monitor is not available, at least an electrocardiogram tracing must be procured as it may act as an important tool to rule out any cardiac problem.

Specific Management

Specific management will be dependent on the cause. However, in these situations most of the times the cause is difficult to identify and generally supportive treatment is instituted till the cause is pinpointed which may take sometime.

AMNIOTIC FLUID EMBOLISM (ANAPHYLACTOID SYNDROME OF PREGNANCY)

Amniotic fluid embolism is a rare life threatening complication of pregnancy with high mortality rates. The mortality rates have fortunately decreased from 80 to 90 percent in the 1970s to less than 30 percent in the more recently reported Western studies.[1]

It commonly occurs in late pregnancy during labor, delivery or immediate postpartum; however it can occur during termination of early pregnancy. Amniotic fluid may gain access into maternal circulation as a result of a breach in the physiological barrier between maternal and fetal compartments. This can happen at any time during spontaneous labor and delivery, at amniotomy or at cesarean section. Conditions such as abruptio placentae, intrauterine fetal death, intrauterine pressure catheter insertion, amnioinfusion and operative delivery are associated risk factors.[2] The exposure to liquor amnii containing fetal epithelial squames, fat, lanugo hairs and meconium lead to activation of inflammatory cascades which resemble those seen in an anaphylactic reaction and hence, it is now also referred to as anaphylactoid syndrome of pregnancy.[3]

The initial phase consists of pulmonary and systemic hypertension. This phase is transient and is soon followed by left ventricular failure leading to profound hypotension and shock. Damage to alveoli and pulmonary capillary endothelium due to inflammatory reaction along with pulmonary vasoconstriction results in ventilation perfusion imbalance leading to severe hypoxia, cyanosis, convulsions and coma.[4] Disseminated intravascular coagulation may occur within hours if patient survives initial insult due to release of thromboplastins from placental or decidual tissue into the maternal circulation. This activates maternal coagulation factors which results in widespread intravascular coagulation and depletion of coagulation factors. In response to intravascular coagulation, fibrinolytic system gets activated resulting in hemorrhage and this in turn leads to formation of fibrin degradation products (FDP). There is high incidence of neurological impairment in those who survive because of severe hypoxia.

Diagnosis

Diagnosis is made by exclusion. No specific tests are available to diagnose amniotic fluid embolism. Classically, a women in late stages of labor or immediate postpartum starts gasping, then suffers seizures or cardio respiratory arrest followed by consumptive coagulopathy, massive hemorrhage and death. However, clinical presentation is variable. Disseminated intravascular coagulation is suggested by low platelet count and increased fibrin degradation product levels along with prolonged prothrombin time.

Four of following criteria should be present to diagnose amniotic fluid embolism:

- Acute hypotension or cardiac arrest
- Acute hypoxia
- Consumptive coagulopathy (DIC)
- Absence of any other explanation for the manifestation observed
- Onset during labor or within 30 min of delivery
  Postmortem finding of amniotic fluid contents such as meconium, mucin, epithelial squames in the pulmonary vessels is perhaps the best proof of the diagnosis of amniotic fluid embolism.

Treatment

No form of therapy has been found to improve outcome consistently. Hence, treatment is mainly supportive.
- Immediate administration of oxygen and intravenous fluids are most important measures. Blood component therapy should be started
- Appropriately used low doses of heparin, i.e. 5000 U twice or thrice daily, can block further consumption of clotting factors, thereby slowing the cycle of consumption and fibrinolysis. Heparin should be given only if the patient is not actively bleeding.
- If the fetus is undelivered, immediate delivery should be undertaken. If early delivery is not possible vaginally, cesarean section should be performed.
- These efforts for salvaging the fetus should not interrupt maternal resuscitation.
- Recently, plasma exchange and hemofiltration have been used in selected cases with some benefit, probably by washing out inflammatory mediators.[5]

PULMONARY THROMBOEMBOLISM

Pregnant women are at higher risk because of physiological changes in pregnancy which causes hypercoagulability of blood and promotes venous stasis. Risk further increases in postpartum

Table 19.1: Predisposing factors for thromboembolism[6]	
Obstetrical	*General*
• Cesarean delivery	• Age 35 yrs or more
• Gestational Diabetes	• Obesity
• Hemorrhage	• Prior thromboembolism
• Hyperemesis (dehydration)	• Smoking
• Immobility (prolonged bed rest)	• Sickle cell disease
• Multifetal gestation	• Thrombophilia
• Multiparity	• Oral contraceptive use
• Pre-eclampsia	• Orthopedic surgery
	• Connective tissue disorders
	• Myeloproliferative disease
	• Nephrotic syndrome
	• Cancer

period due to endothelial damage during delivery especially in high-risk situations which are enumerated in (Table 19.1).

Clinical Presentation and Diagnosis

Severity of symptoms depends upon size of vessel blocked by embolus. Most acutely symptomatic emboli are large and likely to be a saddle embolus which causes increased vascular resistance and pulmonary hypertension followed by acute right ventricular dilatation eventually leading to cardiac failure. Smaller emboli travel deep into terminal branches of pulmonary vascular system affecting a lesser area and are therefore less symptomatic.
* Signs and symptoms include
    – Sudden onset dyspnea
    – Chest pain
    – Cough
    – Hemoptysis and
    – Features of collapse like tachycardia, cold clammy skin and syncope.
* There may be clinical features suggestive of deep vein thrombosis. These include pain in the leg with swelling, tenderness, edema, elevated temperature and positive Homans' sign.
* When specifically enquired, sometimes there is history of previous transient episodes of chest pain and dyspnea suggestive of mild pulmonary embolism prior to massive one but the problem is rarely diagnosed at this stage.

A High Index of Suspicion is Required to Diagnose Pulmonary Embolism

Imaging

Various imaging investigations used for confirmation are:
* Ventilation perfusion scintigraphy
* Computed tomographic pulmonary angiography
* Magnetic resonance angiography
    Computed tomographic pulmonary angiography is used as a first line evaluation as X-ray exposure is less then ventilation perfusion scan. These are rarely feasible in our setting especially in an acute emergency but can serve as proof of cause of collapse if available.

Management

Management involves supportive treatment and definitive with treatment antithrombotic therapy.

Antithrombotic Therapy

Started immediately without waiting for lab test results
- Unfractioned heparin (UFH):
  - The American Academy of Pediatrics and the American College of Obstetricians and Gynecologists (2007) recommend an initial loading dose of 80 IU/kg (rounded to nearest 100) followed by continuous infusion of 30,000 IU for 24 hrs and titrated to achieve an activated partial thromboplastin time (aPTT) of 1.5 to 2.5 times the control value.
  - Intravenous infusion should be continued for 5 to 7 days after which therapy is converted to subcutaneous heparin injections 8 hourly to maintain aPTT at similar levels.
  - It cannot cross the placenta and is not secreted in milk, so is safe in both pregnancy and lactation.
  - It can result in hemorrhage, heparin induced thrombocytopenia and osteoporosis if used for prolonged duration.
- Low molecular weight heparin (LMWH):
  - Derived from depolymerization of standard heparin.
  - They have more predictable anticoagulant response and fewer bleeding complications because of their better bioavailability, longer half life and decreased interference with platelets.
  - They are also safe in pregnancy and lactation.
  - Preferred over unfractioned heparin for treatment of deep vein thrombosis but in hemodynamically unstable patient with massive pulmonary embolism, unfractioned heparin is the first choice.
  - Dose:
    - Enoxaparin is administered subcutaneously 1mg/kg twice daily based on early pregnancy weight.
    - Dalteparin is given subcutaneously 90 U/kg every 12 hourly.
  - The American Academy of Pediatrics and the American College of Obstetricians and Gynecologists (2007) recommend that anti factor Xa levels be periodically reevaluated in a women anticoagulated with these agents. Dosing should be enough to achieve a peak anti factor Xa level of 0.5 to 1.2 U/mL. Platelet count should be checked one week after initiating therapy. However, it is not essential to do this monitoring and is therefore an advantage over unfractioned heparin though cost is a constraint to widespread usage of low molecular weight heparin.
- Warfarin:
  - Therapy should be converted to warfarin once the acute phase is over.
  - Warfarin is contraindicated in first trimester of pregnancy as it can cross placenta and can cause fetal death and congenital malformations but is safe in lactation.
  - To avoid paradoxical thrombosis and skin necrosis from early anti-protein C effect of warfarin, these women are maintained on therapeutic doses of UFH or LMWH for 5 days until the international normalized ratio (INR) is in the therapeutic range (The American Academy of Pediatrics and the American College of Obstetricians and Gynecologists,2007).
  - The initial dose of warfarin is usually 5 to 10 mg for the first 2 days. Subsequent doses are titrated to achieve an INR of 2 to 3.
  - Anticoagulation should be continued for at least 6 months.

OTHER CAUSES OF POSTPARTUM COLLAPSE

AIR EMBOLISM

- Air embolus may be introduced into circulation during intrauterine manipulation or during cesarean section.
- Typical symptoms include tachypnea, chest pain and gasping.
- An immediate first aid procedure is to place the patient in head down, lateral position in hope of displacing air embolus towards apex of right ventricle. From here, air may be passed piecemeal into pulmonary circulation to get diffused out in pulmonary alveoli.

- Nitrous oxide should be discontinued and 100 percent oxygen must be started.
- Surgical site should be flooded with saline to avoid further air entry.

OBSTETRIC SHOCK

- Obstetric shock used to be the name given to those patients who went into shock immediately postpartum where the reason could not be ascertained and was not of hemorrhagic nature.
- The precipitating factors are operative vaginal delivery or intrauterine manipulation. Stretching of the parts may be a factor in susceptible individuals. Therefore, it is also considered a variety of neurogenic shock which accounts for its high mortality.
- Most of the times, etiology is not identifiable unless autopsy is performed and sometimes even then cause may not be identified.

UTERINE RUPTURE

Uterine rupture is a life-threatening complication for both mother and fetus. In developing countries, maternal mortality from uterine rupture may be 5 to 15 percent and fetal loss can exceed 80 percent as limitation of health services is a major contributing factor.[7] In developed countries, maternal mortality is rare but morbidity associated with hemorrhage and emergency hysterectomy is common.

Clinical Features and Diagnosis

Classically, patient with a previous uterine scar presents with sudden feeling of something giving way, cessation of uterine contractions, abnormal abdominal contour, severe abdominal pain, hemorrhage and collapse. Tenderness over scar site is often cited as sign of impending rupture.

Where rupture follows obstructed labor, patient becomes exhausted along with rise of temperature, rapidity of pulse and respiration, dry tongue, edema and arrest of secretions of vaginal glands with formation of large caput and excessive moulding of fetal head. Bladder involvement may present with hematuria and tenesmus.

Treatment

Irrespective of cause, supportive treatment should be started immediately. Laparotomy constitutes definitive treatment. After delivery of fetus and securing hemostasis, the choice of surgery depends upon extent of rupture. If the laceration is reparable, repair the uterus along with tubal ligation provided that patient has no desire to retain her fertility. Hysterectomy is required if there is extensive involvement. In most cases of previous scar, repair is possible but a rupture following obstructed labor generally ends up in hysterectomy.

BROAD LIGAMENT/RETROPERITONEAL HEMATOMA

These are paradoxical situations because bleeding is occurring but is not revealed. Large quantities of blood can collect intraperitoneally without producing local physical signs, although general signs of shock are obvious.

Cause

These hematomas may be associated with deep cervical lacerations extending in lower uterine segment or with rupture of lateral aspect of lower uterine segment. Rarely episiotomy or perineal tear may extend through vagina, cervix and reach up to lower uterine segment to form a broad ligament hematoma.

Diagnosis

This can be diagnosed on bimanual examination in which a large hematoma displacing uterus to one side may be felt. Ultrasonography may aid in diagnosis.

Management

- If patient is hemodynamically stable, patient can be managed conservatively with intravenous fluids, blood transfusion and observation.
- Angiographic embolization is a good therapeutic modality if available.
- If patient is unstable, laparotomy should be performed followed by evacuation of hematoma and ligation of bleeding points. In some situations this can be tricky and internal iliac artery ligation may be all that is possible, though it is usually successful.

ACCIDENTS TO OVARIAN CYSTS

Torsion of cyst may occur in labor and occasionally cyst may rupture if it is in path of presenting part resulting in shock. Immediate surgical correction is indicated.

ANESTHETIC ACCIDENTS

Anesthetic complications are notorious in obstetric patients but fortunately are fewer in the current era of safe anesthetic agents. As these patients are directly under close monitoring, they are generally identified early and appropriate management is instituted.

It must be emphasized that postpartum collapse is an uncommon event. This itself means that an individual obstetrician may not see too many cases during their career. Its seriousness merits immediate management but the critical situation may preclude clarity of thought in management Therefore, a suggested algorithm for approach to such a patient is presented below (Flow chart 19.1).

Flow chart 19.1: Algorithm for approach to a case of postpartum collapse

KEY POINTS

- Postpartum collapse is hemodynamic instability of a patient who has recently delivered.
- In the majority of patients revealed hemorrhage is the cause.
- In those without hemorrhage important causes include internal blood loss (uterine rupture, broad ligament hematoma) and pulmonary embolism (thromboembolism, amniotic fluid embolism).
- Resuscitation along with a quick diagnosis of the cause of collapse is essential for optimal management. However, the cause is often difficult to identify and supportive treatment is instituted till the cause is pinpointed.

REFERENCES

1. Tuffnell DJ. Amniotic fluid embolism. Curr Opin Obstet Gynecol 2003;15:119-22.
2. Davies S. Amniotic fluid embolus: a review of the literature. Can J Anaesth 2001;48:88-98.
3. Benson MD. Anaphylactoid syndrome of pregnancy. Am J Obstet Gynecol 1996;175:749.
4. Clark SL. New concepts of amniotic fluid embolism: a review. Obstet Gynecol Surv 1990;45:360-68.
5. Kaneko Y, Ogihara T, Tajima H, Mochimaru F. Continous hemodiafilteration for disseminated intravascular coagulation and shock due to amniotic fluid embolism: report of a dramatic response. Intern Med 2001;40:945-47.
6. Thromboembolic disorders. In: Cunningham F. Gary, Lenevo Kenneth J, Bloom Steven L, Hauth John C, Rouse Dwight J, Spong Catherine Y (eds). Williams's obstetrics. 23rd edn. McGraw-Hill, 2010.pp. 1014.
7. Hofmeyr GJ, Say L, Gülmezoglu AM. WHO systematic review of maternal mortality and morbidity: the prevalence of uterine rupture. BJOG 2005;112:1221-8.

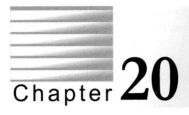

Chapter **20**

Puerperal Sepsis

YM Mala, Parul R

INTRODUCTION

Pelvic infections are the most common serious complications of puerperium, and along with pre-eclampsia and obstetric hemorrhage, have formed the lethal triad of causes of maternal death for many decades.[1] Puerperal fever is technically defined as temperature of 38°C (100.4°F) or higher, occuring on any 2 of the first 10 days postpartum, exclusive of the first 24 hours, and to be taken by mouth by a standard technique at least 4 times daily.[1] Though most persistent fevers associated with childbirth are caused by genital tract infections, extragenital causes must be excluded.

Causes of Puerperal Pyrexia

*   Breast infection and milk engorgement.
*   Puerperal sepsis.
*   Urinary tract infections, e.g. pyelonephritis or cystitis.
*   Deep venous thrombosis.
*   Respiratory infection, e.g. influenza, tonsillitis, pneumonia.
*   General diseases, e.g. typhoid or malaria.
*   Complications in an associated pelvic tumor like degenerated fibroid (rare).

Every case of puerperal pyrexia should be regarded as a case of puerperal sepsis until proven otherwise.

Source of Infection

Bacteria may be either endogenous or exogenous.

*   *Endogenous bacteria:* These are bacteria which normally live in the vagina and rectum without causing harm (e.g. some types of Streptococci and Staphylococci, *E.coli, Clostridium welchii*). Even when a clean technique is used for delivery, infection can still occur from endogenous bacteria. Endogenous bacteria can become harmful and cause infection if:
    *   They are carried into the uterus from the vagina by the examining finger or by instruments during pelvic examinations.
    *   There is tissue damage, i.e. bruised, lacerated or dead tissue (e.g. after a traumatic delivery or following obstructed labour).
    *   There is prolonged rupture of membranes because micro-organisms can then enter the uterus.

- *Exogenous bacteria:* These are bacteria which are introduced into the vagina from the outside (streptococci, staphylococci, *clostridium tetani*, etc.). Exogenous bacteria can be introduced into the vagina:
  - By unclean hands and unsterile instruments.
  - By droplet infection (e.g. a health provider sneezing, coughing onto own hands immediately prior to examination).
  - By foreign substances that are inserted into the vagina (e.g. herbs, oil, cloth).
  - By sexual activity.

Causative Organisms

- *There is usually a mixed infection of gram -ve, gram +ve and anaerobic organisms:*
- *Anaerobic streptococci*—This is the most common cause, usually causing a mild infection.
- Group-A hemolytic streptococci—are responsible for severe cases.
- Staphylococci, usually present in infected perineal or episiotomy wounds- cause suppuration and pus formation.
- *E. Coli* and other nonhemolytic streptococci.
- Specific organisms—*Clostridia welchii* and tetani, gonococci, and Chlamydia.

Risk Factors for Puerperal Sepsis

Antepartum Factors

- Malnutrition and anemia
- Preterm labour
- Premature rupture of membranes
- Prolonged rupture of membranes >18 hrs
- Chronic debilitating illness
- Immunodeficiency

Intrapartum Factors

- Repeated vaginal examinations
- Traumatic operative delivery
- Dehydration and ketoacidosis during labour
- Hemorrhage – antepartum or postpartum
- Retained bits of placental tissue or membranes
- Placenta previa – placental site lying close to vagina
- Cesarean delivery

Clinical Features

Various presentations of puerperal sepsis depend on site of infection:

Primary Sites of Infection

- *Perineum:* Lacerations of the perineum are likely to be infected by organisms of low virulence. There may be collections of seropurulent discharge or pus which results in complete disruption of the wound.
- *Vagina and cervix:* Vaginal lacerations may be infected directly or by extension of the perineal lacerations. Infected lacerations of vagina cause mild pyrexia, local discomfort or pain, tenderness, edema and congestion and are relieved by drainage of the pus. Cervix also gets lacerated frequently.

- *Uterus (Endomyometritis):* The incidence is about 1 to 3 percent following vaginal delivery and 10 percent following cesarean delivery.

Secondary Sites of Infection

- *Parametritis:* It occurs about the 10th day after delivery.
  Patient may have a rise of temperature and pulse, vague abdominal pain, backache but there is no abdominal rigidity.
  Vaginal examination: Uterus may be pulled to one side or fixed.
  Per rectal examination: A firm tender mass extending from the uterus to the lateral pelvic wall on one or both sides. Softening in the mass usually indicates suppuration (parametric abscess).
- *Salpingo-oophoritis*
  Patient presents with fever, rigors, vomiting and lower abdominal pain.
  Abdominal examination: Tenderness and rigidity in the iliac fossa.
  Vaginal examination: There is tenderness, fullness in both fornices and bilateral lower abdominal pain on moving the cervix.
- *Pelvic peritonitis:* It usually develops as a complication of salpingitis.
  Patient presents with pyrexia, tachycardia and lower abdominal pain.
  Abdominal examination: Tenderness and rigidity on lower abdomen.
- *Pelvic abscess:* Pelvic peritonitis may result in a pelvic abscess.
  Patient presents with diarrhea and rectal tenesmus.
  Vaginal examination: Tender fluctuant swelling in the pouch of Douglas (POD) felt through the posterior fornix.

Generalized Spread, Septicemia and Pyemia

- *Generalized peritonitis:* Patient presents with toxic general condition, generalized abdominal pain, continuous vomiting and may be dehydrated, there may also be rigors and high fever.
  On examination there is tachycardia, abdominal tenderness and distension but rigidity may not be marked (due to the previous stretch of the abdominal muscles during pregnancy).
- *Septicemia:* It usually occurs about the 3rd or 4th day after delivery secondary to virulent uterine infection. There is a more marked rise of temperature and increase of pulse rate (120 or more) which is raised out of proportion to pyrexia, rigors, severe headache and abdominal pain. Sometimes erythematous skin eruptions occur.
  Diagnosis is based on positive blood cultures.

CASE SCENARIO-1

A 23-yr-old P2L2 presented to the emergency with complaints of feeling unwell since her delivery (a week ago). She gave history of high-grade fever for past 4 days lower abdominal pain and foul smelling discharge per vaginum for 2 days.

> **Comments:** In this patient diagnosis of puerperal sepsis should be considered since she complained of lower abdominal pain, fever ≥100.4°F for more than 24 hours and foul smelling lochia.

POINTS TO BE NOTED IN THE HISTORY

- Time of onset of fever following delivery
- Method and place of delivery and the person who conducted it (trained/untrained)
- Time of rupture of membranes in relation to delivery
- Any problem encountered during delivery (retained products, manual removal of placenta, postpartum hemorrhage (PPH), suturing of lacerations (cervical, vaginal, perineal)
- Urinary catheterization during delivery

- Fatigue, loss of appetite
- Abdominal pain (localized or all over the abdomen). Onset of pain, duration and site
- Nausea, vomiting and diarrhea
- Breast (inability to feed the baby, breast pain, breast swelling)
- Sore throat
- Burning micturition
- Lower limb pain or swelling
- History of diabetes
- Whether known HIV positive
- Past history (fever, tuberculosis, anemia).

> **History in this case:**
> Patient gave history of leaking per vaginum for 2 days prior to delivery. There is history of fever >100.4°C for 2 days, lower abdominal pain and foul smelling lochia. There was no history of retained products, manual removal of placenta or PPH.

POINTS TO BE NOTED IN EXAMINATION

General Examination

- Pulse rate, temperature, respiratory rate and blood pressure (BP)
- Anemia
- Tonsils and pharynx
- Breast engorgement, tender swelling or breast abscess, pallor, skin eruptions or jaundice (due to hemolysis in *Clostridia welchii* septicemia).
- Axilla- Axillary tail/abscess
- Lower limbs for evidence of thrombophlebitis (swollen, painful, tender legs).

Cardiovascular and Respiratory System Examination

Abdominal Examination

- Tenderness in the abdomen, suprapubic (uterus) or loins or iliac fossa
- Distension, rigidity and guarding
- Presence of free fluid
- Height of the fundus and any abdominal masses in relation to the uterus
- Intestinal sounds may be absent or sluggish in case of peritonitis.

Pelvic Examination

Per Speculum (P/S) Examination

- Lochia (amount, character, color and odor).
- Perineal or vaginal lacerations (tender, swollen).

Per Vaginal (P/V) Examination

- Size and mobility of the uterus
- Tenderness on moving the cervix in case of salpingo-oophoritis
- Any pelvic swelling with associated tenderness in fornices.
- Bogginess or fullness of POD in case of pelvic abscess
- Uterus is fixed in case of parametritis

Per Rectal Examination

In case of parametritis, tender swelling extends from sides of the uterus to pelvic bones depending on the severity.

> **Examination in this case:**
> She was febrile (101°F), pulse—114/min, BP—100/70, mild pallor present.
> Abdominal examination—A soft abdomen with normal bowel sounds and tenderness in infraumbilical region.
> P/S—Lochia was foul smelling, purulent discharge coming through os.
> P/V—External os patulous, internal os closed and uterus 12-14 weeks size, tender on movement. Bilateral forniceal tenderness was present. No fullness in POD

Diagnosis

Puerperal sepsis

INVESTIGATIONS

- Complete hemogram—Hb, total and differential leukocyte counts
- Midstream urine specimen for culture.
- Swab from the upper vagina or cervix for culture and sensitivity for bacteriologic examination.
- Blood cultures taken at the height of the fever.
- Other investigations if necessary such as Widal test for typhoid, X-ray chest, blood film for malaria.
- Ultrasound is important to detect uterine collection, tubo-ovarian swelling, pelvic abscess and peritoneal collections of pus.
- Doppler ultrasound is of great value in cases of suspected pelvic thrombophlebitis.

TREATMENT

- Broad spectrum antibiotics should be started immediately, covering gram +ve, gram -ve and anaerobic organisms. One of the commonly used regimens is
  - Ampicillin 1 gm intravenous (IV) every 6 hours.
  - Gentamycin 80 mg or Amikacin 0.5 gm intramuscular (IM) or IV every 8 hours.
  - Metronidazole 500 mg IV every 8 hours.
- After 48 hours same drugs may be continued or changed to another drug regimen according to the clinical response (temperature, pulse, abdominal and vaginal examination) and the sensitivity test result.
- In cases of *Cl. welchii* infection anti-gas gangrene serum is also given.
- If patient is not responding (high temperature, vomiting, abdominal pain) to the previous measures—pus collection is suspected.

Promotion of Drainage

- Semi-sitting (Fowler's) position.
- Small doses of ergot to increase the tone of the uterus may be used.
- Removal of sutures in infected episiotomy or cesarean section wound sites.
- Drainage of pelvic abscess by posterior colpotomy.
- Gentle removal of any piece of retained placental cotyledon if felt bulging from the cervix during vaginal examination or suction curettage of retained placental bits in the uterus.
- Drainage of uterine collections by dilatation of cervix in case of pyometra (ultrasound shows fluid collection).

- Presence of pyoperitoneum needs a laparotomy followed by drainage of pus and thorough abdominal lavage. If the condition of the patient does not permit so, a closed drainage under ultrasound guidance may be considered.

> **Management in this case:**
> All investigations were sent
> Ultrasound imaging did not show any retained POCs.
> She responded well to IV broad spectrum antibiotics.

CASE SCENARIO-2

A 26-yr-old primigravida underwent a cesarean section for meconium stained liquor with non – reassuring fetal heart pattern. Patient was well for first 3 days of the post-operative period. On the 4th post-operative day she developed high-grade fever, associated with chills. Despite 3 days of IV antibiotics her fever did not subside. On examination, a tender fluctuant mass was felt in the POD. She responded to continued IV broad spectrum antibiotic coverage and drainage by posterior colpotomy incision.

> **Conmments:**
> Diagnosis of pelvic abscess was considered because of:
> a. High-grade fever not responding to routine IV antibiotics.
> b. A tender fluctuant mass in the POD.
> c. Patient responded after drainage of abscess.

MEDICAL AND SURGICAL COMPLICATIONS OF PUERPERAL SEPSIS

Wound Infections

The incidence of abdominal incisional infections following cesarean delivery ranges from 3 to 15 percent,[2] with an average of 6 percent.[3] When prophylactic antimicrobials have been given, the incidence is less than 2 percent.[4] Risk factors are obesity, diabetes, corticosteroid therapy, immunosuppression, anemia and poor hemostasis with hematoma formation.

Clinical Features

- Fever which develops around the 4th postoperative day. If there is accompanying uterine infection then fever may persist from the 1st or 2nd postoperative day.
- Wound becomes swollen and red.
- Pus may form which leads to disruption of wound.

Treatment

Antimicrobials and surgical drainage with careful inspection to ensure that abdominal fascia is intact.

Wound Dehiscence

Disruption or dehiscence refers to separation of the fascial layer. Treatment includes secondary closure under anesthesia.

Necrotizing Fascitis

Fortunately this most serious of all wound infections is rare, but it is associated with high mortality. These infections may involve abdominal incisional infections, or may complicate episiotomy or perineal lacerations. Diabetes and obesity predispose to it. Infection may be caused by a single virulent bacterial species such as group A β–hemolytic streptococci, but more commonly infections are polymicrobial.

Treatment

Clindamycin given with β–lactam antibiotic is the most effective regimen. Adjunctive treatment includes promptly debriding wide margins of the fascial incision. With extensive resection, synthetic mesh may be required to close the fascial incision.

Peritonitis

Occasionally, this condition is encountered following cesarean delivery complicated with metritis and uterine incisional necrosis and dehiscence. Likewise, a parametrial or adnexal abscess may rupture to produce generalized peritonitis.

Clinical Features

Abdominal rigidity may not be a prominent feature because of the abdominal wall laxity due to pregnancy. Pain may be severe. Paralytic ileus may be a feature. Thus, there may be marked bowel distension.

Treatment

Antimicrobial therapy may suffice in most cases. Conversely, peritonitis caused by uterine incisional necrosis or by a bowel lesion is treated surgically along with antimicrobial therapy.

Adnexal Infections

An ovarian abscess rarely develops from puerperal infection, presumably from bacterial invasion through a rent in the ovarian capsule. The abscess is usually unilateral and patient typically presents 1 to 2 weeks after delivery.

Parametrial Phlegmon

In some women who develop metritis following cesarean delivery, parametrial cellulitis is intense forming an area of induration, termed a *phlegmon*, within the leaves of the broad ligament. These infections should be suspected when fever persists for longer than 72 hours despite IV antibiotics.[5] These are usually unilateral and frequently limited to the base of the broad ligament. Most commonly, they extend laterally to the lateral pelvic wall. Posterior extension may involve the rectovaginal septum, forming a firm mass posterior to the cervix.

Clinical Features

Pain is a common feature due to necrosis and separation. Peritonitis may develop due to extrusion of purulent material. On examination a woody, indurated mass is felt unilaterally.

Treatment

In most women with a phlegmon clinical improvement follows continued treatment with a broad-spectrum antimicrobial regimen. Complete absorption may take several days to weeks. Surgery is reserved for women in whom uterine incisional necrosis is suspected. Hysterectomy and surgical debridement are usually difficult, & there is often appreciable blood loss. In rare cases, uterine debridement and resuturing of the incision are feasible. Sometimes the intense inflammatory process extends to the pelvic side wall and may involve the ureters. Adnexa are seldom involved, and one or both ovaries usually can be conserved.

Abscess Formation

Rarely, a parametrial phlegmon suppurates, forming a fluctuant mass that may point above the Poupart's ligament. They may dissect posteriorly to involve the rectovaginal septum. Sometimes, a psoas abscess may form following delivery.

Treatment

These abscesses may be amenable to CT guided needle drainage. A rectovaginal abscess may be drained by a colpotomy incision. Psoas abscess is easily accessible percutaneously.

Septic Pelvic Thrombophlebitis

Puerperal infection may extend along venous routes and cause thrombosis. Lymphangitis often co-exists. The ovarian veins may become involved because they drain the upper uterus, which often includes veins draining the placental site.[6,7] Overall incidence is 1:2000 to 1:3000.[8]

Clinical Features

These women continue to have fever despite antimicrobial coverage. They may be asymptomatic except for chills. In some women, the cardinal feature is pain typically manifested on the 2nd or 3rd postpartum day.

Diagnosis

Diagnosis is by computerized tomography (CT) or magnetic resonance imaging (MRI). Doppler will detect the site of the thrombosed vessel.

Treatment

- Continue the use of antibiotics.
- Anticoagulation (parentral heparin). Before imaging modalities were available, heparin challenge test was used for diagnosis. However, in a follow-up randomized study it was concluded that the addition of heparin to antimicrobial therapy did not hasten recovery or improve outcome.[9] Therefore, the use of heparin is controversial.
- Immobilization of the limb until temperature subsides.

PREVENTION

Antenatal

- Improve the general condition by proper diet, vitamins and minerals.
- Treat diseases which lower resistance such as anemia, toxemia or diabetes.
- Treat vaginal discharge (high vaginal swab culture) or any septic focus.

Intranatal

Proper management of delivery including strict asepsis for the patient, instruments and attendants, and avoidance of unnecessary vaginal examination.

Postnatal

- Maintenance of aseptic precautions.
- Minimize visitors particularly those showing any infection.
- Early isolation of suspected cases.

KEY POINTS

- Puerperal sepsis is an important cause of maternal death
- Every case of puerperal pyrexia should be regarded as a case of puerperal sepsis until proven otherwise.

- The incidence is more common with operative delivery.
- Broad spectrum antibiotics should be started immediately, covering gram +ve, gram -ve and anerobic organisms.
- In case of pelvic abscess drainage should be performed.
- Doppler study is helpful in diagnosing septic pelvic thrombophlebitis.

REFERENCES

1. Puerperal Infection. In: Cunningham FG, Leveno KJ, Bloom SL, Hauth JC, Gilstrap LC III, Wenstrom KD (eds). Williams Obstetrics. 22nd edn. New Delhi:Mc Graw Hill, 2005.pp. 711-24.

2. Chaim W, Bashiri A, Bar-David J, Shoham-Vardi I, Mazor M. Prevalence and clinical significance of postpartum endometritis and wound infection. Infect Dis Obstet Gynecol 2000;8:77-82.

3. Owen J, Andrews WW. Wound complications after cesarean sections. Clin Obstet Gynecol 1994;37:842-55.

4. Andrews WW, Hauth JC, Cliver SP, Savage K, Goldenberg RL. Randomized clinical trial of extended spectrum antibiotic prophylaxis with coverage for ureaplasma urealyticum to reduce postcesarean delivery endometritis. Obstet Gynecol 2003;101:1183-9.

5. DePalma RT, Cunningham FG, Leveno KJ, Roark ML. Continuing investigation of women at high-risk for infection following cesarean delivery. Three-dose perioperative antimicrobial therapy. Obstet Gynecol 1982;60:53-9.

6. Witlin AG, Sibai BM. Postpartum ovarian vein thrombosis after vaginal delivery: a report of 11 cases. Obstet Gynecol 1995;85:775-80.

7. Brown CE, Dunn DH, Harrell R, Setiawan H, Cunningham FG. Computed tomography for evaluation of puerperal infections. Surg Gynecol Obstet 1991;172:285-9.

8. Dunnihoo DR, Gallaspy JW, Wise RB, Otterson WN. Postpartum ovarian vein thrombophlebitis: a review. Obstet Gynecol Surv 1991;46:415-27.

9. Brown CE, Stettler RW, Twickler D, Cunningham FG. Puerperal septic pelvic thrombophlebitis: incidence and response to heparin therapy. Am J Obstet Gynecol 1999;181:143-8.

Chapter 21

Abnormal Behavior in a Postpartum Patient

Chandan Dubey

INTRODUCTION

Abnormal behavior in a postpartum patient could be due to postpartum psychosis, pre-existing psychiatric disorder or an organic cause like a neurological or endocrinological disease.

Postpartum psychosis is an obstetric emergency which occurs in 1-2/1000 women within 2 to 4 weeks of delivery.[1] It may start as early as 2 to 3 days after delivery. There is a dramatic change in behavior, with the patient experiencing mood swings, bizarre and grandiose delusions and hallucinations, confusion and extremely disorganized behavior. It is the most severe form of postpartum psychiatric disorder but fortunately the rarest, with the less severe ***postpartum depression*** and ***maternity blues*** occurring in 10 percent and 80 percent of new mothers respectively. It is critical to identify and treat women with postpartum psychosis as it may lead to grave consequences affecting the health and wellbeing of mothers and their infants.

According to the *Diagnostic and Statistical Manual of Mental Disorders,* 4th ed. (DSM-IV)[2] postpartum psychosis is a severe form of major depression or the onset/recurrence of a primary psychotic disorder like schizophrenia. There is evidence to suggest that 72 to 88 percent of patients with postpartum psychosis have bipolar or schizoaffective disorder and around 12 percent have schizophrenia.[3] Other possible contributing factors are postpartum hormonal changes and psychosocial stressors like lack of financial and emotional support or marital discord.[4] Women with bipolar disorder or a personal or family history of postpartum psychosis are at substantial risk and should be screened throughout pregnancy and puerperium using tools like Edinburgh Postnatal Depression Scale (EPDS) or advised psychiatry referral.

Postpartum psychosis is an emergency in which patient needs to be hospitalized and urgently evaluated. A psychiatry referral should be taken. The initial evaluation should include a thorough history and examination and investigations to rule out an organic cause for postpartum psychosis. Women with untreated psychosis are at risk of suicide and infanticide.[5,6]

CASE SCENARIO-1

Mrs. X, a 28-year-old G2 P1 had a full term normal vaginal delivery of a healthy baby. She was discharged after 24 hours. On the 4th postpartum day she was brought to the gynecological emergency by her husband in a disoriented state. She was well for 3 days after delivery and was breastfeeding her baby. On the 4th day she complained of insomnia, developed paranoid delusions and auditory hallucinations and stopped breastfeeding her baby. She also complained of feelings of intense dislike for the baby.

> **Comment:** This patient has presented with abnormal behavior postpartum. While a provisional diagnosis of postpartum psychosis is made, any organic cause must be ruled out.

Differential Diagnosis of Postpartum Psychosis and Relevant Investigations

Psychiatric Disorders

- Bipolar disorder
- Unipolar depression
- Schizophrenia or
- Obsessive compulsive disorder.
  Patient's past history of psychiatric disorder, past or family history of postpartum psychosis needs to be taken.

Medical Causes

- Cerebrovascular:
  - Ischemic stroke (arterial or venous) secondary to pre-eclampsia, eclampsia, severe hemorrhage or cerebral vein thrombosis.
  - Hemorrhagic stroke due to uncontrolled hypertension, aneurysm, arteriovenous malformation, disseminated intravascular coagulation. History of hypertension, pre-eclampsia, headache, unilateral weakness, new onset sensory deficits or seizures should be taken. Blood pressure should be taken. In suspected cases magnetic resonance imaging (MRI) or computerized tomography (CT) head should be done along with neurology consultation.
- Metabolic or nutritional:
  - Hyponatremia or hypernatremia. Serum electrolytes should be checked
  - Diabetic ketoacidosis or hypoglycemia. Fasting blood glucose and HbA1C should be checked in patients with diabetes mellitus or gestational diabetes
  - Uremic encephalopathy. Blood urea and creatinine levels are checked in patients with renal dysfunction
  - Hepatic failure. Liver function tests are done in patients with hepatitis or liver disease
  - Thyrotoxicosis or myxedema. Thyroid function tests are done in suspected cases
  - Vitamin B_{12}, folate or thiamine deficiency. Serum B_{12}, RBC folate and thiamine levels are checked in anemic and malnourished women.
- Medications:
  - Corticosteroids, narcotics, benzodiazepines and barbiturates. History to rule out any such drug intake should be taken.
- Immunological:
  - Systemic lupus erythematosus needs to be ruled out in the medical history.
- Infectious:
  - Sepsis
  - Meningitis or encephalitis
  - HIV
    Complete blood count, HIV test, lumbar puncture and CT head may be done in suspected cases.

> **History in this case:**
> - There was no history suggestive of organic disease like fever, headache, neurological deficits, and seizures.
> - Her present pregnancy had been uneventful.
> - She had been treated for depression following her last delivery 5 years back for 6 months, after which she had discontinued medication on her own. She had not revealed this history in the present antenatal follow up.
> - There was no other significant past medical history of hypertension, diabetes mellitus, liver or renal disorder or thyroid disease.

Risk factors in this case: Past history of postpartum depression puts this patient at a high-risk of developing similar problem in future pregnancies. If she had revealed the history antenatally, the treating obstetrician could have prophylactically taken a psychiatry consultation earlier and screened her using EPDS.

Examination in this case:
Patient was conscious but disoriented.
She was afebrile with pulse—78/minute; BP—110/70 mm Hg and respiratory rate—12/minute.
There was no pallor, icterus or cyanosis.
Thyroid was not enlarged.
Neurological, chest, cardiovascular, abdominal and pelvic examination was normal.

Diagnosis

Psychiatry consultation was taken and diagnosis of postpartum psychosis was made.

Investigations in this case:
Hemogram, blood sugar, serum electrolytes, renal and liver function tests and TSH levels were normal.

TREATMENT

The various treatment modalities are:
• Psychotherapy
• Pharmacotherapy
• Electroconvulsive therapy (ECT)
Acute treatment includes:
• A mood stabilizer like lithium, valproate or carbamezapine.
• Antipsychotics and benzodiazepines.
• If pharmacotherapy is not enough ECT is well tolerated and rapidly effective.

Antipsychotics used are the older group called "typical antipsychotics "or the newer "atypical antipsychotics "(Table 21.1 and 21.2)

The older antipsychotics act by blocking action of dopamine in the brain while the atypical ones have less dopamine blocking property but act on other chemical messengers like serotonin and hence have lesser Parkinsonian side-effects and tardive dyskinesia.

Table 21.1: Typical Antipsychotics

Tablets	Trade name	Usual daily dose (mg)
Chlorpromazine	Largactil	75-300
Haloperidol	Haldol	3-15
Pimozide	Orap	4-20
Trifluoperazine	Stelazine	5-20

Table 21.2: Atypical Antipsychotics

Tablets	Trade name	Usual daily dose (mg)
Clozapine	Clozaril	200-450
Olanzapine	Zyprexa	10-20
Risperidone	Risperidal	4-6
Zotepine	Zoleptil	75-200

Care of Baby

Help of social worker, patient's husband and relatives needs to be taken to ensure that baby is well cared for and attended at all times. Antipsychotic drugs are secreted in breast milk and baby should be under followup of pediatrician for symptoms of toxicity.

Treatment in this case:
The patient was admitted and started on haloperidol, sodium valproate and lorazepam by the psychiatrist. Later on sertraline was added for persistent depression.
Her mood and symptoms improved and she was discharged on the above medication after 10 days, with advice to follow up in psychiatry clinic.

CEREBRAL VEIN THROMBOSIS

Clinical Presentation

Cerebral vein thrombosis can occur any time in pregnancy but is most commonly seen in second or third week after delivery.[7] The patient may present with varied symptoms and signs ranging from headache, seizures, focal neurologic deficits, aphasia, visual disturbances, papilledema, lethargy, confusion or coma.

Predisposing Factors

Apart from the fact that puerperium is a hypercoagulable state, other predisposing factors for postpartum cerebral vein thrombosis are anemia, infection, dehydration, hemoglobinopathies, hyperviscosity syndromes, leukemia, collagen vascular disease and thrombophilias.[8,9] In the present case anemia and dehydration due to gastroenteritis could have contributed.

Investigations

Magnetic resonance venography is the most sensitive investigation and the test of choice.[10]

Treatment

Systemic anticoagulation with heparin is the treatment of choice.[11] Long-term anticoagulation is needed with warfarin after the acute phase is over.

Prognosis

The prognosis is good in the absence of coma, recurrent seizures or declining neurological status.

CASE SCENARIO-2

A 28-year-old lady was brought to gynecological emergency 10 days after delivery with the complaint of severe headache, disorientation and confused behavior and history of one episode of seizure at home.

Comments: Complains of severe headache and seizures should raise the suspicion of an organic cause of abnormal behavior in this patient.

History in this case:
She had delivered her second baby by a normal vaginal delivery ten days earlier in the same hospital. There were no antepartum or intrapartum complications except anemia. Her hemoglobin was 8.4 gm% before and 7.6 gm% after delivery. She had been discharged 48 hours after delivery on iron tablets.
She developed gastroenteritis at home on the 7th day which was treated by a physician and improved on the 9th day.

Examination in this case:
She was irritable and disoriented.
She was afebrile with pulse—90/ minute and BP—120 /70 mm Hg
There was mild pallor and dehydration.
There were no sensory neurological deficits but some motor weakness of left side was evident.
Respiratory, cardiovascular, abdominal and pelvic examination was normal.

Diagnosis

Cerebral vein thrombosis

Investigations in this case:
Presence of neurological deficit was suggestive of an intracranial event in this patient.
Urgent neurology consultation was taken and magnetic resonance (MR) venography was done.
MR venography—superior sagittal sinus thrombosis.
Hemogram, blood sugars, liver and renal function tests were normal.

Treatment in this case:
Patient was admitted in neurology ward and started on heparin infusion. Clinical improvement was seen after 10 days of therapy and she was switched over to warfarin. Repeat MRI showed resolving thrombus.

KEY POINTS

- Abnormal behavior in a postpartum patient could be due to psychiatric disorder or an organic cause.
- Thorough history, examination and necessary investigations will help to arrive at the correct diagnosis.
- Multidisciplinary input from neurologist, psychiatrist and physician may be needed.

REFERENCES

1. Kendell R, Chalmers J, Platz C. Epidemiology of puerperal psychoses. Br J Psychiatry 1987;150:662.
2. American Psychiatric Association. Diagnostic and statistical manual for mental disorders, 4th edn. Washington, DC: American Psychiatric Press, 1994.
3. Brockington IF: Puerperal psychosis. Motherhood and mental health. New York: Oxford University Press, 1996:200.
4. Sharma V, Smith A, Khan M: The relationship between duration of labour, time of delivery, and puerperal psychosis. J Affective Disord 2004;83:215.
5. Kumar R, Marks M, Platz C, Yoshida K: Clinical survey of a psychiatric mother and baby unit: Characteristics of 100 consecutive admissions. J Affective Disord 1995;33:11.
6. CEMD. Confidential inquiries into maternal deaths: Why mothers die, 1997–99. London: Royal College of Obstetricians and Gynaecologists, 2001.
7. Srinivasan K. Cerebral venous and arterial thrombosis in pregnancy and puerperium: A study of 135 patients. Angiology 1983;34:731-74.
8. Wozniak AJ, Kitchens CS. Prospective hemostatic studies in patient with paroxysmal nocturnal hemoglobinuria, pregnancy and cerebral venous thrombosis. Am J Obstet Gynecol 1982;142:591-93.
9. Bousser MG, Chiras J, Bories J, et al. Cerebral venous thrombosis- A review of 38 cases. Stroke 1985;16:199-213.
10. Carhuapoma JR, Tomlinson MW, Levine SR. Neurologic Disorders. In: James DK, Steer PJ, Weiner CP, Gonik B (eds). High Risk Pregnancy: Management Options. 3rd edn. Philadelphia PA: Elsevier Saunders, 2006. pp. 1061-97.
11. Einhaupl KM, Villringer A, Meister W, et al. Heparin treatment in sinus venous thrombosis. Lancet 1991;338:597-600.

Chapter 22

Resuscitation of the Depressed Neonate in Delivery Room

Siddarth Ramji

INTRODUCTION

There are about 26 million births each year in India (which is almost one-fifth of the global burden) and of these 1.2 million infants die before the age of one month (India's share of neonatal deaths is almost one-third of the global neonatal deaths). Asphyxia at birth contributes to approximately 25 percent of these deaths.

BIRTH ASPHYXIA

Apgar score has been traditionally used to identify birth asphyxia (Table 22.1). Birth asphyxia has been defined variously as Apgar score < 7 at 1-min, no breathing at birth or gasping respiration at birth. The more appropriate term for these infants is *nonvigorous depressed* infants since not all neonates who are unable to breath at birth have antecedent intrapartum hypoxia, e.g. extremely preterm infants, those with malformations of the thoracic cage/respiratory system or where there has been maternal narcotic administration have usually no associated intrapartum hypoxia.[1] It is the commonest neonatal emergency in the delivery room. It is estimated that about 10 percent newborn infants do not establish adequate breathing efforts at birth and need assistance to establish adequate breathing/ventilation. Table 22.2 lists the risk factors associated with the need for neonatal resuscitation; however, it is important to remember that not all infants born depressed at birth have one or more of these associated risk factors. Thus, all personnel in the delivery room must be trained in basic neonatal resuscitation and every birth must be treated as a potential emergency needing resuscitation at birth.

IDENTIFICATION OF NEWBORNS WHO NEED RESUSCITATION AT BIRTH

To identify neonates who would need resuscitation at birth, one needs to identify if the baby is depressed/nonvigorous at birth. Ask the following 2 questions:
1. Is the baby crying or breathing? (*Identified by observing chest rise which should be visible and regular*)
2. Is there good muscle tone? (*Identified by noting the posture which should show generalized flexion at upper and lower limbs*)

If the answer to both the questions is "**Yes**", then the newborn needs to be dried and kept warm. Both these actions can be performed with the newborn lying on the mother's chest and should not require separation of mother and baby.

Table 22.1: Apgar score			
Parameters	*0*	*1*	*2*
Respiratory effort	Absent	Gasping	Good cry
Heart rate	Zero	< 100/min	>100/min
Color	Central cyanosis	Peripheral cyanosis	Pink
Tone	Flaccid	Partial flexion of extremities	Complete flexion
Response to nasal catheter	None	Grimace	Sneeze

Table 22.2: Risk factors associated with need for neonatal resuscitation	
Antepartum factors	*Intrapartum factors*
• Maternal diabetes • Pregnancy induced hypertension • Anemia • Antepartum hemorrhage • Maternal infection • Maternal cardiac, renal or pulmonary disease • Polyhydramnios • Oligohydramnios • Premature rupture of membranes • Post-term gestation • Multiple gestation • Fetal malformation • Maternal substance abuse • Diminished fetal activity • No antenatal care • Maternal age < 16 or > 35 years	• Emergency cesarean section • Forceps or vacuum assisted delivery • Breech or other abnormal presentation • Premature labor • Chorioamnionitis • Prolonged labor (> 24 hours) • Fetal bradycardia • Use of general anesthesia • Narcotics administered to mother within 4 hours of delivery • Meconium stained amniotic fluid • Abruptio placentae or placenta previa

If the answer is "**No**" to any of these questions, then the neonate is depressed/non-vigorous and needs resuscitation. The newborn must be assessed to determine their need for one or more of the following actions in sequence:

• Initial steps for stabilization (dry and provide warmth, position, assess airway, stimulate to breathe)
• Ventilation
• Chest compression
• Medications

Progression to the next step is initially based on the simultaneous assessment of respiration and heart rate. Progress to the next step occurs only after the successful completion of the preceding step. Approximately 30 seconds is allotted to complete each of the first 2 steps successfully, reevaluate and decide whether to progress to the next step. This "**golden minute**" is critical to minimize postnatal hypoxia to the neonate (Figure 22.1 summarizes the steps of neonatal resuscitation).[2] Table 22.3 provides a list of equipment that must be available in the delivery room for resuscitation of the newborn infant.

Initial Assessment and Intervention

• Dry all babies soon after birth.
• Assess for the breathing and tone of the baby while drying is done.

Vigorous babies: Neonates who are vigorous should not be separated from the mother and should be kept warm by placing on mother's chest and covering the baby with a sheet of cloth. In vigorous

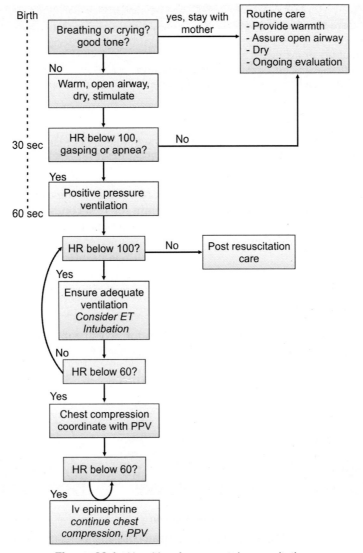

Figure 22.1: Algorithm for neonatal resuscitation

babies cord clamping should be delayed for at least 1 minute, as there is strong evidence of the benefit of the additional transfer of blood to the baby in preventing anemia in the latter months of infancy.[3]

Nonvigorous babies: For nonvigorous babies who need resuscitation, clamp and cut the cord immediately and place the baby under a radiant warmer to provide warmth.

- Open airway and position the head – To open the airway, slightly extend the neck and maintain this position by placing a folded towel (about 1 inch thick) under the shoulder (Figure 22.2).
- Apply suction to the baby's mouth and then the nose using a mucous extractor or Dee Lee trap. There is no evidence that peripartum suctioning benefits neonates who are vigorous irrespective of whether the amniotic fluid is meconium stained or not.[2]

  If amniotic fluid is meconium stained and the baby is not vigorous, suction the baby's mouth and nose. If one has the expertise, then the trachea may also be cleared by suctioning under direct laryngoscopy.
- Tactile stimulation – If the infant is not breathing even after suction, provide tactile stimulation by flicking the sole or gently rubbing the back (Figure 22.3). *Do not slap the back or squeeze the rib cage.*

Table 22.3: List of resuscitation equipment

- Radiant warmer
- Oxygen (central supply or cylinder)
- Suction device (mucus extractor or central suction facility)
- Self-inflating resuscitation bag (250-500 ml) with oxygen reservoir and pop-off valve·Face masks (sizes 0 and 1)
- Laryngoscope (straight blade No. 0,1)
- Endotracheal tubes (sizes 2.5 mm, 3 mm, 3.5 mm ID)
- Drugs – Adrenaline (1:1000), Naloxone, Normal saline and Ringer's lactate
- Intravenous cannula, umbilical catheters, syringes, needles

- Re-assess the neonate. A prompt increase in heart rate remains the most sensitive indicator of resuscitation efficacy. Auscultate over the precordium for 10 seconds and multiply by 10 to get the infant's heart rate. *If the heart rate is below 100 or the neonate is gasping/apneic it is indication to initiate positive pressure ventilation.*

VENTILATION

Positive Pressure Ventilation (PPV)

It can be provided with bag and mask, or bag and endotracheal tube. A small towel 1" thick is placed under the infant's shoulder. The self-inflating bag used for neonates must have a volume

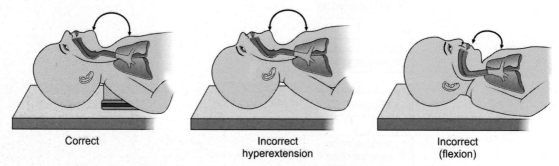

| Correct | Incorrect hyperextension | Incorrect (flexion) |

Figure 22.2: Correct and incorrect head positions for resuscitation

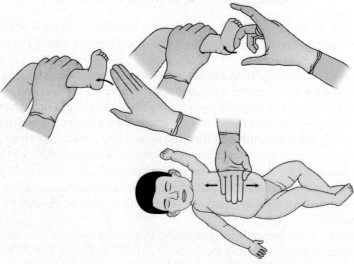

Figure 22.3: Methods to provide tactile stimulation

between 250-500 ml, with an oxygen reservoir. One must select the correct sized mask (zero size for preterm and size one for term infants) for resuscitation. The correct fit mask when placed over the infant's face should cover the chin, mouth and nose and *not the eyes* (Figure 22.4).

Ensure that the mask makes a good seal around the mouth and nose such that when the bag is inflated there is visible chest rise in the infant. If the chest does not rise the possible reasons could be:

- The seal is inadequate
- Airway is blocked
- Insufficient inflation pressure

Rate of Ventilation

If adequate chest rise has been established, the rate of ventilation must be sufficient to provide 40-60 breaths/min. Figure 22.5 provides the rhythm that would enable one to sustain the desired breath rate.

Initiate Ventilation with 21% Oxygen (Room Air)

Current evidence strongly supports initiating resuscitation with room air rather than 100% oxygen.[4] Oxygen may be supplemented if there is access to pulse oximetry in the delivery room and the SaO_2 is < 75%. *Infant color in the delivery room is a poor marker of hypoxia and should not be used for providing supplemental oxygen.*

Good response to assisted ventilation after 30 seconds of ventilation is indicated by:

- Appearance of spontaneous breathing efforts
- Rise in heart rate to more than 100/min

CHEST COMPRESSION

Chest compression (cardiac massage) *is indicated when the heart rate <60/min after 30 seconds of assisted ventilation.* Chest compression requires two personnel – one to continue assisted ventilation and the other to perform chest compressions. The thumb for compression is placed over the lower third of the sternum. Assisted ventilation and chest compression are coordinated in a ratio of 30 ventilation to 90 chest compressions (1:3). Chest compression is discontinued when heart rate rises to above 60/min.

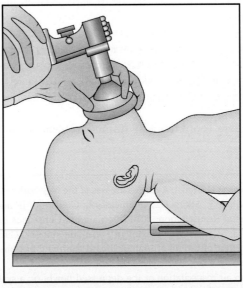

Figure 22.4: Correct position of face mask

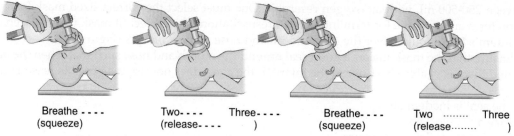

| Breathe - - - -
(squeeze) | Two- - - -
(release- - - -) | Three- - - - | Breathe- - - -
(squeeze) | Two ....
(release........) | Three |

Figure 22.5: Rhythm for maintaining breath rate of 40-60 per minute

MEDICATIONS

Adrenaline—It is indicated whenever the heart rate remains <60/min in spite of chest compression. The dose is 0.1-0.3 ml/kg of 1:10,000 solution given intravenously or intratracheal. The dose may be repeated after 3 to 5 minutes as indicated.

Naloxone—It is a narcotic antagonist. It is indicated to reverse respiratory depression in an infant whose mother has received narcotics within 4 hours of delivery. The dose is 0.1 mg/kg given intravenously, intratracheal or if perfusion is adequate, intramuscular or subcutaneously.

Volume expanders—It is indicated in neonates in shock – poor pulses, pale and cold extremities. Dose is 10 ml/kg of normal saline or Ringer's lactate given by intravenous push over for 5 to 10 minutes. Nonresponse to volume expansion with 20 ml/kg of crystalloid would be indication for ionotropes such as dopamine or dobutamine.

At present there isn't sufficient evidence to recommend use of sodium bicarbonate in the delivery room.

When to Discontinue Resuscitation

It may be appropriate to consider discontinuing resuscitation if no heart rate is detected for 10 minutes.[2]

KEY POINTS

- About 10 percent newborn infants do not establish adequate breathing efforts at birth and need assistance to establish adequate breathing/ventilation.
- Every birth must be treated as a potential emergency needing resuscitation at birth.
- Apgar score used traditionally to identify birth asphyxia, is not a good tool for deciding resuscitative interventions.
- Resuscitation of a nonvigorous baby is performed in a step-wise manner; the first step being positioning the baby's head, opening the airway and suction of baby's mouth and nose.
- If the neonate is not breathing even after suction, tactile stimulation is provided by flicking the sole or gently rubbing the back. Do not slap the back or squeeze the rib cage.
- Subsequently positive pressure ventilation, chest compression and medications may be required.
- All personnel in the delivery room must be trained in basic neonatal resuscitation.

REFERENCES

1. Taeusch HW, Ballard RA, Gleason GA (eds). Avery's Diseases of the Newborn.8th edn. Philadelphia: Saunders, 2005.
2. Perlman JM, Wyllie J, Kattwinkle J, Atkins DL, Chameides L, Goldsmith JP and Neonatal Resuscitation Chapter collaborators. Part 11: Neonatal Resuscitation: 2010 International Consensus on Cardiopulmonary Resuscitation and Emergency cardiovascular Science With Treatment Recommendations. Circulation 2010;122:S516-38.
3. McDonald SJ, Middleton P. Effect of timing of umbilical cord clamping of term infants on maternal and neonatal outcomes. Cochrane Database Syst Rev 2008:CD004074.
4. Rabi Y, Rabi D, Yee W. Room air resuscitation or the depressed newborn: a systematic review and meta-analysis. Resuscitation. 2007;72:353-63.

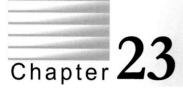

Chapter **23**

Cardiopulmonary Resuscitation of a Pregnant Patient

Anju Bhalotra, Raktima Anand, Gunjan Manchanda

INTRODUCTION

Cardiopulmonary resuscitation (CPR) of a pregnant patient requires special consideration since one is dealing with two potential patients, the mother and the fetus and the best hope for fetal survival is maternal survival. Although pregnant patients are usually younger than other cardiac arrest patients, the survival rates are lower.

Conditions where a Pregnant Patient May Require CPR

1. *Cardiac disease:* The risk of myocardial infarction in pregnancy is 3 to 4 times that of nonpregnant women of reproductive age. Increasing maternal age increases chances of atherosclerotic heart disease and aortic dissection. Also, more women with congenital heart disease are surviving to have children.
2. *Magnesium sulfate toxicity:* Pregnant patients with renal/metabolic derangements may develop toxicity after relatively lower magnesium doses. Empirical calcium administration may be lifesaving.
3. *Pre-eclampsia/Eclampsia:* Severe hypertension with diffuse organ-system failure.
4. *Life-threatening pulmonary embolism/Amniotic fluid embolism.*
5. *Anesthetic complications:* Spinal shock as a result of regional anesthesia; loss of airway control/pulmonary aspiration during general anesthesia; hypoventilation or airway obstruction during emergence from anesthesia; tachyarrhythmias due to bupivacaine toxicity (best treated by electrical cardioversion/bretylium/lipid emulsion).
6. *Concealed/overt hemorrhage:* Uterine atony, abruptio placentae, placenta previa, DIC.
7. Pre-existing anemia.
8. *Trauma/drug overdose.*

Precautions to Prevent Cardiac Arrest in a Critically ill Pregnant Patient

- Nurse in the complete left-lateral position.
- Give 100% oxygen.
- Secure intravenous access above the diaphragm.
- Treat any hypotension aggressively (leads to reduced placental perfusion).
- Detect and treat any reversible causes of critical illness early.

Resuscitation of a pregnant patient is based on the considerations of the physiological changes of pregnancy.

Physiological changes of Pregnancy which Influence CPR

Respiratory	↑alveolar ventilation, intrapulmonary shunting, oxygen consumption, oxygen demand and ↓chest compliance and functional residual capacity → *develop hypoxemia rapidly.* In order to meet increased oxygen needs, a pregnant woman breathes more rapidly -Mild respiratory alkalosis (pH 7.50) and slightly ↑PO_2. Kidneys excrete bicarbonate at increased rate so the pregnant woman is *less able to cope effectively with respiratory compromise or acidosis.*
Airway	Vascular engorgement, edema and soft tissue hypertrophy of the airway and the trachea may be displaced forward → *Difficult intubation* Diabetes, PIH, use of steroids and tocolytics cause further airway edema.
GIT	Incompetent gastroesophageal sphincter, increased intragastric pressure, increased acidity of gastric contents - *increased risk of regurgitation and aspiration*
CVS	Compression of IVC and aorta by pregnant uterus impedes venous return, reduces stroke volume and cardiac output leading to *supine hypotension syndrome (aortocaval compression)* Physiological anemia → *reduced O_2 carrying capacity*
Anatomical	Obesity and breast hypertrophy cause difficulty in laryngoscopy and interfere with effective chest compressions and defibrillation.

CARDIOPULMONARY RESUSCITATION

The terminology commonly used is:

Basic Life Support (BLS): Comprises a series of sequential assessments and actions provided by a rescuer with no/minimum equipment.

Advanced Cardiovascular Life Support (ACLS): The subsequent life support provided by trained ACLS providers presumed to be equipped with advanced methods of assessment and management.
(These actions are presented as a sequence of distinct steps to help a single rescuer prioritize actions, but whenever there is a team of providers different actions should be performed simultaneously).

Primary CABD Survey: To assess and manage circulation, airway, breathing, and defibrillation

Chain of Survival: A set of coordinated actions required to be done rapidly and sequentially and is formed by the following links.
- Immediate recognition of cardiac arrest and activation of emergency response system (EMS)
- Early CPR with emphasis on chest compressions
- Rapid defibrillation
- Effective advanced life support
- Integrated postcardiac arrest care

The steps for cardiopulmonary resuscitation of a pregnant woman follow the ACLS guidelines, but with a few additional measures.

CASE SCENARIO

A 25-year-woman with 8 months pregnancy presents to the casualty with history of bleeding per vaginum for 4 hours. She is restless and irritable and then suddenly collapses.

BASIC LIFE SUPPORT

Determine whether the Patient is in Cardiac Arrest

- Ensure that the scene is safe to approach the patient, i.e. wear gloves etc.
- Check for a response by tapping the patient on the shoulder and shouting.

Recognition of Arrest and Activation of Emergency Response

- If patient does not respond, activate the institutional emergency team and call for a defibrillator and emergency cart. *CALL FOR HELP!*
- If the patient is not breathing or is gasping, assume the patient is in cardiac arrest.
- If patient has an obviously gravid uterus activate protocol for emergency cesarean delivery.

Begin Early CPR

- Place the patient supine on a firm surface and kneel at the level of her chest.
- Before initiating chest compressions, displace the gravid uterus.
- Perform manual left uterine displacement from either the patient's left side with the 2-handed technique or the patient's right side using a 1-handed technique.
- If this is unsuccessful, and an appropriate wedge is readily available, use a firm wedge to support the pelvis and thorax and maintain a left-lateral tilt of 27 to 30°.
- A human wedge may be used by turning the patient on to a rescuer's knees to provide a stable position for BLS.

C-A-B-D SEQUENCE OF ACTIONS

C-Circulation

Perform Pulse check;

- Feel Adam's apple/thyroid notch
- Slide your fingers into the groove between trachea and strap muscles of neck and palpate the carotid pulse on the ipsilateral side for 5 to 10 seconds.
- If strong and easily palpable pulses are felt, proceed to steps A and B.
- If no pulse is definitely felt, start chest compressions.

Perform High Quality Chest Compressions

Forceful rhythmic application of pressure over the lower half of the sternum increases intrathoracic pressure and directly compresses the heart to generate blood flow and oxygen delivery to the heart and brain.

- Place the heel of one hand on the center of the patient's chest slightly above the level of a line joining the nipples. In the pregnant patient, chest compressions are performed slightly higher on the sternum to adjust for elevation of the diaphragm and abdominal contents caused by the gravid uterus.
- Place the heel of the other hand on top of the first so that the hands are overlapped and parallel and fingers are lifted off the chest wall.
- Lean over the patient with arms straight and elbows locked so that your shoulders are directly over patient's sternum and your entire body weight is transmitted to the patient.
- Provide high-quality chest compressions consisting of;
  - Compressions at a rate of *at least* 100/minute
  - Depth of compressions should be *at least* 2 inches (5 cm)
  - Allow complete chest recoil after each compression (allows heart to fill)
  - Equal chest compression and relaxation times
  - Minimize any interruptions in compressions
  - Avoid excessive ventilations
  - Rotate compressor every 2 mins

After giving a set of 30 compressions, assess for A and B.

If chest compressions remain inadequate after lateral uterine displacement, consider immediate emergency cesarean section.

If untrained as a rescuer you may continue with chest compressions only (Hands-Only CPR, Compression Only CPR) until an AED arrives or trained persons take over as airway maneuvers are technically challenging and may delay or interrupt chest compressions.

Airway and Breathing (A - B)

After giving 30 chest compressions:

A—Open the Airway

- Use the head tilt– chin lift (HTCL) maneuver.
- Place fingers of one hand on the patient's forehead and gently tilt the head back. Place index and middle finger of the other hand below the chin and lift the chin up.
- If a cervical spine injury is suspected, open the airway using jaw thrust maneuver without head extension.
- However maintaining a patent airway and providing adequate ventilation are priorities in CPR, so HTCL maneuver should be used if jaw thrust does not open the airway.

B—Give Rescue breaths in sets of 2 breaths.

Ventilate the patient using a bag valve mask assembly (Ambu bag) ie. BMV (bag mask ventilation). Stand at the head end of the patient and place the mask on the patient's face. Hold the mask in your dominant hand in the *C-E grip* to create an airtight seal. Place your thumb and forefinger on the body of the mask to form a C and compress the mask down on the patients face. Place the other three fingers on the ramus of the patient's mandible to firmly elevate the jaw. Tilt back the patient's head to achieve HTCL and compress the bag with the other hand to push air into the chest to achieve visible chest rise. The characteristics of each rescue breath are:
- Deliver each rescue breath over 1 second.
- Give tidal volume adequate to just produce visible chest rise.
- If there is no chest rise with the first breath, reposition the head and try to reopen the airway by HTCL before giving the second breath.
- Provide supplemental oxygen at a rate of 10 to 12 liters per minute as soon as possible
- Avoid excessive ventilation*

* Excessive ventilation may be detrimental during CPR

1. During CPR, cardiac output is only 25 to 33 percent of normal so a lower tidal volume and respiratory rate is enough to maintain adequate oxygenation and ventilation
2. Larger tidal volumes run risk of gastric insufflation, pulmonary aspiration and splinting and elevation of the diaphragm with reduced pulmonary compliance
3. Rise in intrathoracic pressure leads to decrease in venous return and cardiac output.

- Until an advanced airway is inserted, continue resuscitation with 30:2 compression ventilation ratio.

Other Means of Providing Rescue Breaths; Expired Air Ventilation

Mouth-to-Mouth Breathing	Maintain HTCL and pinch the patient's nose. Take a normal* breath, open your mouth and make an airtight mouth-to-mouth seal around the patients mouth and blow, keeping eyes on the patient's chest to see for chest rise. Then remove your mouth and keep looking at the patient's chest while passive expiration occurs. In the same manner give a second rescue breath. (*Taking of a deep breath by the rescuer leads to rescuer getting lightheaded and tired and may lead to over inflation of the victim's lungs).

Contd...

Contd...

Mouth-to-Nose Breathing	If ventilation through the patient's mouth is not possible.
Mouth-to-Stoma Breathing	In patients with tracheal stoma.
Mouth-to-Mask Device Breathing	A pocket mask is a small portable device with a one way valve so that the victims expired breath is directed away from the rescuer. Place the pocket mask firmly onto the patient's face and open the patient's airway using HTCL. Blow into a port on the mask and give rescue breaths.

A set of 30 Compressions followed by 2 Rescue Breaths Completes 1 Cycle of CPR

CPR is continued in sets of 5 cycles. If a cardiac monitor has been attached, rhythm check is done after 5 cycles and if an organized rhythm is found, pulse check is performed. If no cardiac monitor has been attached, pulse check is to be done after every 5 cycles.

If multiple rescuers are available, they should rotate the task of compressions after every 5 cycles or 2 minutes. This switch should be accomplished in <5 seconds.

D-Early Defibrillation

- As soon as a defibrillator arrives and rhythm check reveals a shockable rhythm, defibrillation should be performed
- Defibrillation should be performed at recommended ACLS defibrillation doses and is considered safe at all stages of pregnancy
- Any internal or external fetal monitors should be removed prior to defibrillation
- Defibrillation may be performed using a manual defibrillator or an AED (Automated External Defibrillator)
- Using a monophasic defibrillator, a shock of 360 J is given for a shockable rhythm, i.e. ventricular fibrillation (VF)/ pulseless ventricular tachycardia (VT). Shock delivery should be immediately followed by 5 cycles of CPR starting with chest compressions after which rhythm check is done. As long as a shockable rhythm persists, shocks of 360 J are given
- If a nonshockable rhythm (pulseless electrical activity PEA, asystole) is seen on the monitor, CPR should be resumed immediately
- For biphasic defibrillators, the manufacturer's recommended energy dose (120 to 200 J) should be used. If the manufacturer's recommended dose is not known, defibrillate at the maximal dose

1. VF is the most common and treatable rhythm in adults with sudden cardiac arrest and survival rates are highest when immediate CPR is provided and defibrillation occurs within 3 to 5 minutes of collapse.
2. AED is a sophisticated, reliable computerized device that uses voice and visual prompts to guide defibrillation in VF and pulseless ventricular tachycardia (VT). An AED may be used on a pregnant patient.
3. Defibrillators may be monophasic or biphasic.

Recovery Position

If the patient is unresponsive, but has normal breathing and effective circulation, she should be placed on the side with the lower arm in front of the body. The position should be stable, with the head dependent and no pressure on the chest to impair breathing. This recovery position is designed to maintain a patent airway and reduce the risk of airway obstruction and aspiration.

EFFECTIVE ADVANCED CARDIOVASCULAR LIFE SUPPORT (ACLS)

Once the emergency response team arrives, interventions must be made to treat cardiac arrest and improve the outcome of patients who have achieved a return of spontaneous circulation (ROSC) after cardiac arrest.

Already the patient should be receiving cycles of chest compressions and rescue breathing (30:2).

- Certain adjuncts may be used to improve airway control and ventilation which include oropharyngeal airway (OPA), nasopharyngeal airway (NPA), suction devices, supraglottic devices and endotracheal intubation
- Placement of an advanced airway should not cause undue interruptions in CPR
- Any interruptions in chest compressions should be minimized and <10 seconds
- BMV may be continued if successful
- If the rescuer is unable to do BMV adequately, an advanced airway is urgently required
- Pregnant patient are more susceptible to regurgitation and aspiration and early endotracheal intubation should be considered if the rescuer is suitably trained
- Rapid intubation will maximize oxygenation and decrease the risk of aspiration
- Pregnancy results in a difficult airway. Intubation with an endotracheal tube or supraglottic airway should be performed only by experienced providers if possible
- Because of the pregnancy-related changes in airway anatomy, intubation equipment should include small endotracheal tubes, short laryngoscope handles, and instruments for cricothyrotomy
- Oxygen desaturation in pregnancy is significantly faster during a period of apnea and preoxygenation with 100% oxygen by bag-mask ventilation prior to attempting intubation is especially important.

OPA, NPA	May be used to facilitate delivery of ventilations with a bag-mask device and relieve upper airway obstruction
Suction Devices	Portable and installed suction devices should be available to provide adequate vacuum and flow for pharyngeal suction.
Advanced Airways: **Endotracheal tube/ Supraglottic airway**	**Supraglottic airways** that may be inserted in cardiac arrest include laryngeal mask airway (LMA), the esophageal-tracheal tube (combitube) and the laryngeal tube or King LT. *Endotracheal Intubation;* Keeps airway patent, allows suctioning of secretions and delivery of a high concentration of oxygen, provides a route for administration of emergency drugs and delivery of a selected tidal volume and protects the airway from aspiration. Attempts at intubation by unskilled rescuers can lead to trauma of upper airway, interruptions in CPR and hypoxemia from many/prolonged intubation attempts or tube displacement.
Oxygen	100% should be provided

Verify position of advanced airway: Once an advanced airway is inserted, its proper positioning must be verified. This assessment should not interrupt chest compressions.

1. Visualization of bilateral chest expansion and auscultation over the epigastrium (breath sounds not heard) and the lung fields bilaterally (breath sounds equal and adequate)
2. Additional confirmation of placement by;
   a. Waveform capnography
   b. Esophageal detector device
   c. Laryngoscopy to visualize the tube passing through the vocal cords.
   d. If still in doubt about correct placement, remove the tube and provide BMV until the tube is replaced

Once confirmed, the depth of the endotracheal tube should be recorded and marked. It should be well secured with tape/commercial device.

Quantitative Waveform Capnography

1. Used as early as possible after placement of an advanced airway to confirm correct device placement.
2. If end tidal CO_2 is less than 10 mm Hg, try to improve CPR quality
3. An abrupt sustained increase in end tidal CO_2 > 40 mm Hg may indicate a return of spontaneous circulation (ROSC)

Once an advanced airway is in place, CPR is no longer delivered in cycles (30 compressions: 2 breaths).

One rescuer gives continuous chest compressions at a rate of at least 100 per minute while another provides ventilation at 8 to 10 breaths per minute.

EKG Rhythms in Cardiac Arrest

1. Cardiac arrest is associated with 4 EKG rhythms: VF, pulseless VT, PEA and asystole, none of which generate a cardiac output.
2. The presence of 3 or more sequential ventricular premature beats defines VT. Diagnostic criteria include the presence of fusion beats, capture beats, and AV dissociation.
3. VF is an irregular rhythm that results from a rapid discharge of impulses from one or more ventricular foci or from multiple wandering reentrant circuits in the ventricles. Ventricular contractions are erratic and represented on ECG by bizarre patterns of various size and configuration. P waves are not seen.
4. PEA includes a heterogeneous group of organized electric rhythms associated with mechanical ventricular activity inadequate to generate a clinically detectable pulse.
5. Asystole is an absence of any detectable ventricular electric activity with a flat line on ECG.

VF/Pulseless VT

- When a rhythm check shows a VF or VT, **immediate defibrillation** is recommended
- CPR is continued while the defibrillator is readied for use and should be resumed immediately after the shock is delivered
- If VF or pulseless VT persists after at least 1 shock and 2-minutes of CPR, a **vasopressor** should be given
- **Amiodarone** may be considered in VF/VT is unresponsive to CPR, defibrillation, and vasopressor therapy
- If amiodarone is unavailable, **lidocaine** may be given
- **Magnesium sulfate** should be considered only for torsades de pointes associated with a long QT interval.

PEA/Asystole

- If the rhythm is asystole or carotid pulse is absent, i.e. PEA, no shock is indicated
- **CPR** should be resumed immediately and continued for 2 minutes before rhythm check is repeated
- A **vasopressor** can be given as soon as feasible
- When an organized rhythm is found, a pulse check is performed
- PEA is often caused by reversible causes. Recall the H's and T's.
- Asystole is commonly the end-stage rhythm that follows prolonged VF or PEA, and thus the prognosis is much worse.

CONSIDER AND TREAT POTENTIALLY REVERSIBLE CAUSES

While resuscitating the patient, recall the 5 H's and T's to identify a factor that may have caused the arrest and may be complicating resuscitation.

5 H's	5 T's
Hypoxia	Toxins
Hypovolemia	Tamponade (cardiac)
Hydrogen ion (acidosis)	Tension pneumothorax
Hypo-/hyperkalemia	Thrombosis, pulmonary
Hypothermia	Thrombosis, coronary

ACCESS FOR PARENTERAL MEDICATIONS DURING CARDIAC ARREST

- Secure adequate and immediate IV access in any obstetric hemorrhage and commence appropriate fluid resuscitation.
- In a cardiac arrest situation, after beginning CPR and attempting defibrillation, intravenous (IV) or intraosseous (IO) access should be secured.
- After giving any drug by the peripheral venous route during CPR, follow it by a 20-mL bolus of IV fluid and briefly elevate the limb to facilitate drug flow into the central circulation.
- Naloxone, atropine, vasopressin, epinephrine and lidocaine (NAVEL) are absorbed via the trachea. If IV or IO access cannot be established, these drugs may be administered by the endotracheal route during cardiac arrest. The optimal endotracheal dose is 2 to 2.5 times the recommended IV dose diluted in 5 to 10 mL of sterile water or normal saline and injected directly into the endotracheal tube.

Use vasopressors as per standard ACLS protocols. Even though fetal blood flow is reduced and increase in glomerular filtration and plasma volume are reported during normal pregnancy, current medications and doses need not be altered.

Medications during Cardiac Arrest

Drug	Action	Dose
Vasopressors		
Epinephrine	Alpha adrenergic receptor-stimulator; increases coronary and cerebral perfusion pressure	1 mg IV/IO every 3 to 5 mins
Vasopressin	Nonadrenergic peripheral vasoconstrictor; coronary and renal vasoconstriction	Single dose 40 units IV/IO to replace first or second dose of epinephrine
Antiarrhythmics		
Amiodarone	Affects sodium, potassium, calcium channels; has alpha and beta adrenergic blocking properties; in VF or pulseless VT unresponsive to CPR, defibrillation, and vasopressors	300 mg IV/IO followed by 1 dose 150 mg IV/IO
Lidocaine	If amiodarone unavailable	1 to 1.5 mg/kg IV; then 0.5 to 0.75 mg/kg IV every 5 to 10 mins to a max dose 3 mg/kg
Magnesium Sulfate	VF/pulseless VT cardiac arrest associated with torsades de pointes	1 to 2 g diluted in 10 mL D5W.

MATERNAL CARDIAC ARREST NOT IMMEDIATELY REVERSED BY BLS/ACLS

Consider Emergency Cesarean Section

As soon as cardiac arrest is identified in a pregnant woman with an obviously gravid uterus, regardless of fetal viability, the protocol for an emergency cesarean delivery should be activated at the onset of maternal cardiac arrest. In the meantime, standard CPR is started.

Emergency cesarean section may be considered at 4 minutes after onset of maternal cardiac arrest if there is no return of spontaneous circulation.

Potential Benefits of Perimortem Cesarean Section

1. Relief of aorto-caval compression and improvement in maternal hemodynamics
2. Improved chest mechanics/improved thoracic compliance/improved efficacy of chest compressions
3. Decreased maternal oxygen demand
4. Improved chance of fetal survival

Perimortem cesarean was initially popularized by Katz, et al in 1986 and a "four minute rule" from the onset of maternal arrest to initiation of cesarean delivery was advocated. At 24 to 25 weeks of gestation, the best survival rate for the infant occurs when the infant is delivered no more than 5 minutes after the mother's heart stops beating. Typically, this requires that the hysterotomy begins about 4 minutes after cardiac arrest

This time frame presents a significant challenge and even in well-trained teams it can be very difficult to meet this benchmark. Transfer to an operating theatre is usually not possible and hence plans need to be in place to be able to perform the cesarean at the scene of the arrest. Team planning should be done in collaboration with the obstetric, neonatal, emergency, anesthesiology, intensive care, and cardiac arrest services.

Management of cardiac arrest in a pregnant patient a summarized in Flow chart 23.1.

Flow chart 23.1: Cardiac Arrest in a Pregnant Patient[1,2,3]

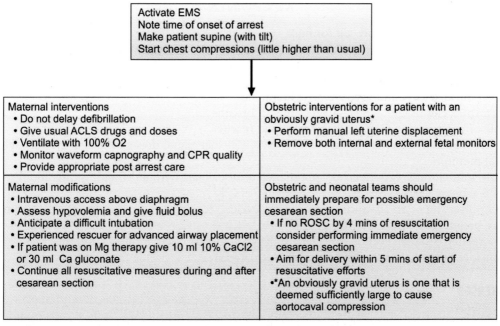

(Adapted from 2010 American Heart Association guidelines for Cardiopulmonary Resuscitation and Emergency Cardiovoscular care)

SUBSEQUENT RESPONDERS

Search for and Treat Possible Contributing Factors (BEAU-CHOPS)

B	Bleeding/DIC
E	Embolus-coronary/pulmonary/amniotic fluid
A	Anesthetic complications
U	Uterine atony
C	Cardiac disease- MI/ischemia/aortic dissection/cardiomyopathy
H	Hypertension/pre-eclampsia/eclampsia
O	Others- differential diagnosis as ACLS guidelines
P	Placenta abruptio/previa
S	Sepsis

POSTCARDIAC ARREST CARE

- If there is ROSC, postcardiac arrest care should be initiated.
- Treat hypoxemia and hypotension.
- Strive for early diagnosis and treatment of the underlying cause.
- Therapeutic hypothermia may be considered on an individual basis after cardiac arrest in a comatose pregnant patient.
- The fetus should be continuously monitored for bradycardia as a potential complication, and obstetric and neonatal consultation sought.

KEY POINTS

- Identify cardiac arrest and call for help
- Activate protocol for emergency cesarean section if obviously gravid uterus
- Make supine and displace gravid uterus
- If no pulse start effective chest compressions C
- Open the airway A and give 2 rescue breaths B
- Perform cycles of CPR – 30 compressions : 2 breaths
- Role of compression-Only CPR in untrained rescuer
- Perform Early Defibrillation and Effective ACLS – use usual doses of drugs and remove any fetal monitors
- Early intubation if experienced - pregnancy is associated with a difficult intubation. Provide 100% oxygen early
- After insertion of an advanced airway – no cycles ; continue compressions at > 100/min and give breaths 8-10/min
- Emergency cesarean section if no return of spontaneous circulation in 4 minutes
- Consider possible causes- BEAU-CHOPS- treat early

REFERENCES

1. 2010 American Heart Association. Guidelines for Cardiopulmonary Resuscitation and Emergency Cardiovascular Care: International consensus on science. Circulation 2010 circulation 2010;122:S250-75.
2. Morris S, Stacey M. Resuscitation in pregnancy. BMJ 2003;327:1277-9.
3. Luppi CJ. Cardiopulmonary resuscitation: pregnant women are different. AACN Clin Issues 1997;8:574-85.

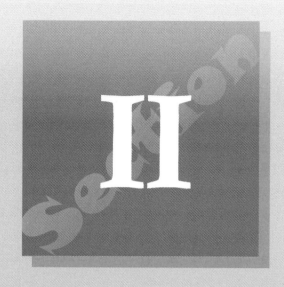

Gynecological Emergencies

Chapter 24

Acute Pelvic Inflammatory Disease

Madhavi M Gupta, Garima Sharma

INTRODUCTION

Pelvic Inflammatory Disease (PID) is described by the Centres for Disease Control and Prevention (CDC) as a spectrum of inflammatory disorders of the upper female genital tract, including any combination of endometritis, salpingitis, tubo-ovarian abscess, and pelvic peritonitis.[1]

It is generally due to the ascending infection from the vagina and endocervix to the endometrium, fallopian tubes or contiguous structures. Sexually transmitted organisms, especially *N. gonorrhoeae* and *C. Trachomatis* [2,3] are implicated in many cases; however, microorganisms that comprise the vaginal flora (e.g., anaerobes, *G. vaginalis*, *Haemophilus influenzae*, enteric gram-negative rods, and *Streptococcus agalactiae*) also have been associated with PID. In addition, cytomegalovirus (CMV), *M. hominis*, *U. urealyticum*, and *M. genitalium* might be associated with some cases of PID.

By definition, PID is an acute infectious process. *Acute salpingitis is the most important component of the PID spectrum.* Chronic refers to the sequelae of the acute process such as adhesions, scarring, and tubal obstruction.

PID is a common cause of morbidity and accounts for 1 in 60 consultations by women under the age of 45.[4] Delays of only a few days in receiving appropriate treatment markedly increases the risk of sequelae, which include infertility, ectopic pregnancy and chronic pelvic pain.[5] PID causes approximately 30 percent of infertility cases, and 50 percent of ectopic pregnancies.[6]

CDC DIAGNOSTIC CRITERIA FOR THE DIAGNOSIS OF PID[7]

Minimal Criteria

- Lower abdominal tenderness
- Uterine/adnexal tenderness
- Cervical motion tenderness

Additional Criteria

- Oral temperature >38.3°C (101°F).
- Abnormal cervical or vaginal mucopurulent discharge.
- Presence of white blood cells (WBCs) on saline microscopy of vaginal secretions.
- Elevated erythrocyte sedimentation rate (ESR).

- Elevated C-reactive protein level.
- Laboratory documentation of cervical infection with *Neisseria gonorrhoeae* or *Chlamydia trachomatis*.

Definitive Criteria

- Histopathologic evidence of endometritis on endometrial biopsy.
- Transvaginal sonography or magnetic resonance imaging techniques showing thickened, fluid-filled tubes with or without free pelvic fluid or tubo-ovarian complex.
- Laparoscopic abnormalities consistent with PID.

CASE SCENARIO-1

A 23-year-lady para 3 from low socio-economic status presented to the emergency with acute pain lower abdomen, vomiting and high-grade fever (>101°) for 2 days.

> **Comments:** Acute PID should be considered in the differential diagnosis since she has lower abdominal pain along with high-grade fever.

Differential Diagnosis

This would include any other cause, gynecological or otherwise presenting with acute pain lower abdomen, high-grade fever and tenderness on examination.

a. *Pregnancy-related causes*
   - Ruptured ectopic pregnancy
   - Spontaneous, threatened or incomplete abortion
   - Intrauterine pregnancy with corpus luteum hemorrhage
b. *Gynecologic disorders.*
   - PID
   - Endometriosis
   - Ovarian cyst hemorrhage or rupture
   - Adnexal torsion
   - Mittelschmerz
   - Uterine leiomyoma torsion
   - Primary dysmenorrhea.
c. *Nonreproductive tract causes*
   - Gastrointestinal
     - Appendicitis
     - Inflammatory bowel disease
     - Mesenteric adenitis
     - Irritable bowel syndrome
     - Diverticulitis
   - Urinary tract.
     - Urinary tract infection (cystitis)
     - Renal calculus

POINTS TO BE NOTED IN THE HISTORY

- Age: Age is inversely related to PID rates and directly correlated with PID sequelae, (e.g., tubal damage and infertility).[8] Sexually active teenagers are three times more likely to be diagnosed as having PID than are 25- to 29-year-old women.[9]
- Pain: Characteristics of pain onset, duration, and palliative or aggravating factors .Bilateral lower abdominal and pelvic pain which is dull in nature is characteristic of PID. The onset of pain is more rapid and acute in gonoccocal infections (3 days) than in chlamydial infections (5-7 days).

- Fever, lassitude and headache—Whether associated with chills, general malaise.
- Irregular and excessive vaginal bleeding is usually due to associated endometritis.
- Abnormal vaginal discharge which is purulent and/or copious.
- Nausea and vomiting
- Dyspareunia
- Pain and discomfort in the right hypochondrium due to concomitant perihepatitis (Fitz-Hugh-Curtis syndrome) may occur in 5 to 10 percent of cases of acute salpingitis. The liver is involved due to transperitoneal or vascular dissemination of either gonoccocal or chlamydial infections.
- Associated symptoms like urinary or gastrointestinal symptoms.
- Socio-economic status—Low levels of education, unemployment, and low income as measures of socioeconomic status have been associated with increased risk of PID.[10]
- Sexual behaviour—Several dimensions of sexual behaviour, however, have been associated with increased risk of PID. These include young age at first sexual intercourse, multiple sex partners[11], high frequency of sexual intercourse,[12] and increased rate of acquiring new partners within the previous 30 days.[13]
- Contraceptive practice. Contraceptive choice affects risk of PID as well as risk of STD and tubal infertility. Because of complex interrelationships, precise etiologic associations are difficult to unravel.
  - Barrier methods.
    When properly used, mechanical and chemical barriers decrease the risk of STD, PID, and tubal infertility.
  - Oral contraceptives.
    Current data on use of oral contraception (OC) and risk of lower- and upper-genital-tract infection and sequelae are inconsistent. Women who use OC have an increased risk of *C. trachomatis* infection of the cervix[14], but lower risk of symptomatic, clinically overt PID.[15,16] No substantial increase or decrease in risk of tubal infertility occurs among women using OC.
  - Intrauterine devices.
    Women who use intrauterine devices (IUDs) are probably at increased risk of PID that may not be STD-related. Most of this increased risk occurs in the first month after insertion of an IUD. Lower risks of PID have been reported with the current generation of IUDs than with types used in earlier years.
- Other risk variables: Vaginal douching, menses, cigarette smoking, and substance abuse have also been suggested as variables influencing the risk of PID. Data from several reports suggest that women with acute PID are more likely to have a history of douching than women without PID.[17,18] Current data, however, do not provide sufficient information to determine whether positive associations are attributable to characteristics of the women who douche, or to douching itself.
- Menstrual history: Last menstrual period (LMP) (rule out ectopic gestation), irregular and excessive bleeding is associated with PID.
- Obstetric history: History of minor procedures like dilatation and curettage (D&C), suction evacuation, manual removal of placenta (associated with increased risk of PID), history of ectopic pregnancy in the past.
- Past medical history: Surgical history, gynecologic history in particular of sexually transmitted diseases should be determined. Current sexual activity and practices should be assessed.
- History of the partner: Profession, whether into a polygamous relationship, any previous sexually transmitted infection.

History in this case:
History of acute lower abdominal pain, vomiting and fever for 2 days. She had an IUCD inserted 3 months back. Her menstrual cycles were regular with her last menstrual period being 14 days back.

POINTS TO BE NOTED IN EXAMINATION

General Examination

- General condition
- Temperature, pulse, respiratory rate (RR) and blood pressure (BP)
- Pallor, icterus

Cardiovascular and Respiratory System Examination

Abdominal Examination

- Location and severity of pain
- Tenderness, guarding, rigidity and rebound tenderness
- Any palpable hepatomegaly
- Presence of free fluid in the peritoneal cavity.

Pelvic Examination

Local Examination

- Any growth, ulceration, abnormality should be noted on vulva, perineum, urethra (congested in PID), sub urethral region and anus.
- Vaginal discharge: Color, smell, amount, consistency

Per Speculum (P/S) Examination

- Cervical discharge: Amount, color, and smell. Cervical swab is sent for gram's stain, culture and sensitivity.
- Condition of cervix—cervix is congested in PID
- Presence of foreign body, IUCD thread

Per Vaginum (P/V) Examination

- Uterine size and position
- Tenderness on palpation of the uterus, adnexae or when uterus is moved.
- Pelvic mass (there may be thickening or a definite mass felt through one of the fornices in PID)—its size, shape, position, consistency, mobility and whether tender.

> **Examination in this case:**
> Pulse—110/min, BP—110/70 mm of Hg, Temp—102° F, RR 20/min
> General physical and systemic examination unremarkable
> Abdominal examination reveals tenderness in both the lower quadrants
> Local Examination: Purulent discharge present, external urethral meatus congested.
> P/S -Purulent discharge present, cervix hypertrophied, congested, vagina normal, IUCD thread seen.
> P/V- Cervix backward with cervical motion tenderness, uterus is anteverted, multiparous size, firm in consistency, mobile with movements tender and all fornices clear but adnexal tenderness present.

Diagnosis

Acute Pelvic Inflammatory Disease

INVESTIGATIONS

- Urine pregnancy test (UPT) to check for ectopic pregnancy
- Hemoglobin, hematocrit, complete blood counts and ESR

- Urine—Albumin, sugar, microscopy and culture & sensitivity (C/S)
- Cervical swab for culture and sensitivity
- Test for HIV, HBsAg and syphilis
- Transvaginal ultrasound scan (TVS).

Investigation in this case:
Urine pregnancy test (UPT)—Negative
Hemoglobin—10 gm %, Hematocrit—30%
Complete blood count (CBC)- 18,000/cu mm with 90 percent polymorphs, ESR—30 mm in the first hour
Urine albumin, sugar and microscopy—Normal, sample sent for C/S
Cervical swab sent for culture and sensitivity
Test for HIV, HBsAg and syphilis—Negative in both partners
TVS—Uterus was bulky (9.5x6.8x5.2 cm), endometrium was triple layer, both the ovaries were normal. No free fluid, no pelvic mass.

MANAGEMENT OF ACUTE PID

There is a wide variation in the symptoms and signs of PID. Many women with PID have subtle or mild symptoms. Sometimes it presents as an emergency. Treatment mainly involves administration of broad spectrum antibiotics against common pathological organisms causing PID, supportive therapy (hydration, analgesics, antipyretics) and close monitoring of the clinical course.

1. Assess for Need for Hospitalization

Not all patients with the diagnosis of acute PID need to be admitted. There are certain set criteria for in patient management (Sexually transmitted treatment guideline 2006).
The criteria for hospitalization of patients with acute PID:
- Surgical emergencies (such as appendicitis) cannot be excluded
- The patient is pregnant
- The patient does not respond clinically to oral antimicrobial therapy
- The patient is unable to follow or tolerate an outpatient oral regimen
- The patient has severe illness, nausea and vomiting, or high fever
- A tubo-ovarian abscess.

2. Antibiotics

All antibiotic regimens used to treat PID should be effective against *N. gonorrhoeae* and *C. Trachomatis*. Negative endocervical screening for these organisms does not rule out upper-reproductive-tract infection.

Recommended Parenteral Regimen A

Cefotetan 2 g IV every 12 hours
OR
Cefoxitin 2 g IV every 6 hours
PLUS
Doxycycline 100 mg orally or IV every 12 hours
Parenteral therapy may be discontinued 24 hours after a patient improves clinically, and oral therapy with doxycycline (100 mg twice a day) should continue to complete 14 days of therapy. Because of the pain associated with infusion, doxycycline should be administered orally whenever possible, even when the patient is hospitalized. Oral and intravenous (IV) administration of doxycycline provides similar bioavailability. When tubo-ovarian abscess is present, many health-care providers use clindamycin or metronidazole with doxycycline for continued therapy, rather than doxycycline alone, because it provides more effective anaerobic coverage.

Antibiotics need to be changed if the patient does not improve within 48 hours. If fever persists, patient should also be investigated for other causes of fever (typhoid, malaria).

Clinical data are limited regarding the use of other second-or third-generation cephalosporins (e.g., ceftizoxime, cefotaxime, and ceftriaxone), which also might be effective therapy for PID and may replace cefotetan or cefoxitin. However, these cephalosporins are less active than cefotetan or cefoxitin against anaerobic bacteria

Recommmended Parenteral Regimen B

Clindamycin 900 mg IV every 8 hours
PLUS
Gentamicin loading dose IV or IM (2 mg/kg of body weight), followed by a maintenance dose (1.5 mg/kg) every 8 hours.

Parenteral therapy can be discontinued 24 hours after a patient improves clinically; Oral therapy is continued and it should consist of doxycycline 100 mg orally twice a day or clindamycin 450 mg orally four times a day to complete a total of 14 days of therapy. When tubo-ovarian abscess is present clindamycin is preferred over doxycycline for continued therapy as it provides more effective anaerobic coverage.

Alternative Parenteral Regimens

Limited data support the use of other parenteral regimens, but the following three regimens have been investigated in at least one clinical trial, and they have broad spectrum coverage.

Levofloxacin 500 mg IV once daily*
WITH OR WITHOUT
Metronidazole 500 mg IV every 8 hours
OR
Ofloxacin 400 mg IV every 12 hours*
WITH OR WITHOUT
Metronidazole 500 mg IV every 8 hours
OR
Ampicillin/Sulbactam 3 g IV every 6 hours
PLUS
Doxycycline 100 mg orally or IV every 12 hours
* Quinolones should not be used in persons with a history of recent foreign travel or partners' travel to areas with increased Fluoroquinolone-resistant *Neisseria gonorrhoeae* (QRNG) prevalence.
- IV ofloxacin has been investigated as a single agent; however, because of concerns regarding its spectrum, metronidazole may be included in the regimen.
- Levofloxacin is as effective as ofloxacin and may be substituted; its single daily dosing makes it advantageous from a compliance perspective.
- One trial demonstrated high short-term clinical cure rates with azithromycin, either alone for 1 week (atleast one IV dose followed by oral therapy) or with a 12-day course of metronidazole.
- Ampicillin/sulbactam plus doxycycline is effective coverage against *C. trachomatis, N. gonorrhoeae,* and anaerobes and for patients who have tubo ovarian abscess.

(The out patient treatment of milder cases of PID is discussed in Chapter 30)

3. Management of Sex Partners

Male sex partners of women with PID should be examined and treated if they had sexual contact with the patient during the 60 days preceding the patient's onset of symptoms.

4. Follow-up and Counseling to Adopt Safe Sex Practices

All women diagnosed with acute PID should be offered HIV testing.
No evidence suggests that IUCDs should be removed in women diagnosed with acute PID. Surgical intervention may be needed in cases not responding to medical therapy, as in pelvic abscess.

Treatment in this case:

The patient was hospitalized as she had severe illness.

Antibiotics:
- Cefotaxime 2 g intravenous (IV) every 12 hours
- Doxycycline 100 mg orally every 12 hours
- Metronidazole 500 mg twice a day for 14 days

Supportive therapy:
- Paracetamol 500 mg was given when the fever was ≥ 100° F
- Diclofenac sodium 100 mg 12 hourly as an anti-inflammatory
- Pantoprezole 40 mg once daily was also given
- Hydration was taken care of by encouraging the patient to accept orally

Close monitoring was done for fever, pulse rate and symptomatic improvement.

Parenteral therapy was discontinued 24 hours after the patient improved clinically, and oral therapy with doxycycline (100 mg twice a day) along with metronidazole (500 mg twice a day) was continued to complete 14 days of therapy.

The patient's husband was also given oral antibiotic treatment on an outpatient basis.

CASE SCENARIO-2

A 27-year-old para 1 attended the casualty complaining of pain lower abdomen for 12 days which has increased in severity for two days, high-grade fever >102 ° F for four days, malaise, and irregular bleeding for last 15 days. History of surgical medical termination of pregnancy (MTP) at 2 months amenorrhea by a local doctor two weeks back

Comment: Pain and irregular bleeding soon after the MTP may be due to endometritis and post abortion PID. However other differential diagnosis, particularly ectopic pregnancy must be ruled out.

Differential Diagnosis

- Septic Abortion
- Incomplete abortion
- Ectopic pregnancy
- Any surgical cause

History in this case: MTP by a local doctor 2 weeks back. She developed pain 2 days later along with high grade fever and malaise.

Examination in this case:

General condition was stable.

Pulse—104/min, BP—100/66 mm Hg, RR—18/min, Temperature—102.4 ° F

No pallor or jaundice

Respiratory system—Normal

Cardiovascular system—Tachycardia

Abdominal Examination—Soft with lower abdominal tenderness present, no guarding or rigidity, no free fluid, no mass palpable, bowel sounds normal

P/S: Slight bleeding through os

P/V: Os closed, uterus normal size, firm, mobile, an elongated soft to cystic tender mass ~5x4 cm, with restricted mobility was palpable in the left fornix, right fornix free but there was generalized tenderness.

Diagnosis

Acute pelvic inflammatory disease with left tubo-ovarian abscess following an unsafe abortion.

Investigations in this case:
Urine pregnancy test (UPT) - Negative
Hemoglobin—9 gm %, hematocrit—28 %
Complete blood count (CBC)- 20,000/cu mm with 92 percent polymorphs
ESR—25 mm in the first hour
Urine—albumin, sugar and microscoy—normal; sample sent for C/S
Cervical swab sent for culture and sensitivity
Test for HIV, HBsAg and syphilis done for both partners—Negative in both
TVS—Uterus was normal size (8.5x6.1x5.2 cm), endometrium—6 mm, a retort shaped 5.8x4.7 cm mass of mixed echogenicity in the left fornix with no vascularity, left ovary not seen separately from the mass. Right ovary normal. Small amount of free fluid in the pouch of Douglas.

Treatment and clinical course in this case:
Since the patient had a tubo- ovarian abscess she was admitted and started on IV broad spectrum antibiotics. Supportive management in the form of NSAIDS for pain and fever, stress ulcer prophylaxis was same as in the previous case
Parenteral therapy was discontinued 24 hours after the patient improved clinically, and oral therapy with doxycycline (100 mg twice a day) along with metronidazole (500 mg twice a day) was continued to complete 14 days of therapy.
Treatment of the husband and contraceptive counseling was done.
A repeat bimanual pelvic examination after two-weeks revealed significant decrease in the size of the tubo-ovarian abscess. The same was confirmed on an endovaginal scan. By six weeks posttreatment the tubo-ovarian abscess disappeared completely.

SPECIAL CONSIDERATIONS

Pregnancy

Because of the high-risk for maternal morbidity and preterm delivery, pregnant women who have suspected PID should be hospitalized and treated with parenteral antibiotics.

HIV Infection

Differences in the clinical manifestations of PID between HIV infected women and HIV negative women have not been well-delineated. In previous observational studies, HIV infected women with PID were more likely to require surgical intervention. More comprehensive observational and controlled studies have demonstrated that HIV infected women with PID had similar symptoms when compared with uninfected controls. They were more likely to have a tubo-ovarian abscess but responded equally well to standard parenteral and oral antibiotic regimens when compared with HIV negative women.[19] The microbiologic findings for HIV positive and HIV negative women were similar, except HIV infected women had higher rates of concomitant *M. hominis*, candida, streptococcal, and HPV infections and HPV-related cytologic abnormalities. Whether the management of immunodeficient HIV infected women with PID requires more aggressive interventions (e.g., hospitalization or parenteral antimicrobial regimens) has not been determined.

IUCD

The risk of PID associated with IUD use is primarily confined to the first 3 weeks after insertion and is uncommon thereafter. Given the popularity of IUDs, practitioners might encounter PID in IUD users. *No evidence suggests that IUDs should be removed in women diagnosed with acute PID*. However, caution should be exercised if the IUD remains in place, and close clinical follow-up is mandatory. The rate of treatment failure and recurrent PID in women continuing to use an IUD is unknown. No data exist on antibiotic selection and treatment outcomes according to type of IUD (e.g., copper or levonorgestrel).

PREVENTION

Prevention of chlamydial infection by screening and treating high-risk women reduces the incidence of PID. Theoretically, the majority of cases of PID can be prevented by screening all women or those determined to be at high-risk (based on age or other factors) by using DNA amplification on cervical specimens (in women receiving pelvic examinations) and on urine specimens (in women not undergoing examinations). Although bacterial vaginosis is associated with PID, whether the incidence of PID can be reduced by identifying and treating women with bacterial vaginosis is unclear.

KEY POINTS

- Diagnosis of acute PID should be considered when a sexually active reproductive age woman presents with pain lower abdomen, fever with or without irregular bleeding.
- A thorough clinical and investigative work-up is essential to establish the diagnosis and assess the severity of illness.
- Acute ectopic pregnancy and other surgical causes should always be excluded.
- Broad spectrum antibiotics owing to the polymicrobial cause along with anaerobic coverage are to be given either orally or parenterally.
- Patients who are pregnant, who do not respond to or are non-compliant with oral therapy, who are severely ill with nausea, vomiting, high-grade fever, or who have a tubo-ovarian abscess require hospitalization for parenteral antibiotic therapy.
- The patient should be re-evaluated within 48 to 72 hours of initiating outpatient therapy to determine the response of the disease.
- Male sex partners of women with PID should be examined and treated if they had sexual contact with the patient during the 60 days preceding the patient's onset of symptoms.
- All women diagnosed with acute PID should be offered HIV testing.
- No evidence suggests that IUDs should be removed in women diagnosed with acute PID.
- Sequeale includes infertility, ectopic pregnancy and chronic pelvic pain

---

REFERENCES

1. Centres for Disease Control and Prevention. 1993 Sexually transmitted diseases treatment guidelines. MMWR Morb Mortal Wkyl Rep 1993;42:75.
2. Bevan CD, Johal BJ, Mumtaz G, Ridgway GL, Siddle NC. Clinical, laparoscopic and microbiological findings in acute salpingitis: report on a United Kingdom cohort. BJOG 1995;102:407-14.
3. Recommendations arising from the 31st Study Group: The Prevention of Pelvic Infection. In: Templeton A (ed). The Prevention of Pelvic Infection. London: RCOG Press; 1996:267-70.
4. Simms I, Vickers MR, Stephenson J, Rogers PA, Nicoll A. National assessment of PID diagnosis, treatment and management in general practice: England and Wales. Int J STD AIDS 2000;11:440-4.
5. Hillis SD, Joesoef R, Marchbanks PA, Wasserheit JN, Cates W, Jr., Westrom L. Delayed care of pelvic inflammatory disease as a risk factor for impaired fertility. Am J Obstet Gynecol 1993;168:1503-9.
6. Eschenbach DA. Epidemiology of pelvic inflammatory disease. In: Landers DV, Sweet RL (eds). Pelvic inflammatory disease. New York: Springer-Verlag, 1997. pp. 1-20.
7. Centres for Disease Control and Prevention. 1993 Sexually transmitted diseases treatment guidelines. MMWR Morb Mortal Wkyl Rep 2006;55(RR-11):56.
8. Cates W, Rolfs RT, Aral SO. Sexually transmitted diseases, pelvic inflammatory disease, and infertility: an epidemiologic update. Epidemiol Rev 1990;12:199-220.
9. Bell TA, Holmes KK. Age-specific risks of syphilis, gonorrhea, and hospitalized pelvic inflammatory disease in sexually experienced U.S. women. Sex Transm Dis 1984;11:291-5.
10. Washington AE, Aral SO, Wolner-Hanssen P, Grimes DA, Holmes KK. Assessing risk for pelvic inflammatory disease and its sequelae. In: Joint Meeting of the Centers for Disease Control and National Institutes of Health about Pelvic Inflammatory Disease Prevention, Management, and Research in the 1990s, Bethesda, Maryland, September 4-5, 1990.

11. Marchbanks PA, Lee NC, Peterson HB. Cigarette smoking as a risk factor for pelvic inflammatory disease. Am J Obstet Gynecol 1990;162:639-44.

12. Lee NC, Rubin GL, Borucki R. The intrauterine device and pelvic inflammatory disease revisited: new results from the Women's Health Study. Obstet Gynecol 1988;72:1-6.

13. Wolner-Hanssen P, Eschenbach DA, Paavonen J, et al. Association between vaginal douching and acute pelvic inflammatory disease. JAMA 1990;263:1936-41.

14. Platt R, Rice PA, McCormack WM. Risk of acquiring gonorrhea and prevalence of abnormal adnexal findings among women recently exposed to gonorrhea. JAMA 1983;250:3205-9.

15. Washington AE, Cates W Jr, Wasserheit JN. Preventing pelvic inflammatory disease. JAMA 1991;266:2574-80.

16. Wolner-Hanssen P, Eschenbach DA, Paavonen J, et al. Decreased risk of symptomatic chlamydial pelvic inflammatory disease associated with oral contraceptive use. JAMA 1990;263:54-9.

17. Forrest KA, Washington AE, Daling JR, Sweet RL. Vaginal douching as a possible risk factor for pelvic inflammatory disease. J Natl Med Assoc 1989;81:159-65.

18. Rice PA, Schachter J. Pathogenesis of pelvic inflammatory disease caused by *Chlamydia trachomatis* and *Neisseria gonorrhoeae*: where should research efforts focus? In: Joint Meeting of the Centers for Disease Control and National Institutes of Health about Pelvic Inflammatory Disease Prevention, Management, and Research in the 1990s, Bethesda, Maryland, September 4-5, 1990.

19. Irwin KL, Moorman AC, O'Sullivan MJ, Sperling R, Koestler ME, Soto I, et al. Influence of human immunodeficiency virus infection on pelvic inflammatory disease. Obstet Gynecol 2000;95:525-34.

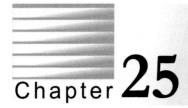

Chapter 25

Bartholin Abscess

Madhavi M Gupta, Garima Sharma

INTRODUCTION

Bartholin abscesses and cysts account for 2 percent of all gynecological visits per year.[1] Most cases occur 'out of the blue' in women aged between 20 and 30. However, they can occur in older or younger women.

Bartholin Glands

The Bartholin glands are a pair of pea-sized, vulvovaginal, mucrus-secreting vestibular glands that are located in the labia minora in the 4- and 8-o'clock positions, beneath the bulbospongiosus muscle.

Bartholin Cyst

A Bartholin cyst is a fluid-filled sac that develops in one of the Bartholin glands or ducts when the duct that drains the fluid from the gland becomes blocked and causes the duct and gland to swell.

Bartholin Abscess

A Bartholin gland abscess develops either when a Bartholin cyst becomes infected or when the Bartholin gland itself becomes infected.[2] Bartholin gland abscesses were thought to develop mainly from gonococcal or chlamydial infections. However, Brook reported 67 different bacterial isolates similar to the natural vaginal flora in a series of Bartholin gland abscesses.[3]

The differences between Bartholin abscess and cyst are described in Table 25.1.[4]

CASE SCENARIO

A 32-year-old para 2 presented to the emergency with complaints of vulval pain and swelling and fever over the past 2 to 3 days, making walking and sitting very uncomfortable.

Comments: Bartholin cyst and abscess are a common cause of vulval swelling.

Table 25.1: Differentiation between Bartholin abscess and Bartholin cyst	
Bartholin Abscess	*Bartholin Cyst*
Erythema present in skin overlying and surrounding the gland	Erythema absent
Skin overlying the gland typically warm to the touch	No increase in temperature
Fever present, especially with tachycardia	Fever absent
Advancing cellulitis can be present	Cellulitis absent
WBC count elevated	WBC count not elevated
Bacteria and WBCs are present in the fluid (pus) contained within the Bartholin gland	No bacteria or WBCs present in (serous) fluid contained within the cyst
Enlarged gland	Enlarged gland

Table 25.2: Differential diagnosis of Bartholin gland abnormalities	
Vulval lesions	*Vaginal lesions*
Sebaceous cyst	Vaginal inclusion cyst
Dysontogenetic cyst	Endometriosis
Hematoma	Adenosis
Fibroma	Gartner duct cyst
Lipoma	Leiomyoma
Hidradenoma	Inguinal hernia
Syringoma	
Endometriosis	

Differential Diagnosis

See Table 25.2

POINTS TO BE NOTED IN HISTORY

- History of swelling -a lump develops and quickly gets bigger, typically over a few hours or days.
- *Pain:* Site, character, duration, relation of pain with sitting or walking, micturition, coitus, how is the pain relieved
- Any similar swelling in the past, and how did it resolve
- History of fever
- Muco-purulent cervical discharge, dysuria
- Sexual practices—previous sexually transmitted infections, pelvic inflammatory disease
- Male sex partner—profession, whether into a polygamous relationship, any previous sexually transmitted infection.
- Date of last menstrual period to determine if the patient is pregnant.

> **History in this case:**
> History of vulval pain and a tender swelling locally.

POINTS TO BE NOTED IN EXAMINATION

General Examination

- General condition
- Temperature, pulse, respiratory rate and blood pressure
- Pallor, icterus

Cardiovascular and Respiratory System Examination

Abdominal Examination

Pelvic Examination

Local Examination

- Swelling:
  - Inspection—Situation, colour, shape, size, surface, edge, number, skin over the swelling (red and edematous in inflammatory).
  - Palpation—Temperature, tenderness, size, shape, extent, surface, consistency, reducibility, compressibility.
- Any growth, ulceration, abnormality should be noted on vulva, perineum, urethra, sub urethral region and anus.

Per Speculum (P/S) Examination

- Cervical discharge—Amount, color, and smell. Cervical swab is sent for gram's stain culture and sensitivity.

Per Vaginum (P/V) Examination

- Uterine size and position
- Tenderness on palpation of the uterus, adnexae or when uterus is moved.
- Pelvic mass

> **Examination in this case:**
> Pulse -100/min, BP-120/70 mm Hg, temperature-100°F, respiratory rate-16/min
> General and systemic examination unremarkable
> Abdominal examination unremarkable
> Local examination- There is a 5×5 cm, tender, fluctuant, erythematous swelling at 5 o'clock position within the left posterior labium minus.
> P/S – Profuse mucopurulent discharge.
> P/V—Uterus is anteverted, normal size, mobile, adnexal tenderness present.

Diagnosis

Bartholin abscess.

INVESTIGATIONS

- Hemoglobin, total and differential leukocyte counts
- Blood sugar
- Urine albumin, sugar , microscopy, culture and sensitivity
- Cervical swab for culture and sensitivity

> **Investigations in this case:**
> Hemoglobin—11gm%, Hematocrit—32%
> Complete blood count—15,000/cu mm with raised neutrophils
> Blood sugar (random)—99 mg%
> Urine routine and microscopy—Normal, a sample was sent for culture and sensitivity
> Cervical swab was sent for culture and sensitivity

TREATMENT

- *Conservative*—Treatment of Bartholin abscess is similar to that of symptomatic cysts. If an abscess points and ruptures spontaneously, the patient may need only sitz baths, antibiotics and pain medication. In fact, it is prudent to treat early abscesses with sitz baths until the abscess points, making incision and definitive treatment easier.
- *Infection control*—Cultures for Chlamydia and gonococcal organisms should be obtained and a course of oral broad-spectrum antibiotics prescribed. Diabetic patients need careful observation due to their susceptibility to necrotizing infections, and consideration should be given to inpatient management of these patients.
- *Surgical*—There are several treatments for Bartholin duct cysts and abscesses.[5] Marsupialization or "window" procedure, placement of a word catheter, application of silver nitrate to the abscess cavity, carbon dioxide laser excision and surgical excision are all acceptable options for treatment of a Bartholin gland abscess, although excision would not be the primary choice because of the risk of hemorrhage.

Marsupialization

A marsupialization procedure can be performed for a Bartholin abscess or if a cyst recurs despite treatment with a word catheter or if the physician prefers it as a first-line technique. It can be performed in the emergency department or outpatient surgical set up under local anesthesia. The recurrence rate after marsupialization is about 10 percent.

Procedure

After sterile preparation of the cyst and surrounding area, a no. 11 scalpel is used to make a vertical elliptic incision just inside or outside the hymenal ring, but not on the outer labium majus. The incision should measure about 1.5× 3 ×1.0 cm and should be deep enough to include both the vestibular skin and the underlying cyst wall. The cyst or abscess will drain. An oval wedge of vulval skin and underlying cyst wall should be removed. Loculations are broken if necessary; the cyst wall is sewn to the adjacent vestibular skin using interrupted 3-0 or 4-0 delayed-absorbable sutures on a small needle. The new tract will slowly shrink over time and epithelialize, forming a new duct orifice.

Treatment in this case:
- Marsupialization was done. Although it can be done under local anesthesia but since the patient was very apprehensive a saddle block was given.
- Fluid drained was sent for culture for *Neisseria gonorrhoeae*, *Chlamydia*, and aerobic and anerobic bacteria.
- Broad spectrum antibiotics- In this case, Cefotaxime 1 gm intravenous (IV) 12 hourly was given.
- Other medications :
  - Paracetamol 500 mg was given when the fever was ≥ 100° F. (patient was afebrile after marsupialization)
  - Diclofenac sodium 100 mg 12 hourly as an anti-inflammatory and analgesic.
  - Pantoprazole 40 mg once daily was also given.
- Hot sitz bath

Outcome in this case: The patient recovered fully and was discharged after 24 hours on oral antibiotics anti-inflammatory agent diclofenac sodium with specific advice to use safe sex practices.

Complications

The procedures that have been described are safe and effective; however, complications can occur. Septic shock has been reported after drainage of a Bartholin gland abscess.[3] Other potential complications include excessive bleeding, cellulitis and dyspareunia.

Prognosis

The chance of full recovery is excellent. About 10 percent of the time, abscesses recur. It is important to treat gonorrhea or any other infection that causes abscesses.

Prevention

Safer sex behaviours (especially condom use) and good personal hygiene may decrease the risk of developing a Bartholin abscess.

BARTHOLIN ABSCESS IN A PREGNANT PATIENT

Pregnancy

Although none of the treatment methods discussed is contraindicated in pregnant women, the increase in blood flow to the pelvic area during pregnancy may lead to excessive bleeding when Bartholin cysts or abscesses are treated. For this reason, surgical treatment for asymptomatic cysts should probably be withheld until after delivery. If treatment is necessary because a cyst becomes infected or the patient presents with an abscess, local anesthesia is not contraindicated, and most broad-spectrum antibiotics appear safe for use during pregnancy.

Labor

Occasionally, patients present with symptomatic Bartholin gland abscesses during labor. In this situation, it seems wise to withhold treatment until after delivery if possible, since an open labial abscess theoretically places the patient at risk for endomyometritis. Unless the abscess obstructs the vagina (soft tissue dystocia), cesarean section is not indicated.

KEY POINTS

- Bartholin abscess presents as a tender, angry looking swelling in the posterior aspect of either side of the vulval area which makes even walking and sitting painful.
- *N. gonorrhoea* and *Chlamydia* are the most commonly implicated organisms.
- Mainline treatment is incision and marsupialization along with broad spectrum antibiotics and pain relief.
- Recurrent cyst and abscess formation mandates excision of the gland.

REFERENCES

1. Pundir J, Auld BJ. A review of the management of diseases of the Bartholin's gland. J Obstet Gynecol 2008;28:161-5.
2. Singh N, Thappa DM, Jaisankar TJ, Habeebullah S. Pattern of non-venereal dermatoses of female external genitalia in South India. Dermatol Online J 2008;14:1.
3. Lopez-Zeno JA, Ross E, O'Grady JP. Septic shock complicating drainage of a Bartholin gland abscess. Obstet Gynecol 1990; 76:915-6.
4. Faro S. Vulvovaginal infections. In: Bieber EJ, Sanfilippo JS, Horowitz IR, (eds).Clinical Gynecology. Pennsylvania: Churchill Livingstone Elsevier, 2006.pp.249-58.
5. Wechter ME, Wu JM, Marzano D, Haefner H. Management of Bartholin duct cysts and abscesses: a systematic review. Obstet Gynecol Surv 2009;64:395-404.

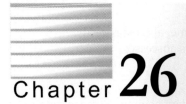

Chapter 26

Abnormal Uterine Bleeding in Gynecology

Raksha Arora, Vidhi Choudhary

INTRODUCTION

Abnormal and excessive bleeding per vaginam from childhood to menopause is a common problem which is encountered by gynecologists. The main objective of discussion in this chapter is the management of severe vaginal bleeding in adolescent, perimenopausal and reproductive age groups. However, bleeding prior to menarche should be investigated and managed as an abnormal finding.

CASE SCENARIO-1

Miss X, a 16-yr-old girl presented to gynae casuality with heavy menstrual bleeding for one week. It was associated with dysmenorrhea and breathlessness. On examination, she was pale and had a pulse of 102/min. No abnormal findings on systemic examination; per abdomen—soft, no mass palpable. Vulval pad showed few clots.

> **Comment:** Heavy bleeding in adolescents results from anovulation and coagulation defects.[1,2] However, pregnancy and sexual abuse should always be considered in differential diagnosis.

POINTS TO BE NOTED IN HISTORY

- Age at menarche
- Duration, amount of bleeding
- Cycle length to know whether they are ovulatory or anovulatory
- History of preceding amenorrhea which may point towards anovulatory cycles or abortion if she is sexually active (history of sexual contact should be elicited in private in young girl)
- History of dysmenorrhea whether spasmodic or congestive. In anovulatory cycles dysmenorrhea is usually absent
- History of easy bruisability/prolonged bleeding from wounds/heavy bleeding after any surgery or history of epistaxis which may be suggestive of coagulation disorder
- History of low-grade fever, night sweats or chest pain suggestive of tuberculosis
- History of weight gain, cold intolerance, fatigue or constipation suggestive of hypothyroidism
- History of jaundice may be suggestive of chronic liver disease.

History in this case:
She came to the casualty at midnight with excessive menstrual bleeding for the last one week. It was associated with passage of clots. She also gave history of breathlessness and fatigue. There was no history suggestive of TB, hypothyroidism or coagulopathy.
She had menarche at the age of fourteen years her previous cycles were 3-4/30 days but for last one year 5-6/40-45 days.

Points to be Noted in Examination

General Examination

- Vitals—Pulse rate, blood pressure (BP), respiratory rate (RR), temperature
- Pallor, pedal edema, icterus
- Palpation of lymph nodes for TB, lymphoma and leukemia
- Thyroid swelling
- Petechial hemorrhage at different sites or bleeding gums

Respiratory and Cardiovascular Examination

Abdominal Examination

- Hepatosplenomegaly
- Any abdominal mass to rule out fibroid or ovarian mass

Pelvic Exam

Local Examination

Foreign body, evidence of any injury, hymen intact or torn, amount of bleeding.

Per Rectal (P/R) Examination

Size of uterus, its mobility, whether tender on movement, presence of any mass in the lateral fornices, condition of rectovaginal septum.

Per Vaginum (P/V) Examination

It should be avoided unless necessary.

Examination in this case:
She was very pale and thin built. She had tachycardia (pulse 104/min).
Thyroid was not enlarged, there was no lymphadenopathy.
CVS and respiratory examination were normal.
No abdominal mass palpable.
On examination of vulva few clots were seen. Patient did not allow P/R examination.

Investigations

Following investigations should be done in cases of puberty menorrhagia:
- Complete hemogram and peripheral smear
- Bleeding and clotting time
- Prothrombin time (PT)/Activated partial thromboplastin time (APTT)
- ESR, Mantoux test and chest X-ray if suspicion of tuberculosis (TB)
- Thyroid function tests (TFT) if symptoms suggestive of hypothyroidism are present

- USG pelvis for uterine size and endometrial thickness, for any adnexal mass and to rule out any congenital malformation
- Special hematological investigations where needed
  - Bone marrow aspiration
  - Platelet function study
  - Factor VIII and IX study
- Menstrual blood for PCR tuberculosis if strong suspicion of TB.

> **Investigations in this case:**
> Hb—6.5 gm%
> Peripheral smear—Microcytic hypochromic anemia
> Blood group—B +ve
> Coagulation profile—Normal
> Urine routine and microscopy (R/M)—Normal
> Chest X-ray—Normal
> Transabdominal USG scan—Normal study.

Diagnosis

A provisional diagnosis of anovulatory dysfunctional uterine bleeding was made.
Dysfunctional Uterine Bleeding (DUB) is the abnormal interine bleeding after exclusion of pregnancy of tumor and any other organic causes.
Anovulatory DUB is common in this age group because of immature hypothalamic pituitary axis.
Ovulatory DUB is due to change in endometrial hemostasis and alteration in synthesis and release of prostaglandin. A change in the ratio of endometrial vasoconstrictor PGF2 Alpha and PGE2 (Endometrial vasodilator) and increase in total prostaglandin may be the cause.

MANAGEMENT

Immediate Treatment

It is directed towards controlling acute bleeding by high doses of hormones and blood transfusion if Hb < 7gm%. Coagulopathy and pregnancy should be excluded.
Following hormones are used to arrest an acute episode of bleeding:[3-6]
1. Tab norethisterone 10 to 20 mg 8 hourly till bleeding stops and dose is tapered off to 10 mg 12 hourly for 7 to 10 days and then once daily for 10 days.
2. Combined oral contraceptive (COC) pills (Ovral-G, Mala –N) 2 to 4 tablets per day till bleeding stops followed by one tab daily over 3 to 4 weeks.
3. Another regime described but not commonly used—Intravenous Conjugated equine estrogens (Premarin) 25 mg intravenously (IV) every 4 hrs till bleeding stops or decreases significantly followed by oral progesterone (medroxyprogesterone 20 mg BD or norethisterone 5- 10 mg BD for 10 days) or COC pills can be given for 3 to 6 months to regularize menstrual cycles.
   Most of the times bleeding stops by any of the above regimes and dilatation and curettage (D&C) is required very rarely.

Maintenance Therapy

1. Cyclical progesterone (medroxyprogesterone acetate) 5 to 10 mg BD from 15th to 26th day of menstrual cycles for 3 to 6 months.
2. COC pills for 21 days every month for 3 to 4 months.
3. Tranexamic acid 50 mg three times a day during periods.
4. Hematinics and calcium supplementations.
5. Exercise and dietary advice.
   Treatment can be stopped after 3 to 4 months or can be continued longer if needed. On stopping treatment patient should be reassessed to ascertain if cycles are regular with normal flow.

Treatment in this case:
Patient was admitted and was transfused 2 units packed cells.
She was given COC pills with 50 μg of ethinyl estradiol (e.g. Ovral G) daily with tranexamic acid 500 mg three times a day.
Bleeding stopped after 3 days. She was discharged with advice to continue COC pills for 21 days and to start again after next period for 3 cycles.

CASE SCENARIO-2

A 27-years-old multiparous woman presented to the gynae casualty with complaints of excessive bleeding per vaginum for last 10 days with history of passage of clots. There was no associated dysmenorrhea. Menstrual history revealed that the duration of bleeding was for 8 to 10 days occurring at an interval of 28 to 30 days for the last 4 cycles.

Comment: This patient in reproductive age group has menorrhagia which is generally caused by pathology in the uterus or any vascular abnormality.
Complications of pregnancy should always be ruled out

Differential Diagnosis

Different causes of excessive bleeding in this age group are anatomical, hormonal, and systemic or drug related (Table 26.1).

POINTS TO BE NOTED IN HISTORY

- Detailed menstrual history eliciting the amount, duration of bleeding and cycle length. The cycle length should be considered from first day of last menstrual bleeding. For example if a

Table 26.1: Causes of excessive menstrual bleeding in reproductive age group	
Anatomical causes	**Systemic causes**
• Submucous fibroid	• Thrombocytopenia
• Adenomyosis	• Leukemia
• Endometriosis	
• Pelvic inflammatory disease (PID)	
• Tubercular endometritis	
• Intrauterine contraceptive device (IUCD)	
• Functioning ovarian tumor	
• Uterine arteriovenous malformations	
Hormonal causes	**Drugs**
• Hypothyroidism	• Warfarin
• DUB which may be classified as:	• Heparin
Ovulatory –It can be irregular ripening due to	• Aspirin
corpus luteal deficiency leading to premenstrual	• Herbal medicines rich in estrogen
breakthrough bleeding. Other type is due to	
persistent corpus luteum (Halban's disease)	
resulting in prolonged and heavy bleeding due	
to irregular shedding.	
Anovulatory – Ovulation does not occur; as a	
result proliferative endometrium persists due to	
unopposed estrogen secretion. Continued growth	
without any periodic shedding of endometrium	
leads to breakdown of endometrial tissue causing	
episodes of amenorrhea followed by acute heavy	
bleeding. Histopathology can be proliferative	
endometrium, simple/complex hyperplasia with	
or without atypia.	

woman has menstrual bleeding for 7 days and the next period is after 15 days the menstrual cycle is 22 days and not 15 days. The patient will give history that she has bleeding twice a month and one may wrongly think that she is having polymenorrhea.

- History of postcoital bleeding which is suggestive of polyp, fibroid, ectropion and cancer of cervix.
- History of intermenstrual bleeding, which may be due to polyp or submucous fibroid or even carcinoma cervix
- Pain abdomen with discharge per vaginum suggests PID.
- History of weight gain, lethargy, constipation suggest hypothyroidism
- History of dysmenorrhea, dyspareunia, dysuria, dyschezia, or infertility is suggestive of endometriosis.
- History of IUCD Insertion
- History of drug intake or any other herbal medicine
- History of bleeding diathesis.
- History of preceding amenorrhea to rule out pregnancy and history of recent delivery, abortion or ectopic to evaluate for PID.

History in this case:
This patient had excessive bleeding with increased duration of flow for 4 cycles. She changed 7-8 pads / day. However, periods were regular.
Previous cycles 4-5/28-30 days.
Menarche was at 13 yr of age. No history of bleeding diathesis.
There was no history of intermenstrual bleeding, postcoital bleeding or dyspareunia.

POINTS TO BE NOTED IN EXAMINATION

General Examination

Look for anemia, lymphadenopathy, thyroid and do breast examination

Cardiovascular and Respiratory System Examination

Abdominal Examination

For mass in lower abdomen, hepatic and splenic enlargement

Pelvic Examination

Per speculum Examination—Note whether cervix is healthy/unhealthy or presence of endocervical discharge in the vagina, or any other lesion.
Per vaginal Examination—Check for cervical motion tenderness. Size and shape of uterus along with mobility should be noted and finally any mass, thickening or tenderness in fornices should be elicited.

Examination in this case:
The patient's general condition was fair, mild pallor was present and there was no lymphadenopathy. Breasts were normal.
Abdominal examination—No mass palpable
Per speculum examination—Cervix and vagina were healthy; no discharge
Per vaginal examination—On bimanual examination cervix felt normal, pointing downwards and forwards. Cervical movements were not tender. Uterus was multiparous size, mobile, nontender, no mass or thickness or tenderness was felt in fornices.

Diagnosis

A provisional diagnosis of ovulatory DUB[3] was made as patient had heavy bleeding with normal cycle length.

Differential Diagnosis

- PID
- Tuberculous endometritis
- Adenomyosis
- Hypothyroidism

INVESTIGATIONS

- Routine blood and urine examination.
- Other tests—Coagulation profile, TFT on basis of clinical suspicion.
- Pap smear is done when patient is not bleeding.
- Transvaginal sonography (TVS)—To rule out any structural abnormality. Assessment is done regarding endometrial thickness, endometrial polyp, fibroid or adenomyosis, adnexal mass (e.g. tubo-ovarian mass, endometrioma).
- Saline sonohysterography (SIS)—In cases of suspicion of endometrial polyp or fibroid on TVS (more specific).
- Endometrial aspiration by Karman cannula (No. 4) is highly sensitive and specific method of assessing endometrium.
- Hysteroscopy—It is indicated only when less invasive methods, i.e. TVS, SIS or Endometrial biopsy results are inconclusive.

> **Investigations in this patient:**
> Hb—8 gm%, coagulation profile—normal.
> TFT—Normal.
> TVS—Normal study.
> Endometrial aspiration was done as emergency measure as she was bleeding profusely for last ten days. Endometrial tissue was hyperplastic on gross examination and was sent for histopathological examination (HPE).

TREATMENT

Most of the patients respond well to medical treatment. Endometrial ablation techniques, resection or hysterectomy is considered once the medical management fails.

Nonhormonal Methods

1. Nonsteroidal anti-inflammatory drugs (NSAIDS)—inhibit cyclo-oxygenase, thus reducing prostaglandin levels and reduce blood loss by 20 to 50 percent. Mostly mefenamic acid in dosage of 500 mg 8 hourly/day is used during menstruation.
2. Tranexamic acid – 1 gm 4 times daily during menstruation reduces blood loss by 50 percent. It inhibits action of plasminogen activators.

Hormonal Therapy

This consist of progesterone, combined estrogen and progesterone, estrogen and GnRH analogs
1. Progesterone halts the endometrial growth and allows an organized sloughing of the endometrium. They also increase the PGF2 Alpha/PGE ratio stimulating the arachidonic acid formation in the endometrium. Progesterone can be given as cyclical therapy, continuous oral or intramuscular or as intrauterine device (IUD) (Mirena).
   a. Cyclical therapy, given as medroxyprogesterone acetate 5 to 10 mg daily from 15th to 25th day is effective in case of anovulatory cycles. But in case of endometrial hyperplasia, medroxyprogesterone acetate is given from 5th to 26th day for 3 to 6 cycles.
   b. Continuous progesterone may be considered in very anemic patients to avoid menorrhagia in each cycle

   c. Levonorgestrel IUD is effective in both ovulatory and anovulatory bleeding. It reduces blood loss by 94 percent after 3 months. It contains 52 mg of levonorgestrel and releases 20 μg daily 5 years. High cost is a limitation of this effective method.

   d. Depot medroxyprogesterone acetate (DMPA) 150 mg every 3 months is effective for anovulatory bleeding. It causes atrophy of the endometrium leading to amenorrhea and intermittent spotting.

2. Combined estrogen and progesterone—Combined hormones given in form of COC pills (e.g. Mala N) is a very effective therapy both in anovulatory or ovulatory DUB in patients with heavy bleeding episodes.[7] The treatment starts with 3 to 4 tablets (of pills containing 35 μg of ethinylestradiol) per day till bleeding stops and then gradually tapered to 2 tablets per day for the next 3 days followed by one tablet per day until the pack is finished. The patient can be put on COC pills for next 3 to 4 cycles or she can be maintained on cyclical progesterone if estrogen is to be avoided.

3. High-dose estrogen therapy is effective in controlling acute bleeding episodes because it promotes rapid endometrial growth to cover denuded endometrial surfaces. Most of the time it is not a very commonly used method because of side effects of high doses of estrogen. However it may be used if bleeding is not controlled by other methods.
   - Estrogens are given as IV conjugated equine estrogen as discussed earlier
   - Orally 1.25 mg conjugated equine estrogen (Premarin 2 tab) or 2 μg of micronized estradiol every 4 to 6 hours. The dose is tapered down to one tablet daily for 7 to 10 days after the bleeding is controlled
   - After control of acute bleeding, progesterone or combined estrogen and progesterone are given to stabilize the estrogen stimulated endometrial growth.

4. Centchroman—60 mg twice weekly for 3 months can be considered for ovulatory DUB.

5. GnRH analogues—The use of goserelin acetate or leuprolide acetate is limited to achieving a short-term relief of bleeding prior to surgical procedure, i.e. ablation, myomectomy and hysterectomy.

Surgical Methods

These are used in cases refractory to medical management.
- Endometrial ablation
- Hysterectomy.

Role of D & C in such patient is justified only in cases of persistent menorrhagia not responding to medical management or patients presenting with shock due to heavy bleeding. The therapeutic effect of D & C is limited to the current menstrual cycle.

> **Treatment in this case:**
> Endometrial aspiration was done in OPD and patient was put on progesterones (tab medroxyprogesterone 10 mg BD). Bleeding stopped after 5 days and then dose was tapered to 1 OD for total of 10 days.
> Patient came for follow-up after 2 weeks with HPE report showing secretory endometrium.
> She was offered Mirena in view of ovulatory DUB which she declined due to cost factor. She was subsequently put on COC pills for 3 cycles.

CASE SCENARIO-3

A 50-years-old woman postmenopausal for the last 3 years presented to gyane OPD with history of excessive bleeding per vaginum for one week.

> **Comment:** Perimenopausal women usually have anovulation as the cause of such bleeding, however malignancy of cervix and endometrial should always be ruled out.

POINTS TO BE NOTED IN HISTORY

- Ingestion of exogenous hormones
- Itching over vulva to rule out atrophic vaginitis and cervicitis
- Prior history of vaginal discharge
- Pain lower abdomen (Simpson's pain) typical of endometrial cancer
- Coital trauma, postcoital bleeding
- History suggestive of diabetes, hypertension
- Past or family history of cancer of colon, endometrial and breast cancer.

POINTS TO BE NOTED IN EXAMINATION

General Examination

- Body mass index (BMI)
- Blood pressure
- Lymphadenopathy
- Breast examination—To rule out any nodule.

Cardiovascular and Respiratory System Examination

Abdominal Examination

- Mass in lower abdomen
- Hepatic and splenic enlargement.

Pelvic Exam

Local

- Inspection of external genitalia for any growth over vulva, urethral orifice (urethral caruncle may be a cause of bleeding) and note for any discharge.

Per Speculum Examination

- Check for any growth on cervix or any bleeding or discharge coming through the os. A bulky cervix with foul smelling discharge mixed with blood may be suggestive of cervical growth
- Thorough inspection of the vagina (from fornices to lower vagina) to look for any lesion, rugosity, hemorrhagic spots or atrophic changes.

Per Vaginum Examination

- Feel of cervix is very important since very hard and bulky cervix is suggestive of cervical carcinoma
- Uterus, small or enlarged; firm or soft; mobile or fixed. A multiparous or just bulky uterus may be large for postmenopausal woman
- Fornices are checked for any adnexal mass which will be felt separate from the uterus with a notch in between. The movements of cervix are not conducted to an adnexal mass and conversely gentle pushing of the adnexal mass upwards should not pull the cervix up.

Per Rectal Examination or Combined Vaginal and Rectal Examination (P/V/R)

It is done keeping the index finger in the rectum to look for any involvement of the parametrium, secondaries in pouch of Douglas and involvement of the rectovaginal septum. Any mass in the rectum and involvement of the rectal mucosa should also be ruled out.

Examination in this case:
General condition- fair, BMI-30 kg/m², BP-150/90 mm Hg
Breast examination-normal
P/A—Obesity present
P/S—cervix and vagina healthy
P/V—uterus retroverted, retroflexed, 6-8 weeks, soft, bilateral fornix clear
P/V/R—bilateral parametrium free, rectal mucosa free

INVESTIGATIONS

- Complete blood count, fasting blood sugar, urea, urine R/M , X-ray chest, ECG
- Pap smear may be delayed till the bleeding stops
- Biopsy from the cervix if there is growth
- TVS[10]-for focal lesions and endometrial thickness.
- Endometrial aspiration with a 4 mm cannula and the material should be sent for HPE. Endocervical curettage specimen is likely to be contaminated in the presence of bleeding.

TREATMENT

- Tranexamic acid may be given to stop bleeding
- If bleeding does not stop TVS may be done prior to hysteroscopy directed endometrial biopsy.
- If HPE report is endometrial hyperplasia without atypia 10 to 20 mg of medroxyprogesterone acetate is given for 3 to 6 months and re-evaluation by endometrial aspiration is done after 6 months.
- If HPE shows endometrial cancer, staging laparotomy with extrafascial hysterectomy and lymph node sampling is done.

Investigations in this case:
Hb—10 gm%, platelets—normal.
Fasting blood glucose—180 mg/dL,
Liver and kidney function tests—normal
Paps smear—Inflammatory smear.
TVS—Uterus—Normal size; bilateral ovaries—Normal; endometrial thickness—14mm.
Endometrial aspiration—HPE report of simple focal adenomatous hyperplasia without atypia.

Management in this case:
On the basis of HPE report patient was put on medroxyprogesterone acetate 10 mg three times a day for 6 months. Repeat TVS and endometrial aspiration showed endometrial thickness of 3 mm and normal endometrium. She was kept on strict follow up with strict diabetes and hypertension control.
Two years later the endometrial aspiration revealed endometrial cancer. Extrafascial hysterectomy and bilateral salpingo oopherectomy was done. Pelvic and para aortic lymphadenectomy was not done because on cut section the uterus showed a small growth involving only the endometrium. She was given postoperative irradiation to the vault.
After 3 years of follow-up, she is doing well.

CASE SCENARIO-4

A 5-year-old girl is brought by her anxious mother to gynae OPD with bleeding from vagina.

Comment: Vaginal bleeding in childhood is always of clinical importance, regardless of its duration and quantity.

Common Causes of Bleeding in Children[1]

- Vulvovaginitis
- Foreign body

- Trauma (sexual abuse)
- Tumors
- Urethral polyp
- Vulval skin disorders

Examination of young girl may be difficult and general anesthesia is often required for adequate exposure and proper evaluation. Vagina is examined using small Sims speculum.

> **Treatment in this case:**
> In above case foreign body was lodged high up in vagina which was removed under general anesthesia.

KEY POINTS

- Common causes of vaginal bleeding in a young child are trauma due to foreign body, sexual abuse, tumor and vulvovaginitis. Examination under anesthesia may be required to check for foreign body in the upper part of vagina.
- Coagulopathy and pregnancy must be ruled out in any young adolescent girl presenting with menorrhagia that is severe or does not respond to typical therapy.
- High doses of norethisterone or medroxy progesterone acetate are used to control acute adolescent menorrhagia. Alternately COC pills can be given to control bleeding.
- DUB in reproductive age women is mostly treated medically, resorting to surgical procedures only in cases not responsive to medical management. COC pills, intrauterine progesterones (Mirena) are the ideal options.
- Perimenopausal and menopausal women with abnormal vaginal bleeding may have genital tract malignancy. Endometrial hyperplasia or carcinoma and cervical cancer must be ruled out by endocervical and endometrial biopsy. No treatment should be started without HPE report.

REFERENCES

1. Noorhasan DJ, Weiss G. Perimenarchal menorrhagia: evaluation and management. J Pediatr 2010;156:162.
2. Ahuja SP, Hertweck SP. Overview of bleeding disorders in adolescent females with menorrhagia. J Pediatr Adolesc Gynecol 2010;23:S15-21.
3. Bongers MY, Mol BW, Brölmann HA. Current treatment of dysfunctional uterine bleeding. Maturitas 2004;47:159-74.
4. Marjoribanks J, Lethaby A, Farquhar C. Surgery versus medical therapy for heavy menstrual bleeding. Cochrane Database Syst Rev 2006;2:CD003855.
5. Hickey M, Higham J, Fraser IS.Progestogens versus oestrogens and progestogens for irregular uterine bleeding associated with anovulation. Cochrane Database Syst Rev 2007;4:CD001895.
6. Lethaby A, Irvine G, Cameron I. Cyclical progestogens for heavy menstrual bleeding. Cochrane Database Syst Rev 2008;1:CD001016.
7. Farquhar C, Brown J. Oral contraceptive pill for heavy menstrual bleeding. Cochrane Database Syst Rev 2009;4:CD000154.
8. Bignardi T, Van den Bosch T, Condous G. Abnormal uterine and post-menopausal bleeding in the acute gynaecology unit. Best Pract Res Clin Obstet Gynaecol 2009;23:595-607.
9. Breijer MC, Timmermans A, van Doorn HC, Mol BW, Opmeer BC. Diagnostic strategies for postmenopausal bleeding. Obstet Gynecol Int 2010;850-12.
10. Dreisler E, Sorensen SS, Ibsen PH, Lose G. Value of endometrial thickness measurement for diagnosing focal intrauterine pathology in women without abnormal uterine bleeding. Ultrasound Obstet Gynecol 2009;33:344-8.

Chapter 27

Dysmenorrhea and Cryptomenorrhea

Shikha Sharma

INTRODUCTION

The term dysmenorrhea is derived from the Greek words *dys*, meaning difficult/painful/abnormal, *mens*, meaning month, and *rrhea*, meaning flow. Dysmenorrhea is a gynecological medical condition of pain during menstruation that interferes with daily activities, as defined by ACOG[1] and others.[2] Still, dysmenorrhea is often defined simply as menstrual pain[3], or at least menstrual pain that is excessive. Dysmenorrhea is one of the most common gynecological problems in reproductive age women.

Dysmenorrhea is generally classified as primary or secondary. Secondary dysmenorrhea is diagnosed when symptoms are attributable to an underlying disease, disorder, or structural abnormality either within or outside the uterus. Primary dysmenorrhea is diagnosed when none of these is detected.

PRIMARY DYSMENORRHEA

Primary dysmenorrhea (also described as true, spasmodic, intrinsic, essential and functional) occurs in ovulatory cycles due to secretion and withdrawal of progesterone. Ovulatory cycles are established by 2 years after menarche in 20 to 45 percent teenage and by 4 to 5 years in 80 percent, therefore in nearly 50 percent of cases the pain does not arise until 2 to 4 years after the menarche; in others even though the initial periods may be painful, severe dysmenorrhea appears later. The overall prevalence of primary dysmenorrhea among adolescent girls is between 60 to 90 percent and decreases as age increases, however, only 15 percent seek medical attention. Primary dysmenorrhea reaches a maximum between the ages of 18 and 24 years and then diminishes. It is often relieved by pregnancy.

In primary dysmenorrhea pain sensation arises in the uterus and is related to muscle contractions. It can be excruciating and experienced a few hours before and after the onset of menstruation but rarely lasts in a severe form for longer than 12 hours and seldom beyond 48 hours. It is colicky (intermittent and spasmodic) in type, although the patient may describe it as a constant pain which may even cause her to 'double up'. The pain is felt mainly in the hypogastrium and is often referred to the inner and front aspects of the thighs; it never extends below the level of the knee and is never experienced in the back of the leg. There may be some low backache as well but this is not the dominant sensation.

During a severe attack upset of autonomic nervous system may present as nausea, vomiting, diarrhea, headache, rectal and bladder tenesmus along with vasomotor changes causing pallor, cold sweats and occasional fainting. Rarely there may be syncope and collapse.

CASE SCENARIO-1

An 18-year-old unmarried girl presented to the emergency with history of severe pain in the lower abdomen for last 2 hours associated with headache and two episodes of vomiting. She gave history of starting menstruation half hour back with slight relief in pain.

> **Comments:** Considering the typical history a diagnosis of primary dysmenorrhea should be considered while excluding other differential diagnosis.

Differential Diagnosis

- Secondary dysmenorrhea and its causes like endometriosis, leiomyoma, adenomyosis, ovarian cysts and pelvic inflammatory disease (PID).
- Ectopic pregnancy
- Acute abdomen due to
  - Surgical cause, e.g. acute appendicitis.
  - Nonsurgical cause, e.g. irritable bowel syndrome and inflammatory bowel disease
- Abortion
- Urinary tract infection (UTI).

POINTS TO BE NOTED IN HISTORY

- *Detailed history of pain*
  - Onset, duration, type, severity and location (site).
  - Relationship to the menstrual cycle and its presence at times other than during menses, whether relieved after onset of menses.
  - Associated symptoms such as nausea, vomiting, bloating, diarrhea, fatigue, headache or back pain.
  - Impact on physical and social activity (work, school or exercise)
  - The use of medication and their effectiveness
  - Any progression in severity with time.
- *Menstrual history*
  - Age at menarche
  - Age at the onset of dysmenorrhea
  - Cycle regularity, length, duration and amount of menstrual flow
  - Last menstrual period
  - Intermenstrual or premenstrual spotting or staining.
- *Obstetric history*
  - Gravidity and parity status
  - Previous pelvic infection
  - Infertility
  - Pelvic surgeries.
- *Sexual history*
  - Choice of contraceptive methods and if used, establish the effect of oral contraceptives on relieving dysmenorrhea pain.
  - Dyspareunia
  - Sexual abuse because this is reportedly associated with dysmenorrhea and pelvic pain.
- *Family history*
  - May suggest endometriosis as the cause of dysmenorrhea

POINTS TO BE NOTED IN EXAMINATION

General Examination

- General condition
- Temperature, pulse, respiratory rate (RR) and blood pressure (BP)
- Pallor, jaundice, cyanosis.

Cardiovascular and Respiratory System Examination

Abdominal Examination

- Location and severity of pain
- Tenderness, guarding, rigidity and rebound tenderness
- Presence of free fluid in peritoneal cavity
- Any mass palpable (including uterus)
- Bowel sounds.

Pelvic Examination

For younger adolescents who have never been sexually active, a careful abdominal examination is appropriate. In older adolescents or those known to be sexually active, a pelvic examination is crucial.

Local Examination

- Look for any rashes, swelling and discoloration.
- Make a note of any vaginal discharge, bleeding or foreign body.

Per Speculum (P/S) Examination

- Bleeding—Amount and site
- Cervical discharge – Amount, color and smell

Per Vaginum (P/V) Examination

- Uterine size and position
- Tenderness on palpation of the uterus, adnexae or when uterus is moved, i.e. cervical motion tenderness (differential diagnosis- ectopic pregnancy)
- Pelvic masses—suggest presence of tubo-ovarian masses (differential diagnosis - ectopic pregnancy, endometriosis, fibroid or PID)
- Culdesac—tenderness or nodularity may suggest endometriosis, PID or pelvic mass.

Per Rectal (P/R) Examination

It may be done in patients who are not sexually active to assess for pelvic pathology

Diagnosis

Primary dysmenorrhea
Patients with this diagnosis usually have normal findings on examination.

INVESTIGATIONS

No tests are specific to the diagnosis of primary dysmenorrhea. Diagnosis is made based on clinical findings.
The following can be performed to exclude organic causes of dysmenorrhea:
- Total and differential leukocyte counts to exclude infection.
- Human chorionic gonadotropin (hCG) level to exclude ectopic pregnancy, abortion etc.
- Erythrocyte sedimentation rate
- Pelvic ultrasonography (USG) is indicated to evaluate for other causes of pelvic pain such as ectopic pregnancy, ovarian cysts, fibroids, and intrauterine contraceptive devices. USG is highly sensitive test for detecting pelvic masses which may cause secondary dysmenorrhea.
- Cervical culture to exclude sexually transmitted diseases.
- Intravenous pyelogram is indicated if uterine malformation is confirmed as a cause or contributing factor for the dysmenorrhea.

TREATMENT

Treatment of primary dysmenorrhea is directed at providing relief from the cramping pelvic pain and associated symptoms. Symptomatic relief can be obtained from the agents that inhibit prostaglandin synthesis and have anti-inflammatory and analgesic properties.

Nonsteroidal Anti-Inflammatory Drugs (NSAID)

For both adolescent girls and women, NSAIDs are the treatment of choice. NSAIDs provide effective relief in 70 to 90 percent of patients.

Their efficacy derives from both a decrease in endometrial prostaglandin production and from decreased menstrual flow. NSAIDs treatment can be started at the onset of menses and continued for the usual duration of pain. Women with severe dysmenorrhea might benefit from starting treatment 1 to 2 days before menstrual bleeding begins.
There are numerous NSAIDs to choose from:
- *Proprionic acid derivatives*
  - Ibuprofen—400 mg x QID
  - Naproxen—250 mg x QID
  - Ketoprofen—75 mg x TDS
- *Fenamates*
  - Mefenamic acid—500 mg x TDS
  - Mecloferamate—100 mg x QID

Selective COX-2 Inhibitors

Although some selective COX-2 inhibitors have been approved for treatment of primary dysmenorrhea their higher cost and greater potential risks suggest their use should be limited.

Oral Contraceptives

Oral contraceptives also are effective treatment for dysmenorrhea. They can be considered a first line agent in sexually active women who require contraception or for those who do not tolerate or are not relieved sufficiently from NSAID treatment. They act by inhibiting ovulation, thereby decreasing endometrial prostaglandin production.

Counseling

Explanation of the menstrual process, sex education and reassurance to the patient are an important aspect of therapy.

Others

A wide variety of therapies including heat application, dietary and vitamin or herbal therapies, exercise and behavioural intervention are all under trial without any definitive results.

Women who fail to respond to treatment with NSAIDs and /or hormonal contraceptives and those having recurrent or worsening pain merit re-evaluation to exclude causes of secondary dysmenorrhea.

SECONDARY DYSMENORRHEA

Secondary dysmenorrhea is dysmenorrhea which is associated with an existing condition. The most common cause of secondary dysmenorrhea is endometriosis[4] but there may be many other causes.[5-10]

Causes

Causes of secondary dysmenorrhea include the following:
- Endometriosis
- Uterine myoma (fibroids)
- Uterine polyps
- Pelvic inflammatory disease
- Tubo-ovarian abscesses
- Ovarian cysts/torsion
- Adenomyosis
- Intrauterine contraceptive devices (IUCD)
- Adhesions
- Psychogenic pain.

CASE SCENARIO-2

A 35-year-old married nulliparous woman was brought to the emergency complaining of acute pain in abdomen for two hours while working on the computer in her office. The pain was enough to disrupt her work and was not relieved even after medication taken as soon as the pain had started. She is due for her periods three days after, and has been experiencing such pre-menstrual pains for the last three years, being more severe this time.

Comment: In this case, patient's age, nulliparity and the onset of pain a number of days before periods suggest secondary dysmenorrhea.

Differential Diagnosis

- Ectopic pregnancy
- Surgical and nonsurgical causes of acute abdomen (as mentioned earlier)
- Urinary tract infection (UTI).

Further work up includes a specific history of symptoms and menstrual cycle and a pelvic examination on the pattern mentioned in the previous case scenario. Once a diagnosis of secondary dysmenorrhea is made, further work up is aimed at finding the underlying cause.

History in this case:
Menstrual history and history of pain
Menarche—12 years, regular cycles, last menstrual period—25 days ago
Dysmenorrhea for 3 years progressively increasing in severity and duration; occurs 1 to 2 days before periods and lasts for 4 to 5 days after the onset of periods; associated with lower back pain. Initially responded to medication but with time very little relief occurs with medication. Dyspareunia for 2 years which has also worsened with time.
Obstetric history
Patient is married for 5 years and taking treatment for primary infertility for one year where she has been advised diagnostic laparoscopy.
Other
No history of any abdominal or pelvic surgeries
No history of dysmenorrhea in mother/sister.

Examination in this case:
Pulse—96/min, BP- 140/82 mm Hg, afebrile, RR- 20/min
General and systematic examination—unremarkable
Abdominal examination: Lower abdominal tenderness on deep palpation
P/S—No discharge
P/V—Uterus anteverted, normal size, slight tenderness with restricted mobility, bilateral adnexal tenderness present without any palpable masses.

Diagnosis

Secondary dysmenorrhea possibly due to PID.

INVESTIGATIONS

Based on results from history and pelvic examination, laboratory studies may be indicated to elucidate the causes of secondary dysmenorrhea:

Lab Tests

- Complete blood count (with differential), for evidence of infection or neoplastic process
- Urinalysis, to exclude urinary tract infection
- Quantitative hCG level to exclude ectopic pregnancy
- Gonococcal/chlamydial cultures, enzyme immuno-assay (EIA), and DNA probe testing, to exclude sexually transmitted infections (STIs)/PID.
- Erythrocyte sedimentation rate (ESR) for subacute salpingitis.
  Although these tests can be used as adjuncts in the work up of dysmenorrhea, they may not be very specific and may be misleading sometimes. Therefore, ancillary laboratory testing should not replace a sound clinical basis for diagnosis of dysmenorrhea and its underlying cause.

Imaging Studies

As already mentioned imaging studies are of little value. However, if pelvic pathology is suspected, abdominal and/or transvaginal ultrasonography are inexpensive and effective modalities.
- Ultrasonography is relatively noninvasive, can be easily performed in emergency and reveals most relevant pelvic pathology such as ectopic pregnancy, ovarian cysts, fibroids, IUCD and endometriosis. It is a highly sensitive test for detecting pelvic masses.
- Hysterosalpingogram is used to exclude endometrial polyps, leiomyomas and congenital abnormalities of the uterus
- Intravenous pyelogram is indicated if uterine malformation is confirmed as a cause or contributing factor for the dysmenorrhea

- Although CT scanning is not routinely ordered in emergency for patients with dysmenorrhea, it does have some utility, particularly in identifying ovarian torsion[11-13]
- MRI has some utility to detect adenomyosis and submucous myomas that might otherwise be missed on other imaging modalities.[11]

Diagnostic Procedures

- Other more invasive studies including laparoscopy, hysteroscopy and dilatation and curettage, may be required
- Laparoscopic examination is the single most useful procedure. It involves a complete diagnostic survey of the pelvis and the reproductive organs to ascertain the presence of any pathology that may account for the clinical symptoms
- Hysteroscopy and dilatation and curettage may be indicated to evaluate intrauterine pathology found on imaging
- An endometrial biopsy may be indicated if endometritis is considered likely.

TREATMENT

As has been discussed in the previous case scenario in addition to pain relief, other mainstays of treatment include reassurance and education. In secondary dysmenorrhea, treatment involves correction of underlying organic causes which may necessitate surgical interventions. In refractory cases of dysmenorrhea, laparoscopic pre-sacral neurectomy (PSN) or uterosacral nerve ablation (LUNA) have been efficacious and still under evaluation. A multidisciplinary approach may be indicated in such cases.

> **Treatment in this case:**
> The patient was given antibiotics as per PID protocol to which she responded successfully.

CRYPTOMENORRHEA

Cryptomenorrhea is a condition where menstruation occurs but is not visible (i.e. the menstrual blood fails to come out from the genital tract) due to obstruction of the outflow tract. A patient with cryptomenorrhea will appear to have amenorrhea but will experience cyclic menstrual pain.

Causes (Table 27.1)

The commonest cause is congenital obstruction due to imperforate hymen or vaginal septum. It may rarely occur due to cervical stenosis following amputation, conization or deep cauterization. The condition is surgically correctable.

Complications

- Hematocolpos (collection of blood in vagina)
- Hematometra (collection of blood in uterine cavity)
- Hematosalpinx (collection of blood in fallopian tube)

Table 27.1: Causes of cryptomenorrhea	
Congenital	*Acquired – stenosis of the cervix*
Imperforate hymen (commonest)	Cervical amputation
Transverse vaginal septum	Deep cauterization of the cervix
Atresia of upper- third of vagina and cervix	Conization

- Endometriosis in long-standing cases
- In severe untreated forms, infertility and urinary retention.

CASE SCENARIO-3

A 14-year-old adolescent girl was brought to the emergency with the complaint of pain abdomen for one day which aggravated suddenly at night, so much so that she was unable to sleep and is having difficulty in passing urine. The remarkable information given by her mother was that the girl was having such periodic pain for almost one year, being relieved on medication. The girl had not attained menarche.

Comment: The clinical presentation strongly suggests cryptomenorrhea.

Differential Diagnosis

- Pregnancy
- UTI.

POINTS TO BE NOTED IN HISTORY AND EXAMINATION

- Whether attained menarche or not—should be confirmed
- Periodic pain experienced by the patient
    - Is it a monthly event?
    - Duration, severity and location of pain
    - Fever associated with pain
- Abdominal examination is done after catheterization in case of urinary retention.
- Finding of a bluish bulge at introitus is diagnostic of imperforate hymen, however this finding may be absent in patients with complete or partial vaginal agenesis.

Examination in this case:
General and systemic examination—Unremarkable
Abdominal examination—A uniform globular mass was palpable in the hypogastrium
Local inspection—A tense, bulging, bluish membrane was seen at the level of hymen
Rectal examination—A large bulging mass was felt anteriorly.

INVESTIGATIONS

USG is diagnostic in such cases. The usual findings are:
- Vagina is seen filled with blood
- Uterus is pushed upwards
- Associated hematosalpinx and hematometra may be seen.

TREATMENT

Treatment of cryptomenorrhea depends on the underlying cause
- Imperforate hymen needs a cruciate incision and the retained blood drains out over next few days
- A thickened transverse vaginal septum can be treated with excision or Z-plasty
- A blind vagina will require a vaginoplasty
- Rarely cases of cervical agenesis may be surgically untreatable and require abdominal hysterectomy for relief of symptoms.[14]

KEY POINTS

- Dysmenorrhea is painful menstruation which incapacitates day-to-day activities
- Primary dysmenorrhea occurs in ovulatory cycles and is relieved following pregnancy and vaginal delivery
- Investigation is required if there are atypical symptoms or abnormal findings on pelvic examination
- NSAIDs are effective as first line management of primary dysmenorrhea
- Combined oral contraceptives are preferred when contraception is also required
- Secondary dysmenorrhea occurs due to pelvic pathologies such as PID, endometriosis or uterine polyps etc.
- Ultrasound is a useful noninvasive method for the detection of pelvic abnormalities
- Laparoscopic examination is the single most useful diagnostic procedure
- In secondary dysmenorrhea treatment of the underlying cause may require surgery
- Cryptomenorrhea is a condition where menstruation occurs but is not visible due to an obstruction of the outflow tract; usually presents at the age of puberty when blood gets collected in the vagina and gives rise to symptoms
- Imperforate hymen is the commonest cause of cryptomenorrhea where management is cruciate incision of the hymen and drainage of the blood.

REFERENCES

1. Patient Education Pamphlet: Dysmenorrhea (AP 046) By American Congress of Obstetricians and Gynecologists.
2. The Free Dictionary > dysmenorrhea Citing:
   Jonas: Mosby's Dictionary of Complementary and Alternative Medicine. Copyright 2005
3. The Free Dictionary > dysmenorrhea Citing:
   - Gale Encyclopedia of Medicine, Copyright 2008
   - Dorland's Medical Dictionary for Health Consumers, Copyright 2007
   - The American Heritage Medical Dictionary, Copyright 2007
   - Mosby's Medical Dictionary, 8th edition.
   - McGraw-Hill Concise Dictionary of Modern Medicine, Copyright 2002
4. French L. Dysmenorrhea in adolescents: diagnosis and treatment. Paediatr Drugs 2008;10:1-7.
5. Hilário SG, Bozzini N, Borsari R, Baracat EC. Action of aromatase inhibitor for treatment of uterine leiomyoma in perimenopausal patients. Fertil Steril 2008;91:240.
6. Nabeshima H, Murakami T, Nishimoto M, Sugawara N, Sato N. Successful total laparoscopic cystic adenomyomectomy after unsuccessful open surgery using transtrocar ultrasonographic guiding. J Minim Invasive Gynecol 2008;15:227-30.
7. Hacker NF, Moore JG, Gambone JC (eds). Essentials of Obstetrics and Gynecology. 4th edn. Elsevier Saunders, 2004.
8. Hubacher D, Reyes V, Lillo S, Pierre-Louis B, Zepeda A, Chen PL, et al. Preventing copper intrauterine device removals due to side effects among first-time users: randomized trial to study the effect of prophylactic ibuprofen. Hum Reprod 2006;21:1467-72.
9. Johnson BA. Insertion and removal of intrauterine devices. Am Fam Physician 2005;71:95-102.
10. Cho S, Nam A, Kim H, Chay D, Park K, Cho DJ, et al. Clinical effects of the levonorgestrel-releasing intrauterine device in patients with adenomyosis. Am J Obstet Gynecol 2008;198:373.e1-7.
11. Baines PA, Allen GM. Pelvic pain and menstrual related illnesses. Emerg Med Clin North Am 2001;19:763-80.
12. Kalish GM, Patel MD, Gunn ML, Dubinsky TJ. Computed tomographic and magnetic resonance features of gynecologic abnormalities in women presenting with acute or chronic abdominal pain. Ultrasound Q 2007;23:167-75.
13. Kamaya A, Shin L, Chen B, Desser TS. Emergency gynecologic imaging. Semin Ultrasound CT MR 2008;29:353-68.
14. Rana A, Gurung G, Begum SH, Adhikari S, Neupane BB. Hysterectomy for hematometra in a 15-year-old mentally handicapped girl with congenital cervicovaginal agenesis and concomitant ovarian adenoma. J Obstet Gynaecol Res 2008;34:105-7.

Chapter 28

Ovarian Torsion

Sangeeta Bhasin, Neha Gupta

INTRODUCTION

Ovarian torsion refers to the twisting of the ovary on its ligamentous supports, often resulting in impedance of its blood supply. It is a gynecological emergency with a prevalence of 2.7 percent.[1] It most commonly affects premenopausal women but upto 17 percent of torsions may occur in prepubertal and postmenopausal females. Diagnosis is often challenging due to its nonspecific clinical presentation. It has been attributed to a variety of etiologies.

Common Causes of Ovarian Torsion

- Anatomical changes affecting the weight and size of the ovary may alter the position of the fallopian tube and cause twisting. 50 to 60 percent cases of torsion occur secondary to pathologically enlarged ovaries, usually > 6 cm in size, although there is no specific size threshold below which the ovary precludes any risk of torsion. The common tumors which torse are the dermoid tumour followed by serous/mucinous cystadenoma and fibroma. Malignant tumors are less likely to undergo torsion due to cancerous adhesions with surrounding tissue.
- The normal ovary is at risk of torsion in children due to a long utero-ovarian ligament or due to developmental abnormalities like a long fallopian tube or absent mesosalpinx.
- Pregnancy is responsible for 20 percent of cases of torsion which occurs secondarily to an enlarged corpus luteal cyst or ovarian enlargement following ovulation induction.
- Strenuous exercise or a sudden increase in abdominal pressure may sometimes promote torsion of the ovary around its vascular pedicle.[2]
- History of pelvic surgery especially ligation increases the risk of torsion due to adhesions providing a site around which the ovarian pedicle may torse.
- The right ovary is more likely to torse than the left, suggesting that the sigmoid colon may help to prevent torsion.[3]

Pathogenesis

Compromise of the vascular pedicles in the suspensory ligament of the torsed ovary impedes lymphatic and venous outflow and arterial inflow. However, the arterial supply to the ovary is not interrupted to the same degree as the venous drainage since the muscular arteries are less compressible than the thin-walled veins. Continued arterial perfusion in the setting of blocked outflow leads to marked ovarian enlargement. Ovarian ischemia then occurs and with time, can result in necrosis, infarction, local hemorrhage, and peritonitis, possibly with systemic infection and inflammation.

CASE SCENARIO-1

A 29-year-old P2L2 presented to the gynecology casualty with complaints of acute onset of severe pain in the lower abdomen for two hours associated with nausea and three episodes of vomiting but no fever. There was no history of amenorrhea. Her last menstrual period was normal. She was passing urine and stools normally.

> **Comments:** Diagnosis of adnexal torsion should be considered since she is complaining of acute onset severe pain and vomiting in the absence of amenorrhea and vaginal bleeding.

Differential Diagnosis

Other causes of acute abdomen—Ectopic pregnancy, ruptured or hemorrhagic cyst, appendicitis, pelvic inflammatory disease, degenerating leiomyoma, renal colic.

POINTS TO BE NOTED IN HISTORY

- Site, intensity, duration and radiation of pain. Any aggravating or relieving factors.
  Pain of torsion is classically sudden onset, severe, unilateral, lower abdominal pain which worsens intermittently over a few hours. It is usually localized over the involved site and may radiate to the back, pelvis or thighs.
- Nausea and vomiting may be seen in 70 percent of patients with torsion.
- Fever is a late feature and may signify that the ovary has become necrotic.
- History of bleeding per vaginum
- History of syncopal attack
- History of abnormal bladder or bowel symptoms
- History of persistent discharge per vaginum and lower abdominal pain
- History of prior such episodes – These may indicate partial, spontaneously resolving torsion.
- Menstrual history- date of last menstrual period, cycle regularity and length, presence of menorrhagia/dysmenorrhea.

> **History in this case:**
> History of sudden onset severe nonradiating pain in lower abdomen associated with vomiting. No history of preceding amenorrhea, bleeding per vaginum or syncopal attack. No history of discharge per vaginum. No bladder, bowel complaints.
> Menstrual history: 5/35 days, regular, moderate flow. LMP—10 days back

POINTS TO BE NOTED IN EXAMINATION

General Examination

- General condition
- Vitals—Temperature, pulse, respiratory rate, blood pressure
- Pallor, icterus, dehydration.

Cardiovascular and Respiratory System Examination

Note any murmur, adventitious sound.

Abdominal Examination

- Location and severity of pain
- Tenderness, guarding, rigidity and rebound tenderness
- Free fluid, any features of peritonitis
- Any palpable mass
- Bowel sounds.

Pelvic Examination

Per Speculum (P/S) Examination

- Condition of cervix and vagina
- Presence of bleeding, amount of bleeding if present
- Cervical os, open or closed
- Cervical discharge: Amount, color and smell. Cervical swab should be sent for gram stain, culture and sensitivity.

Per Vaginum (P/V) Examination

- Any cervical motion tenderness
- Uterine position, size, mobility, consistency, tenderness
- Presence of any adnexal mass, size, mobility, tenderness.

A unilateral tender mass may be palpable in the adnexa in 50 percent patients. However, absence of a mass or tenderness does not exclude torsion.

Examination in this case:
She was afebrile. PR—110 per minute, BP—100/60 mm Hg, RR—18/min.
There was mild pallor;
Abdominal examination—The lower abdomen was tender with slight guarding but no rigidity or rebound tenderness. No free fluid.
P/S—Cervix and vagina healthy. No bleeding or discharge
P/V—Uterus normal size, firm, mobile, non-tender. A 10×10 tender cyst with restricted mobility was palpable in right fornix.

Diagnosis

Based on the history and examination of this patient, the most probable diagnosis is ovarian torsion.

EMERGENT CARE

- Admit and assess vital signs
- Establish intravenous (IV) line, start IV fluids as required
- Exclude other causes of acute abdomen
- IV antiemetics – prochlorperazine, metoclopromide, ondansetron
- Early and judicious use of analgesics: Nonsteroidal anti-inflammatory drugs (NSAIDs) or opiates may be used contrary to earlier belief, this does not delay or impede diagnosis.

INVESTIGATIONS

1. *Urine pregnancy test*- To rule out ectopic pregnancy.
2. *Laboratory tests:*
   - White blood cell count, hematocrit, and serum electrolytes.
     Hemorrhage can result in anemia, ovarian necrosis can cause leukocytosis, and persistent vomiting can lead to electrolyte abnormalities. However, laboratory abnormalities may not be present and, when present, are nondiagnostic.

- Ovarian torsion has been associated with increased serum levels of *interleukin-6 (IL-6)*. A level of more than 10 pg/mL is associated with increased risk of torsion.
- Urinalysis, wet mount, *Chlamydia* culture to exclude pyelonephritis and PID respectively.

3. *Radiological imaging*
   - Ultrasonography (USG) with color Doppler analysis is the first line investigation for evaluation of adnexal torsion.
     - Ultrasound features of ovarian torsion include a unilateral enlarged ovary (commonest finding), uniform peripherally located cystic structures, a coexistent mass within the affected ovary, free pelvic fluid, lack of intraovarian arterial or venous flow. However, these findings are all nonspecific and the presence of normal appearing ovaries does not rule out the diagnosis.
     - A ratio of the torsed adnexal volume to the normal adnexal volume greater than 20 is predictive of an ovarian mass within the torsed ovary. Conversely, a ratio less than 20 is predictive of the absence of an ovarian mass.[4]
     - A positive **whirlpool sign** in the twisted vascular pedicle of the ovary (corresponding to the broad ligament, fallopian tube, adnexal and ovarian branches of uterine artery and vein) has been shown to be the most definitive sign of ovarian torsion.[5] On gray scale sonography, the whirlpool sign refers to the hypoechoic band in the twisted pedicle representing the clockwise and anticlockwise wrapping of blood vessels around a central axis.
     - The presence of intraovarian venous flow on color Doppler imaging does not exclude torsion, but may suggest that the ovary may be viable. Lee has reported a 94 percent predictability of viability of the ovary when arterial and venous flow is seen in the twisted pedicle. Absence of flow in the twisted vascular pedicle or visualization of flow in the artery alone are predictive of nonviability.[5,6]
   - Magnetic resonance imaging (MRI) and computerized tomography (CT) may be valuable when Doppler ultrasound findings are equivocal, but the cost and time required for these imaging studies does not justify their routine use.[6] Furthermore, the diagnostic criteria for torsion using these modalities have not been well-defined or validated in large studies.
     - Common CT and MRI features of adnexal torsion include fallopian tube thickening, smooth wall thickening of the twisted adnexal cystic mass, ascites, and uterine deviation to the twisted side.[7,8]
     - Uncommon imaging findings in adnexal torsion that are specific to hemorrhagic infarction include hemorrhage in the thickened fallopian tube, hemorrhage within the twisted ovarian mass, and hemoperitoneum.

     However, the definitive diagnosis of ovarian torsion remains surgical.

DEFINITIVE TREATMENT

The mainstay of treatment is **swift operative evaluation** to preserve ovarian function and prevent infectious complications

- Historically, laparotomy with removal of the affected ovary had been the standard treatment of the torsed ovary because it was believed that restoring normal anatomy via detorsion could dislodge a clot in the ovarian vein or leave a necrotic vestige. *The paradigm has now shifted from one of ovarian removal to one of ovarian evaluation and likely preservation, even in the face of a dusky, seemingly necrotic appearance.* Detorsion and ovarian preservation with cystectomy is a safe operation in premenopausal patients and adnexectomy should be avoided as ovarian function is preserved in 88 to 100 percent of cases.[9-11] The majority of these ovaries regain previous form and function[12], even if they appeared to be ischemic intraoperatively.
- Methods proposed to identify ovaries that are being perfused and therefore may be viable are:
  - *Fluorescein injection:*[13] Intraoperative intravenous fluorescein injection followed by direct visualization of the affected ovary after untwisting under ultraviolet light has been used to assess arterial perfusion. Yellow-green fluorescence is considered a marker for adequate tissue perfusion.

- *Ovarian bivalving:* The ovary can be untwisted and the ovarian cortex incised to relieve the increased pressure exerted by the lymphatic and venous congestion and to confirm tissue reperfusion under direct visualization.[14]
- A laparoscopic approach to detorsion is an effective management strategy if technically feasible, as it is associated with less morbidity than laparotomy.[15] Simultaneous triplication of the utero-ovarian ligament for shortening may be performed to prevent recurrent torsion in young patients.
- While the benefits of conservative surgery appear to outweigh the theoretical risks of detorsion, irreversible ischemic damage can occur and can lead to peritonitis and systemic infection if a necrotic ovary is retained. This rare complication was demonstrated in one case report of a pregnant patient who underwent laparotomy and detorsion of a hyperstimulated ovary with reperfusion of the torsed adnexa observed intraoperatively.[16]
- Salpingo-oopherectomy may be indicated if severe vascular compromise, peritonitis or tissue necrosis is clearly evident.

Investigations in this case:
Hb—10 gm%, TLC—12,000/cu mm,
Serum electrolytes—normal,
Urine routine and microscopy—normal
Urine pregnancy test—negative
USG: 2D USG showed 10×10 cm unilocular cyst in the right adnexa with few internal echoes. Left ovary normal, uterus normal size and echopattern. On color flow Doppler, flow was present in the vascular pedicle

Treatment in this case:
The patient was taken up for an urgent laparotomy. The right ovary was enlarged to 8x10 cm size, hemorrhagic, with a single twist of the ovarian pedicle. The left ovary was normal. After detorsing the ovary a cystectomy was done . The postoperative period was uneventful.

Complications

Infection, sepsis, infarction, peritonitis, adhesions and chronic pain.

PREVENTION OF RECURRENCE

- Unilateral, contralateral, or bilateral **oophoropexy** following ovarian detorsion has been used to prevent recurrence, although the efficacy of this approach has not been evaluated in randomized trials.[17]
- Oophoropexy is recommended in all cases of childhood torsion of normal ovaries, but not routinely in cases of torsion resulting from an ovarian cyst.
- Routine oophoropexy is recommended for girls and young women who have previously undergone an oophorectomy for prior ovarian torsion.

OVARIAN TORSION IN PREGNANCY

- The incidence of ovarian torsion rises 5-fold during pregnancy.
- Luteomas are unique to pregnancy.[18] The most common cause of torsion in pregnancy is a corpus luteum cyst, which usually regresses spontaneously by the second trimester.[19] Ovarian torsion, therefore, occurs most frequently in the first trimester, occasionally in the second, and rarely in the third trimester.[20] It may also occur frequently in early puerperium.
- Clinical features are same as in a torsion without pregnancy, the most common clinical presentation being severe, colicky unilateral pain that is usually nonremitting but can wax and wane in cases of incomplete or intermittent ovarian torsion.

- Ultrasound remains the diagnostic modality of choice though the ovaries may sometimes be difficult to visualize because of the enlarging uterus. If the ovaries are not clearly visualized with vaginal or abdominal ultrasound, magnetic resonance imaging (MRI) can be used.

CASE SCENARIO-2

A 22-year-old primigravida presented to the gynecology casualty with 6 weeks of amenorrhea and persistent pain in the lower abdomen for 2 days. There was no history of bleeding per vaginum, fever or syncopal attack. Her urine pregnancy test was positive.

Comment: Pregnancy with torsion of ovarian cyst should also be considered in the differential diagnosis of this patient.

History in this case:
The patient gave a history of 6 weeks of amenorrhea and sudden onset, persistent pain in the lower abdomen, more on the right side for 2 days associated with increased vomiting for last 1 day. There was no history of bleeding per vaginum, fever or syncopal attack.

Examination in this case:
Patient was afebrile, mildly dehydrated, Pulse—108/min, BP—90/60 mm Hg.
Abdominal examination: A tender mass was palpable in the right lower abdomen. Slight guarding and rebound tenderness was present.
P/S examination: The os was closed, there was no bleeding or discharge.
P/V examination: Cervical motion tenderness was present, uterus was 6 weeks in size and soft in consistency, a tender mass of 5 × 5 cm size was palpable in the right fornix.

Diagnosis

A provisional diagnosis of primigravida with 6 weeks pregnancy with torsion of right ovarian cyst was made.

Investigations in this case:
Urine pregnancy test was positive.
Hb - 9 gm%, Urine for albumin/sugar/ketones - nil
A transvaginal scan done in the emergency showed a single intrauterine gestation sac with a live fetus with CRL 6 weeks 2 days and a 5 × 5 cm sonolucent cyst in the right adnexa. There was minimal free fluid in the pelvis.

MANAGEMENT

- A conservative management approach towards ovarian cysts in pregnancy has been recommended based on sonographic characteristics. Cysts more than 10 cm should be resected because of the increased risk of cancer, rupture, torsion and obstruction of labor. In general, the time of elective surgery should be between 14 and 20 weeks of pregnancy. Management of masses between 6 and 10 cm is controversial and careful ultrasound/MRI evaluation for the possibility of neoplasia should be done. Benign cysts or those less than 6 cm can be managed expectantly with serial ultrasound as most of them undergo spontaneous resolution. Resection is recommended if they grow, display malignant characteristics or become symptomatic.[18]
- Management of torsion in pregnancy is similar to that in the nonpregnant woman, but may be technically more difficult given the size of the gravid uterus.
- The decision to proceed to surgery during pregnancy is somewhat complex, since the well-being of both mother and fetus has to be considered. The risk of any surgery to the pregnancy will depend on the gestational age.
- In the first trimester, when ovarian torsion most often occurs in pregnancy, the risk of fetal loss is the smallest with modern anesthetic techniques.[21] If the corpus luteum is removed before 10

weeks, then 17 α OH progesterone 250 mg intramuscular is given weekly until 10 weeks gestation.[18]

- Surgery during the second or third trimester is associated with the risk of premature labor which may occur in 26 percent of women undergoing surgery during the second trimester and in 82 percent of those undergoing surgery during the third trimester.[21]
- The risk of premature labor can be minimized by
  - Regional anesthesia should be used whenever possible to decrease postoperative pain and the subsequent release of catecholamines, which can stimulate uterine contractility.[22]
  - Continued epidural infusion of narcotics for up to 72 hours is an excellent way to minimize postoperative pain.[23]
  - Uterine monitoring in the immediate postanesthesia period is important for the early detection of regular uterine contractile activity.
- Conservative treatment is recommended with a view to preserve fertility, even for adnexa that initially appear nonviable and purple or black in color.
- Laparoscopic approach remains a safe option even in pregnancy.[24] Researchers have suggested that 26 to 28 weeks be the upper gestational age limit for successful laparoscopy. Beyond 12 weeks some technical modification of standard pelvic laparoscopic entry is required to avoid uterine puncture or laceration. An open entry technique at or above the umbilicus is recommended. In advanced pregnancy, a direct entry through a left upper quadrant port in the midclavicular line 2 cm beneath the costal margin – the palmer point – is described.[25]

Treatment in this case:
The patient was taken up for a diagnostic laparoscopy which revealed minimal amount of clear fluid in the pelvis, a 6 week sized uterus and a 6x 6 cm simple cyst in the right ovary. The ovary appeared congested and hemorrhagic and there was a single twist of its pedicle. The left ovary and both fallopian tubes were normal. The ovary was untwisted and the patient put on micronized progesterone. She was relieved of her symptoms and did well thereafter.

KEY POINTS

- Ovarian torsion can occur in all age groups.
- A clinical diagnosis of ovarian torsion should be considered in women with lower abdominal or pelvic pain and an ovarian cyst/mass, after exclusion of ectopic pregnancy, pelvic inflammatory disease, appendicitis, and leiomyoma-related symptoms.
- Early diagnosis of ovarian torsion is important to preserve ovarian function and prevent adverse sequelae (necrosis, infarction, local hemorrhage, peritonitis, systemic infection).
- Three-dimensional (3D) ultrasound or two-dimensional ultrasound with Doppler for preoperative imaging of the adnexa should be done when torsion is suspected. Diminished or absent blood flow in the ovarian vessels should lead to a high suspicion of ovarian torsion. The presence of hemorrhage further suggests the diagnosis. However, many a times the ovaries continue to have a normal appearance and blood flow.
- A definitive diagnosis of ovarian torsion is based upon surgical findings.
- Women with a possible diagnosis of ovarian torsion should be managed with emergent operative ovarian evaluation and detorsion.
- Detorsion is often possible even in the face of a dusky, seemingly necrotic appearance.
- Oophoropexy is recommended in all cases of childhood torsion of normal ovaries, but not routinely in cases of torsion resulting from an ovarian cyst.
- The incidence of ovarian torsion is increased 5 fold during pregnancy. It occurs most commonly in the first trimester of pregnancy or during early puerperium. Conservative surgery with detorsion and cystectomy (if required) is the treatment procedure of choice.

REFERENCES

1. Sanfillippo JS, Rock JA. Surgery for benign disease of the ovary. In: Rock JA, Jones III HW(eds). Te Linde's Operative Gynecology. 10th edn. Lippincott Williams and Wilkins, 2008:629-47.
2. Littman ED, Rydfors J, Milki AA. Exercise-induced ovarian torsion in the cycle following gonadotrophin therapy: case report. Hum Reprod 2003;18:1641-2.
3. Beaunoyer M, Chapdelaine J, Bouchard S, Ouimet A. Asynchronous bilateral ovarian torsion. J Pediatr Surg 2004;39:746-9.
4. Servaes S, Zurakowski D, Laufer MR, Feins N, Chow JS. Sonographic findings of ovarian torsion in children. Pediatr Radiol 2007;37:446-51.
5. Vijayaraghavan SB. Sonographic whirlpool sign in ovarian torsion. J Ultrasound Med 2004;23:1643-9.
6. Fujii S, Kaneda S, Kakite S, Kanasaki Y, Matsusue E, Harada T, et al. Diffusion-weighted imaging findings of adnexal torsion: initial results. Eur J Radiol 2011;77:330-4.
7. Rha SE, Byun JY, Jung SE, Jung JI, Choi BG, Kim BS, Kim H, Lee JM. CT and MR imaging features of adnexal torsion. Radiographics 2002;22:283-94.
8. Daponte A, Pournaras S, Hadjichristodoulou C, Lialios G, Kallitsaris A, Maniatis AN, et al. Novel serum inflammatory markers in patients with adnexal mass who had surgery for ovarian torsion. Fertil Steril 2006;85:1469-72.
9. Rody A, Jackisch C, Klockenbusch W, Heinig J, Coenen-Worch V, Schneider HP. The conservative management of adnexal torsion—a case-report and review of the literature. Eur J Obstet Gynecol Reprod Biol 2002;101:83-6.
10. Zweizig S, Perron J, Grubb D, Mishell DR Jr. Conservative management of adnexal torsion. Am J Obstet Gynecol 1993;168:1791-5.
11. Oelsner G, Shashar D. Adnexal torsion. Clin Obstet Gynecol 2006;49:459-63.
12. Oelsner G, Cohen SB, Soriano D, Admon D, Mashiach S, Carp H. Minimal surgery for the twisted ischaemic adnexa can preserve ovarian function. Hum Reprod 2003;18:2599-602.
13. McHutchinson L L, Koonings P P, Ballard C A, d'Ablaing G, 3rd. Preservation of ovarian tissue in adnexal torsion with fluorescein. Am J Obstet Gynecol 1993;168:1386-8.
14. Promecene PA. Laparoscopy in gynecologic emergencies. Semin Laparosc Surg 2002;9:64-75.
15. Bottomley C, Bourne T. Diagnosis and management of ovarian cyst accidents. Best Pract Res Clin Obstet Gynaecol 2009;23:711-24.
16. Pryor RA, Wiczyk HP, O'Shea DL. Adnexal infarction after conservative surgical management of torsion of a hyperstimulated ovary. Fertil Steril 1995;63:1344-6.
17. Djavadian D, Braendle W, Jaenicke F. Laparoscopic oophoropexy for the treatment of recurrent torsion of the adnexa in pregnancy: case report and review. Fertil Steril 2004;82:933-6.
18. Reproductive tract abnormalities. In : Cunningham F. Gary, Leveno Kenneth J, Bloom Steven L, Hauth John C, Rouse Dwight J, Spong Catherine Y(eds). Williams Obstetrics; 23rd ed; McGraw- Hill; 2010:912-25.
19. Duic Z, Kukura V, Ciglar S, et al. Adnexal masses in pregnancy: a review of eight cases undergoing surgical management. Eur J Gynaecol Oncol 2002;23:133-4.
20. Hibbard LT. Adnexal torsion. Am J Obstet Gynecol 1985;152:456-61.
21. Visser BC, Glasgow RE, Mulvihill KK, Mulvihill SJ. Safety and timing of nonobstetric abdominal surgery in pregnancy. Dig Surg 2001;18:409-17.
22. Hurd WW, Smith AJ, Gauvin JM, et al. Cocaine blocks extraneuronal uptake of norepinephrine by the pregnant human uterus. Obstet Gynecol 1991;78:249-53.
23. Jayr C, Beaussier M, Gustafsson U, Leteurnier Y, Nathan N, Plaud B, et al. Continuous epidural infusion of ropivacaine for postoperative analgesia after major abdominal surgery: comparative study with i.v. PCA morphine. Br J Anaesth 1998;81:887-92.
24. Mathevet P, Nessah K, Dargent D, Mellier G. Laparoscopic management of adnexal masses in pregnancy: a case series. Eur J Obstet Gynecol Reprod Biol 2003;108:217-22.
25. General Considerations and Maternal Evaluation. In: Cunningham FG, Leveno KJ, Bloom SL, Hauth JC, Rouse DJ, Spong CY (eds). Williams Obstetrics. 23rd edn. McGraw Hill, 2010.pp. 912-25.

Chapter 29

Emergency Contraception

Rachna Sharma

INTRODUCTION

Emergency contraception (EC) refers to a type of contraception that is used as an emergency to prevent pregnancy after an unprotected, possibly fertile intercourse. It is meant for special situations only and not for routine or repeated use.

While knowledge about various temporary and permanent methods among men and women ranges between 45 to 97 percent, knowledge about emergency contraception is only 20 percent in men and 11 percent in women.[1] 11 percent of couples conceive again within 18 months and 28 percent within 24 months of a preceding pregnancy. An additional 11 percent are unwanted.[2] The use of emergency contraception can reduce unintended pregnancies by 1.5 million and abortions by 0.7 million.[3]

The earliest used regimen of emergency contraception was Diethyl stilbestrol for a 13-year-old rape victim.[4] The Yuzpe regimen became the standard course of treatment for postcoital contraception in 1980's.[5]

A "Consortium on National Consensus for Emergency Contraception" was organized by WHO-CCR in AIIMS, to provide recommendations and guidelines for appropriate use and follow up for emergency contraception in India.[6] "Over the counter availability of emergency contraception" came into being in 2005.

CASE SCENARIO-1

A 20-year-old unmarried girl came to family planning department with history of unprotected intercourse with her boyfriend the night before. She wanted advice on chances of becoming pregnant and about contraception.

Comments: The probability of conception after a single act of coitus around midcycle is 8 percent. This girl should be prescribed emergency contraception.

POINTS TO BE NOTED IN HISTORY

- Age of the patient
- Marital status
- Last menstrual period
- Cycle length and duration

- Date of unprotected intercourse
- Dates of any other unprotected intercourses in the same cycle
- Contraceptive history in current and previous cycles
- Risk factors for sexually transmitted infections (STI) , if any
- Obstetric history, particularly history of medical termination of pregnancy (MTP)
- Medical history including current medications
- Reason for emergency contraception – condom failure/forgotten pills/no contraceptive/assault/others.

History in this case:
Unmarried girl who had unprotected intercourse a night before (approx 16 hours before seeking advice). This was her first act of intercourse during this cycle.
Her previous cycles were normal in length and duration and this act of intercourse was performed around midcycle.
No past history of medical disorders, drug intake or STI

POINTS TO BE NOTED IN EXAMINATION

General Examination

- Temperature, pulse rate, blood pressure
- Pallor, icterus

Cardiovascular and Respiratory System Examination

Abdominal Examination

- Any mass, tenderness, organomegaly
- Whether uterus palpable, previous surgery/scar mark

Pelvic Examination

Local Examination

Any signs of forceful coitus, local abrasions/cuts, hymen intact or broken, external genitalia

Per Speculum (P/S) Examination

Any bleeding through os, cervical erosion/discharge, vaginitis, vaginal lacerations

Per Vaginum (P/V)Examination

Cervical motion tenderness, uterine size/consistency/mobility/tenderness, adnexal mass, forniceal tenderness.

Examination in this case:
General condition and systemic examination normal.
Local examination—Hymen ruptured, external genitalia normal
P/S—Cervix and vagina healthy, no discharge, no bleeding
P/V—Uterus normal in size, anteverted, firm, mobile, bilateral fornices free

---

INVESTIGATIONS

- Hemoglobin, blood group and type
- Urine routine and microscopy

- Special investigations: Liver and renal function tests, ultrasound pelvis, X-ray chest, depending on coexisting medical morbidities.

MANAGEMENT

This patient can be prescribed oral emergency contraception using either Yuzpe method or Levonorgestrel emergency contraceptive pill.

1. **YUZPE method:** 100 μg of ethinyl estradiol (EE) and 1 mg of norgestrel or 0.5 mg of levonorgestrel (LNG), given as 2 doses 12 hours apart, first dose within 72 hours of unprotected intercourse.

OR

   4 low dose oral contraceptive pills within 72 hours of unprotected intercourse
   + 4 low dose OCP's 12 hours after first dose.
   - *Efficacy*—prevents 75 percent pregnancies, i.e. 2 of every 8 women may become pregnant.[7]
2. **Levonorgestrel only pills** (E-pill/I-pill/unwanted-72):
   - Available as 2 pill pack (0.75 mg LNG)
   - 0.75 mg of LNG taken within 72 hrs of unprotected intercourse, same dose to be repeated 12 hours apart.
   - *Efficacy*—Prevents 85 percent pregnancies, i.e. 1 of every 8 women may become pregnant.[8]

Counseling

Information to be emphasized at the time of prescribing emergency contraception

- They protect against single act of unprotected intercourse. Multiple acts in the same cycle before or after use of EC will not be protected.
- They are for "one-time use". EC cannot substitute regular contraceptives and should only be used as a back-up method. Benefits of regular contraceptives outweigh EC in terms of dose, safety, efficacy and side effects.
- Appraise the client about existence of a small possibility (1 to 3 percent risk) of failure of EC, but absent fetal risk.

Follow-up

Client should follow-up in the following instances

- Troublesome side effects
- Severe abdominal pain, abnormal bleeding
- Three weeks from taking EC, particularly if menstrual bleeding does not occur, or is unusually light or heavy
- For discussing and receiving regular contraception
- If a woman's menstrual period is delayed by a week or more, urine pregnancy test is indicated.

Menses after EC Pill Use[9]

- 13 percent have a delay of 8+ days
- 15 percent have a delay of 4 to 7 days
- 61 percent have menses within 3 days
- 11 percent have early onset (>3 days early).

Side Effects

- Nausea and vomiting – most common (50.5% - Yuzpe regimen; 23% - LNG users).[9] A repeat dose is recommended if vomiting occurs within 2 hours of taking pill.
- Abdominal pain, fatigue, headache, dizziness, breast tenderness (<20 in LNG users).[8-10]
- Temporary disruption of current menstrual cycle. (if taken before ovulation – withdrawal bleeding; if taken after ovulation – prolong luteal phase).[11]

Contraindications

- Absolute—none
- Relative—severe cardiovascular disease, angina, acute migraine, severe liver disease.

Newer Advances in Emergency Contraception

- Antiprogesterone (Mifepristone): Single dose of 10 mg is as effective as LNG for emergency contraception with no difference in side effects and similar efficacy.[12,13]
- Effective up to 5 days after intercourse
- Yet to be approved in India.

CASE SCENARIO-2

A 30-year-old P3L3 lady presents to family planning OPD with history of rupture of condom during intercourse 4 days back. She wanted advice on chances of becoming pregnant, and method to prevent this and future unwanted pregnancies.

> **Comments:** Since the patient is a multiparous woman and has presented late (>72 hrs), the best method for this patient will be copper releasing intrauterine contraceptive device (IUCD) after ruling out contraindications. IUCD will prevent this as well as future pregnancies.

> **History in this case:**
> 30 yr, multiparous lady, last child birth 3 yrs back. She is midcycle. No history of high-risk behavior/past STD/irregular vaginal bleeding/medical or surgical illness.

> **Examination in this case:**
> General condition fair, no pallor, no icterus
> P/A—Soft
> P/S—Cervix, vagina healthy
> P/V—Uterus normal size, anteverted, mobile, bilateral fornices free and nontender.

Investigations

- Hemoglobin
- Urine albumin, sugar and microscopy
- Special investigations
  - High vaginal and endocervical swab (if suspected PID)
  - Pelvic ultrasonography (USG) – suspected tubo ovarian mass, vaginal bleeding.

Management

IUCD can be used for emergency contraception up to 5 days after unprotected intercourse after ruling out any contraindication to IUCD insertion.

Counseling

Before insertion, every woman should be told about advantages and drawbacks of IUCD.

Advantages

- Only one time motivation needed
- Cost-effective
- Can be continued as a method of regular contraception and gives protection for years
- No systemic side effects.

Disadvantages

- Abdominal pain
- Irregular menses
- Menorrhagia
- Increased chances of ectopic pregnancy
- Increased chances of sexually transmitted diseases.

Follow-up

- Patient should come after next periods or if she misses her periods
- Patient should feel the threads of IUCD following menstruation at least for next 3 periods
- Patient may have heavy menstrual bleeding for next 2 to 3 cycles. She should report back in case of any complication
- Urine pregnancy test (UPT) to be done if >1 week delay in period.

Efficacy of Copper Releasing IUD in Emergency Contraception[14]

- Crude pregnancy rate—0.1 %
- Prevented fraction 99—100 %.

Complications

- Increased bleeding—20 to 30 percent cases
- Lower abdominal pain
- Expulsion 2 to 8 percent cases
- Vaginal discharge
- Perforation 1.2/1000 users
- Infection—PID/STD
- Ectopic pregnancy-1.5/1000 users (30% of contraceptive failures).

Contraindications

Absolute

- Unexplained vaginal bleeding
- Cervical/endometrial cancer
- Current PID

Relative

- Postpartum> 48 hrs to < 4 weeks
- Benign trophoblastic disease
- Nulliparity
- Endometriosis
- Severe anemia.

KEY POINTS

- Emergency contraception (EC) is not effective once the process of implantation has taken place
- Emergency contraceptive should not be used for regular contraception
- Timing of first act of unprotected sexual intercourse is critical in determining eligibility for use of emergency contraceptive
- EC should not be advised in confirmed pregnancies
- Make sure that the client understands that EC does not protect pregnancies from future unprotected sexual intercourse.

REFERENCES

1. American College of Obstetricians and Gynecologists. ACOG Practice Bulletin. Clinical Management Guidelines for Obstetrician-Gynecologists, Number 69, December 2005. Emergency contraception. Obstet Gynecol 2005;106:1443-52.
2. Emergency Contraception and Brief Update on Regular Contraception. Guide Book for Health-Care Providers. Mittal S. WHO-CCR in Human Reproduction, AIIMS. 2003.
3. Trussell J, Ellertson C, von Hertzen H, Bigrigg A, Webb A, Evans M, Ferden S, Leadbetter C. Estimating the effectiveness of emergency contraceptive pills. Contraception 2003;67:259-65.
4. FDA considers DES safe as 'morning-after' pill. JAMA 1973 18;224:1581-2.
5. Yuzpe AA, Thurlow HJ, Ramzy I, Leyshon JI. Post coital contraception—A pilot study. J Reprod Med 1974;13:53-8.
6. Consortium for National Consensus on Emergency Contraception in India. WHO-CCR in Human Reproduction 2001,115.
7. Trussell J, Rodríguez G, Ellertson C. New estimates of the effectiveness of the Yuzpe regimen of emergency contraception. Contraception 1998;57:363-9.
8. Levonorgestrel is more effective, has fewer side-effects, than Yuzpe regimen. Prog Hum Reprod Res 1999;51:3-5.
9. Randomised controlled trial of levonorgestrel versus the Yuzpe regimen of combined oral contraceptives for emergency contraception. Task Force on Postovulatory Methods of Fertility Regulation. Lancet 1998;352:428-33.
10. Faculty of Family Planning and Reproductive Health Care Clinical Effectiveness Unit. FFPRHC Guidance (April 2006). Emergency contraception. J Fam Plann Reprod Health Care 2006;32:121-8.
11. Gainer E, Kenfack B, Mboudou E, Doh AS, Bouyer J. Menstrual bleeding patterns following levonorgestrel emergency contraception. Contraception 2006;74:118-24.
12. Gemzell-Danielsson K, Marions L. Mechanisms of action of mifepristone and levonorgestrel when used for emergency contraception. Hum Reprod Update 2004;10:341-8.
13. von Hertzen H, Piaggio G, Ding J, Chen J, Song S, Bártfai G, et al. WHO Research Group on Postovulatory Methods of Fertility Regulation. Low-dose mifepristone and two regimens of levonorgestrel for emergency contraception: a WHO multicenter randomised trial. Lancet 2002;360:1803-10.
14. Wu S, Godfrey EM, Wojdyla D, Dong J, Cong J, Wang C, von Hertzen H. Copper T380. A intrauterine device for emergency contraception: a prospective, multicentre, cohort clinical trial. BJOG 2010;117:1205-10.

Chapter 30

Acute Complications of Intrauterine Contraceptive Device

Rachna Sharma

Introduction

Intrauterine contraceptive device (IUCD) has been a part of the National Family Planning Programme since the sixties. Different types of copper bearing IUCDs are available in the country. Modern IUCDs are an effective, safe and quickly reversible long-term means of contraception that require little attention after insertion.

Today, almost 153 million women of reproductive age group use the IUCD worldwide.[1] However, some safety concerns like the risk of perforation into the peritoneal cavity which most women erroneously correlate with a lost or missing IUCD thread have held back the IUCD in many countries.

The most commonly encountered complications with the IUCD are a lost or missing IUCD thread, bleeding, lower abdominal pain and perforation.

CASE SCENARIO-1

A 24-year-old female, P2L2 got Cu-T inserted at a primary health center. After 7 days, the patient reported back with complaint of pain lower abdomen for 1 day not relieved by analgesics, increased vaginal discharge and high-grade fever of 101°-102°F

Comment: The woman has most likely developed pelvic inflammatory disease (PID) following IUCD insertion.

Points to be noted in History

- Age of the patient
- Last menstrual period
- Cycle length and & duration
- Risk factors for sexually transmitted infections (STI), if any
- Obstetric history, particularly history of MTPs
- Medical history including current medication

History in this case: There is history of Cu T insertion 7 days back. Patient complains of pain lower abdomen along with increased vaginal discharge and high-grade fever for last 1 day.

Points to be Noted in Examination

General Examination

Temperature, pulse rate, blood pressure

Cardiovascular and Respiratory System Examination

Abdominal Examination

Palpable uterus, previous surgery/scar mark

Pelvic Examination

Local Examination

External genitalia

Per Speculum (P/S) Examination

Cervical erosion/discharge, vaginitis.

Per Vaginum (P/V) Examination

Cervical motion tenderness, uterus size/consistency/mobility/ tenderness, adnexal mass, formiceal tenderness.

> **Examination in this case:**
> General condition—Satisfactory, vitals stable
> Systemic examination—normal.
> Local examination—Unremarkable
> P/S—Cervix and vagina healthy, vaginal discharge present
> P/V—Uterus normal in size, anteverted, firm, mobile, bilateral fornices thickened and tender.

Diagnosis

Post-IUCD pelvic inflammatory disease.

Incidence of PID after IUCD Insertion

- The risk of developing PID after IUCD use is very low—1.4/1000.
- Incidence of PID in IUCD users is almost equal to that in non users. IUCD itself does not cause PID.

High-Risk Factors for Developing PID after IUCD Insertion

- If not inserted under aseptic precautions
- High-risk behavior presence of STIs
- Age < 25 years (2.5 times more as compared to > 25 years)
- Time elapsed since IUCD insertion. Risk is maximum during first 20 days after insertion (6.3 fold rise), decreases thereafter.

Measures to Reduce Risk of Developing PID after IUCD Insertion

- Screen women for high-risk of STIs, e.g. multiple partners etc.
  If present → other method of contraception should be advised OR more careful follow-up
- If PID present → 1st treat PID with Antibiotics
  ↓
  No IUCD for at least 6 weeks

- Insertion under aseptic precautions is very important
- Follow-up after 30 days to check for sign and symptoms of PID clinically and advised to return immediately if fever/lower abdominal pain during 1st month of insertion.
- Prophylactic antibiotics are not recommended but can be given in the setting of high STD prevalence.

MANAGEMENT

Outpatient Treatment of PID following IUCD Insertion

Outpatient oral therapy can be considered for women who develop mild-to-moderately severe acute PID after insertion. Patients who do not respond to oral therapy within 72 hours should be re-evaluated to confirm the diagnosis and should be administered parenteral therapy on either an outpatient or inpatient basis. The IUCD is removed 24 to 48 hrs after starting treatment. If patient wants to keep IUCD, it can be left in place but close follow-up is required.[2]

(The in patient treatment of severe PID is discussed in Chapter 24)

Recommended Regimen (CDC)[2]

1. Ceftriaxone 250 mg IM in a single dose
   PLUS
   Doxycycline 100 mg orally twice a day for 14 days
   with or without
   Metronidazole 500 mg orally twice a day for 14 days
   OR
2. Cefoxitin 2 g IM in a single dose and probenecid, 1 g orally administered concurrently in a single dose
   PLUS
   Doxycycline 100 mg orally twice a day for 14 days
   with or without
   Metronidazole 500 mg orally twice a day for 14 days
   OR
3. Other parenteral third-generation cephalosporin (e.g. ceftizoxime or cefotaxime)
   PLUS
   Doxycycline 100 mg orally twice a day for 14 days
   with or without
   Metronidazole 500 mg orally twice a day for 14 days

Management in this case:
- Antibiotics—Doxycycline 100 mg orally twice a day for 14 days with metronidazole 500 mg orally twice a day for 14 days.
- Analgesics
- IUCD was removed 48 hrs after starting treatment as requested by the patient.
- Husband was advised barrier contraception/abstinence till antibiotic course was completed.
- Couple was screened for STDs.

CASE SCENARIO-2

A 24-year-old female P2L2 comes to the emergency with pain abdomen for last 2 weeks. She gives a history of having got a Cu T inserted 2 weeks back but is unable to feel the IUCD thread.

Comment: Uterine perforation should be kept in mind as her pain coincides with the time of insertion of the Cu T along with the fact that she cannot feel the IUCD thread.

POINTS TO BE NOTED IN HISTORY

- Obstetric history, particularly history of last child birth
- Time of insertion of IUCD with reference to the menstrual cycle
- History of IUCD expulsion
- History of crampy abdominal pain, its location and character
- Sign and symptoms of peritoneal irritation like vomiting, shoulder pain
- History of abdominal distension
- History of constipation/obstipation/any urinary complaint.

> **History in this case:**
> There is history of IUCD insertion 2 weeks back followed by pain in the abdomen soon thereafter. The pain was sudden onset, acute stabbing in nature initially but now of a dull character. There is no urinary or bowel complaint. The patient gives a history of not being able to feel the IUCD thread.

POINTS TO BE NOTED IN EXAMINATION

General Examination

General condition
Vitals—Pulse/BP/respiratory rate/temperature
Pallor, hydration

Cardiovascular and Respiratory System Examination

Abdominal Examination

Presence of distension, tenderness, free fluid, any mass
Presence/absence of bowel sounds

Pelvic Examination

Per Speculum (P/S) Examination

Condition of cervix and vagina, thread seen or not.

Per Vaginum (P/V) Examination

Uterine size, tenderness/mass in any fornix.

> **Examination in this case:**
> The patient's vitals were stable. There was no pallor.
> Her abdomen was soft. There was no distension, no mass palpable. There was tenderness in lower abdomen.
> Bowel sounds were present.
> On pelvic examination the cervix and vagina were healthy, no discharge. IUCD thread was not visible.

Diagnosis

A diagnosis of missing IUCD thread with uterine perforation was made.

Causes of Missing IUCD Thread

Three basic possibilities should be kept in mind on coming across a missing IUCD thread
1. Accidental expulsion of the IUCD with the patient being unaware of it.
2. Perforation of the IUCD into the peritoneal cavity—Perforation rate is higher when the insertion is between 48 hrs and 4 weeks postpartum. Most perforations occur at the fundus at the time of

insertion. If there is suspicion of perforation at the time of insertion, the procedure should be abandoned and the patient observed. Cu-T can then be inserted after 6 weeks or an alternative method of contraception should be advised. Surgical removal of a perforated IUCD becomes necessary because of the intense local inflammatory reaction that it incites.

3. The IUCD[3] is within the uterine cavity, but the thread cannot be seen because either:
   - The thread is coiled up in the cervical canal or uterine cavity or
   - The thread has been cut too short.

MANAGEMENT

- The first step on encountering such a patient is to perform a transvaginal sonography (TVS). In 70 percent cases the IUCD is found inside the uterine cavity and nothing further needs to be done.
- If the IUCD is displaced from its normal position in the uterus, the cervical canal is explored with an artery forceps; the thread located and pulled out. If the thread has receded into the uterine cavity, the cavity is probed with a uterine sound/probe and the IUCD hooked out with a suitable instrument like an endometrial biopsy curette, retreivette, shirodkar hook, ovum forceps, FHI string retriever, Mimark helix, Emmett IUCD retriever. In a few cases, hooking out the IUCD may not be possible and a hysteroscopic-guided removal may be needed.
- If TVS fails to reveal an intrauterine IUCD, straight X-ray of the abdomen and pelvis is done either with a uterine sound or another IUCD in utero serving as a marker. A second radio-opaque shadow of the missing IUCD will show up in the peritoneal cavity if it has perforated through the uterus.[4] The IUCD can then be removed laproscopically by holding with a grasping forceps or sterilization prongs.
- Occasionally the IUCD may be buried amongst dense adhesions, located dangerously close to the gut or bladder or may not be seen at all on laparoscopy, then a laparotomy may be required for removal.

Investigations and Management in this case:
TVS did not show any IUCD in the uterine cavity.
A plain X-ray abdomen showed that the IUCD was in the peritoneal cavity but the exact location of the IUCD could not be made out.
A diagnostic laparoscopy was unhelpful. The patient was then taken up for a laparotomy and the IUCD was found embedded within the omentum from where it was gently released.

KEY POINTS

- Almost 153 million women use the IUCD worldwide
- Common complications encountered with IUCD are a missing thread, vaginal bleeding, lower abdominal pain and perforation.
- Though the incidence of PID in IUCD users is not increased women should be screened for PID before insertion. If present, PID should be treated first and IUCD inserted 6 weeks later.
- If perforation is suspected at the time of insertion, the procedure should be abandoned and IUCD inserted 6 weeks later.
- A plain X-ray abdomen may be required for confirming the presence of a Cu T within the abdominal cavity. It can be taken out laparoscopically or by a laparotomy if required.

REFERENCES

1. Guidelines for IUCD insertion by Deptt.of Family Welfare, India. 2001:8-9.
2. CDC Guidelines 2010. Available at http://www.cdc.gov/std/treatment/2010/pid.htm
3. Gentile GP, Siegler AM. The misplaced or missing IUD. Obstet Gynecol Surv 1977;32:627-41.
4. Badawy S, Iskander S. Omental reaction in cases of uterine perforation by the IUCD. Contraception 1974;10:73-7.

Chapter 31

Ovarian Hyperstimulation Syndrome

Renu Tanwar

INTRODUCTION

The ovarian hyperstimulation syndrome (OHSS) is an iatrogenic complication of the luteal phase or/and early pregnancy after ovulation induction or of ovarian stimulation, in the context of intrauterine insemination (IUI) or *in vitro* fertilization (IVF).[1]

The OHSS is a cystic enlargement of the ovaries with a fluid shift from the intravascular to the third space due to increased capillary permeability and ovarian neoangiogenesis. High concentration of vascular endothelial growth factor (VEGF) has been demonstrated in follicular fluid, making the mediating role of ovarian VEGF in the development of OHSS very plausible.[2]

Time of Onset

Early OHSS: The early form of OHSS occurs <10 days after the ovulation triggering injection of human chorionic gonadotropin (hCG) and is due to an exaggerated ovarian response to gonadotropin stimulation

Late OHSS: The late form occurs ≥ 10 days after hCG administration and is mainly related to secretion of placental hCG.[3]

Risk Factors for OHSS[4]

- Young age <35 years
- Low body weight
- Polycystic ovarian disease (PCOD) or PCO-like ovaries
- Asthenic habitus
- High-serum estradiol (E2)
  - IVF - >3000 pg/mL
  - ovulation induction (OI) - >1700 pg/mL
  - the slope of estradiol rise is the main risk factor and is of more importance than the maximum level
- Multiple follicles (ART >20) (OI >6)
- Pregnancy
- hCG luteal supplementation

Grade	Ovary	Clinical	Lab. Blood
Table 31.1: Classification of OHSS			
Mild	5-10cc	Abdominal distension GIT upset	PCV < 45% TLC < 15,000/cc Normal renal function
Moderate	10-12 cc	Moderate ascites Body weight 2 kg/day	PCV < 45% TLC < 15,000/cc Normal renal function
Severe	> 12cc	Marked ascites Dyspnea Hypovolemia Mild Thromboembolism	PCV > 45% TLC > 15,000/cc Impaired renal function
Critical	Marked enlargement	Tense ascites Hydrothorax Severe thromboembolism. Adult respiratory distress syndrome **Life threatening**	PCV > 55% TLC > 25,000/mm^3 Serum creatinine >1.6 mg%, Creatinine clearance <50mL/min

- GnRH-agonist protocol for pituitary down-regulation
- Previous history of OHSS

Classification of OHSS[5] (Table 31.1)

- Mild
- Moderate
- Severe
- Critical

Mild ovarian hyperstimulation probably occurs in 8 to 23 percent of stimulated cycles, moderate forms in <1 to 7 percent and severe forms in ~0.5 percent of stimulated cycles.[6]

CASE SCENARIO

A 33-yr-old woman presented to emergency with severe abdominal pain and abdominal distention. Patient had undergone an IVF cycle and oocyte retrieval was performed two days back

Comment: A high index of suspicion should be kept for OHSS in patients undergoing IVF, particularly in cases with high-risk factors.

Differential Diagnosis

- Ruptured ectopic pregnancy
- Twisted ovarian cyst/hemorrhage
- Appendicitis
- Intra-abdominal hemorrhage.

POINTS TO BE NOTED IN HISTORY

- Duration of marriage; primary/secondary infertility.
- History of abdominal pain/discomfort/distension.
- History of nausea and vomiting.
- Diarrhea or decreased urinary output.
- Drugs used for ovarian stimulation—oral or injectable gonadotropins.

- Undergoing IUI/IVF cycle; type of stimulation protocol, their dosage.
- Day and time of HCG administration.

POINTS TO BE NOTED IN EXAMINATION

General Examination

- General condition – dyspnea
- Temperature, pulse respiratory rate (RR) and blood pressure (BP)-to rule out hypotension
- Pallor, jaundice
- Weight
- Urinary output.

Cardiovascular and Respiratory System Examination

To rule out pericardial or pleural effusion

Abdominal Examination

- Distention
- Tenderness
- Presence of free fluid in peritoneal cavity(shifting dullness)
- Bowel sounds.

If there is suspicion of OHSS, no speculum examination or palpation of the ovaries and uterus should be performed.

History in this case:
Patient was a case of PCOS and had undergone IVF with oocyte retrieval 2 days back

Examination in this case:
Patient was uncomfortable
Pulse-110/min, BP-100/70 mm Hg, RR-36/min, Temperature- 37⁰ C
Pallor—mild, pedal edema—present, no jaundice or cyanosis
Respiratory and cardiovascular examination—tachypnea and tachycardia
Abdominal examination—distension and tenderness present, free fluid ++, bowel sounds sluggish.
In view of suspected OHSS, pelvic examination was not done.

Diagnosis

Ovarian hyperstimulation syndrome

INVESTIGATIONS

- Hemoglobin and hematocrit, complete blood counts
- Blood group, Rh testing
- Urine for albumin, sugar and ketones
- Random blood sugar
- Urea, creatinine
- Serum electrolytes
- Serum proteins
- Liver function tests
- Coagulation profile—Bleeding time (BT), clotting time (CT), clot retraction time (CRT), prothrombin time (PT), activated partial thromboplastin time (aPTT).
- Chest X-ray—if chest pathology is suspected.
- ECG and echocardiography if pericardial effusion is present.
- Oxygen saturation and arterial blood gases should be monitored if the woman is tachypneic, or dyspneic.

- Transabdominal ultrasound scan to assess ovarian size and degree of ascites.
  Observations and investigation results, recorded on a flow chart will help to identify subsequent trends.

MANAGEMENT

Management depends upon the severity of OHSS.

MILD AND MODERATE OHSS

- Reassurance
- Does not require hospitalization
- Resolves in two weeks
- Outpatient care includes:
  - Limit activity
  - Weigh daily
  - Monitor intake and output
  - Follow up after 2 to 3 days
  - To report if symptoms worsen or weight gain > 2lb/day

Criteria for Hospitalization [1]

- If the patient's compliance or ability to communicate with the caring physician are in doubt or deterioration occurs then hospitalization and inpatient monitoring is recommended
- Hematocrit > 45%

SEVERE OHSS

These patients need to be hospitalized and are usually managed medically under close supervision

Monitoring during Hospitalization

- Vitals every 4 hours
- Fluid intake and output
- Daily weight and abdominal girth
- Daily hematocrit, total and differential leukocyte counts. Hematocrit is one of the best indicators of hemoconcentration and should be taken at least twice a day until stabilization. All the other blood and urine tests are ordered daily, and every 2 to 3 days afterwards.
- Serum electrolyte, liver and renal function tests
- PT, APTT on admission and repeated if necessary.

Patient may require ICU admission in cases of renal failure, adult respiratory distress syndrome (ARDS) and coagulation failure

Fluid Management to Maintain Diuresis

- Choice of fluid:
  - Combination of Ringer lactate + Dextrose 5% solution
    OR
  - NaCl 0.9% + Dextrose 5% solution (crystalloid of choice)
- Rate of administration:
  - First 24 hours: 1500 to 3000 mL.
  - Subsequent days—Fluid volume according to the fluid balance.

- Plasma expander should be utilized when fluid balance cannot be restored by crystalloids alone. Colloid administration should be considered in the following situations: pleural or pericardial effusion, anasarca, ascites, hematocrit above 45 or if the patient is oliguric.
  - Low-salt albumin is the preferred volume expander
  - Intravenous (IV) dextran (Rheomacrodex), fresh-frozen plasma, hemaccel and mannitol have all been utilized successfully as plasma expanders through restoration of oncotic pressure.[5]

Symptomatic Treatment

- *Analgesia*: Paracetamol and opoids, nonsteroidal anti inflammatory drugs are not used
- *Antiemetics:* Metoclopramide
- *Antihistamines:* May cause stabilization of capillary membrane.
- *Dopamine:* Used in oliguric cases to improve perfusion and avoid renal failure.

Anticoagulant Therapy[1]

- Low-molecular weight heparin preparations are given in all cases of severe OHSS particularly if there is presence of:
  - Clinical signs of thromboembolic complications
  - Documented thrombophilia
  - History of hypercoagulability or thromboembolism
  - Uncorrected hemoconcentration after 48 hours of usual intravenous treatment
- Mechanical methods:
  - Encourage to move their legs
  - Antithrombotic stocking may be worn

Diuretics[5]

- Highly controversial
- In case of oliguria, careful hydration of the patient with frequent CVP measurements should be performed. If the CVP rises above 15 cm H_2O and the urinary output is still not satisfactory, IV furosemide (5 to 10 mg) with careful hydration may be recommended until urinary output improves.
- Furosemide should never be used in the presence of hemoconcentration or hypotension.

Ascitic Drainage

- Abdominal paracentesis is recommended for symptomatic relief of abdominal discomfort or dyspnea caused by pronounced ascites.
- Ascitis can be drained both abdominally and vaginally but always under sonographic guidance.[8]
- It should be performed gradually removing a maximum of 4 liters of fluid over 12 hours.
- One liter of ascites fluid contains 3.0 to 3.5 g of albumin; therefore daily administration of 30 to 50 g albumin daily is recommended.
- It is carried out in cases with severe abdominal discomfort and dyspnea.
- It also results in an increased venous return, increased cardiac output, diuresis, creatinine clearance and lung ventilation.

Surgical Treatment

- Surgery is indicated only when ovarian torsion or if rupture of an ovarian cyst occurs
- Both conditions are rare and require surgery by an experienced gynecologist
- Simple unwinding of the ovarian torsion will save the ovary in cases of ovarian torsion
- In cases of actively bleeding ovarian rupture, electrocoagulation will suffice and save the ovary.

Investigations in this case:
Hemoglobin -12.2 gm/dl, hematocrit 44.4%, Total leukocyte count (TLC) – 20,000 with 87% neutrophils, serum creatinine 1.4 mg/dL and serum albumin 2.5 gm/dL.
Ultrasonography (USG):
Uterus—Normal size. Endometrial thickness—14 mm.
Both ovaries were enlarged. Right—12.5 x 8.0 x 11.0 cm, left—11.5 x 12.7 x 8.1 cm. Multiple anechoic structures of variable size, consistent with follicles were seen in both ovaries. Blood flow demonstrated to both ovaries. A moderate-to-severe amount of fluid was seen in the pelvis and abdominal cavity.

Management in this case: This patient had severe OHSS. She was hospitalized and managed medically with close monitoring. She responded well to treatment. Her embryos were cryopreserved with plan to transfer them later.

COMPLICATIONS OF OHSS

- Ovarian torsion[8]—The incidence is 1/5000 stimulation cycles but is more frequent if OHSS and if pregnancy are present.
- Ovarian bleeding—It is caused by ovarian rupture or intraovarian bleeding due to pressure or bimanual examination. It causes signs of acute hemorrhage (hypotension, nausea, sudden drop in hematocrit).
- Thromboembolic symptoms—Both venous (65.7%) and arterial localizations have been described; 83 percent of these occur in neck, arm or head veins (60%); thrombosis also occurs in arteries and veins of the lower body.[9] Pulmonary embolism occurs in 4 to 12 percent of the cases.[10]

PREVENTION

- Patients at high-risk should be identified and informed and lowest dose of gonadotropins should be given
- **Cycle cancellation** by withholding hCG prevents both early and late form of OHSS but it may entail the loss of considerable financial efforts in countries without reimbursement
- **Coasting (soft landing)**
  - When high-risk patients rapidly reach high (>3000 pg/mL) serum estradiol levels with a large number (>20 per ovary) of follicles during stimulation, gonadotropin administration can be decreased or stopped while continuing GnRH agonist administration.[11]
  - It has the advantage that the cycle is brought to its expected end with the replacement of fresh embryos and that no additional technical procedures are needed.
- **Modification of the ovulation triggering agent**
  - Lower doses of hCG than those usually utilized (2000 or 5000 IU) may cause sufficient oocyte maturation while reducing the risk for OHSS
  - Administration of exogenous recombinant LH (5000-30,000 IU), which is now commercially available
  - An endogenous LH surge can be provoked by the administration of a short-acting GnRH agonist (e.g. Luperide 0.5 mg subcutaneous). This is not possible in cycles with pituitary desensitization by a GnRH agonist.[12]
- **Cabergoline**
  - Reverses increased vascular permeability
  - *For prevention of OHSS*—Administer in the last week of stimulation till 1 to 3 week after hCG stimulation
  - *For treatment of OHSS*—Dose 0.05 to1.0 mg/day; continued till symptoms abate.

- **Modified techniques:**
  - *Follicular aspiration* – May be protective against OHSS
  - *Cryopreservation of embryo*—With subsequent replacement in nonstimulated or natural cycle.
  - *In Vitro Maturation (IVM) of immature oocytes*—In PCOS patients, OHSS could be prevented by minimal stimulation and IVM of oocytes.
- **Recent developments:**
  - VEGF receptor antagonist—Prevent increase in capillary permeability
  - Fms like tyrosine kinase (sflt-1) which binds with VEGF and decrease its availability for its endothelial effect
  - These compounds are still preclinical, but may have a role in future.

KEY POINTS

- OHSS is very traumatizing and can be at times life threatening for the patient undergoing fertility treatment.
- Softer stimulation regimes aiming at less oocytes of good quality for ovulation induction are advocated to prevent OHSS.
- In OHSS hematocrit is one of the best indicators of hemoconcentration and should be taken at least twice a day until stabilization. All the other blood and urine tests are done daily, and every 2 to 3 days afterwards.
- At risk patient should be informed about possibilities such as canceling, coasting or freezing for subsequent replacement
- Abdominal paracentesis is recommended for symptomatic relief of abdominal discomfort or dyspnea caused by pronounced ascites.
- Registration of all cases of severe OHSS and their outcome should become compulsory in all ART programs.

REFERENCES

1. Delvigne A, De Sutter P, Dhont M, et al. Ovarian Hyperstimulation Guidelines http://www.eshre.eu/01/default.aspxpageid=372-ohss guideline
2. Garcia-Velasco JA, Pellicer A. New concepts in the understanding of the ovarian hyperstimulation syndrome. Curr Opin Obstet Gynecol 2003;15:251-6.
3. Mathur RS, Akande AV, Keay SD, Hunt LP, Jenkins JM. Distinction between early and late ovarian hyperstimulation syndrome. Fertil Steril 2000;73:901-7.
4. IVF worldwide unit directory Ovarian Hyperstimulation Syndrome. http://www.ivf-worldwide.com/Education/ovarian-hyperstimulation-syndrome-ohss.html
5. Mathur R, Evbuomwan I, Jenkins J. Prevention and management of ovarian hyperstimulation syndrome. Curr Obstet Gynecol 2002;12:111-6.
6. Navot D, Bergh PA, Laufer N. Ovarian hyperstimulation syndrome in novel reproductive technologies: prevention and treatment. Fertil Steril 1992;58:249-61.
7. Padilla SL, Zamaria S, Baramki TA, Garcia JE. Abdominal paracentesis for ovarian hyperstimulation syndrome with severe pulmonary compromise. Fertil Steril 1990;53:365-7.
8. Mashiach S, Bider D, Moran O, Goldenberg M, Ben-Rafael Z. Adnexal torsion of hyperstimulated ovaries in pregnancies after gonadotropin therapy. Fertil Steril 1990;53:76-80.
9. Delvigne A , Rozenberg S. Review of clinical course and treatment of ovarian hyperstimulation syndrome (OHSS). Hum Reprod Update 2003;9:77-96.
10. Stewart JA, Hamilton PJ, Murdoch AP. Thromboembolic disease associated with ovarian stimulation and assisted conception techniques. Hum Reprod 1997;12:2167-73.
11. Delvigne A , Rozenberg S. Preventive attitude of physicians to avoid OHSS in IVF patients. Hum Reprod 2001;16:2491-5.
12. Emperaire JC, Edwards RG. Time to revolutionize the triggering of ovulation. Reprod Biomed Online 2004;9:480-3.
13. The Management of Ovarian Hyperstimulation Syndrome Green Top Guideline No.5 (2006). Royal College of Obstetricians and Gynaecologists. Available at: http://www.rcog.org.uk/files/rcog-corp/uploaded-files/GT5ManagementOvarianHyperstimulation.pdf

Chapter **32**

Sexual Assault

Krishna Agarwal

INTRODUCTION

A woman or a child who has suffered the trauma of sexual assault should be referred to as survivor and not the victim of sexual assault to eliminate the stigma associated with word 'victim'.

Examination of a female survivor of sexual assault is a very sensitive and important issue which should be dealt with an utmost care and in a professional way. The examination findings and the collected specimens make the strongest evidence in court of law in providing justice.

A good job can be done if examination is performed keeping certain goals in mind and carried out in a systematic and stepwise manner.

Goals of Examination

- Medical – Assessment, documentation & treatment of injuries and prevention of pregnancy and sexually transmitted diseases.
- Collection of forensic evidences
- Psychological support

Proper documentation of the findings and collection of the evidences is of utmost importance. It plays an important role later in the court of law to prove or disprove the crime. If the attending doctor fails to collect the evidences properly, he/she may face the charges of destroying the evidences which is punishable in Indian Penal Code.

Every registered medical practitioner should be able to conduct the examination and in emergency even a registered private practitioner may be asked to conduct such an examination. This examination must be part of MBBS teaching curriculum.

The attitude towards patient should be nonjudgmental, empathetic and reassuring. This is of utmost importance and an already suffered person should not undergo further trauma of irrelevant questioning or rough examination.

Examination of the Survivor

- The place of examination must be a separate place ensuring *ABSOLUTE PRIVACY.*
- *If survivor requires urgent medical care, it should take priority over collection of evidence.*
- Examination can be performed on demand of:
  - The police
  - The survivor herself or her relatives

- – Women's right organizations
- – Other law enforcing authorities.
- It should preferably be performed by a female doctor, however if not possible then a female medical attendant must be present at the time of examination and in case of minor her mother or a neutral person must also be present.
- The survivor must be examined immediately without any delay and should be treated as an emergency.
- In case survivor happens to be a child (age less than 12 years), a pediatrician should perform the general examination.
- Psychologist should be always be called for psychological support of the survivor. This is an important aspect of providing holistic care to such a survivor and should never be forgotten.

CASE SCENARIO-1

A 30-year-old woman with history of sexual assault 5 hours back, accompanied by a police constable, presents to the emergency services.

INITIAL CARE

The woman is taken to a separate room with absolute privacy. She is made comfortable and explained about the procedure in her own language.

Written informed consent taken in her native language. She is also assured that all the examination findings and specimen collection would be confidential and would only be handed over to the police. However in spite of explaining everything if survivor denies for examination, then it should be abandoned and reason documented in the register at appropriate place.

All the entries are performed in the Medicolegal Case Register which is to be kept under custody of the staff nurse on duty. The entries are made in duplicate. The accompanying constable's name and number are entered in the register. Copy of the order from the police station requesting for examination should be attached in the Medico Legal Register on the page where the entries are being done.

POINTS TO BE NOTED IN HISTORY

- General medical history and gynecological history is taken.
- Gynecological history should include
  - – The date of last menstrual period
  - – In case of married patient history of prior pregnancies, contraceptive use and last voluntary intercourse, if any is documented
- History of having any bath, defecation, urination, brushing of teeth or changing of her clothes documented
- Detailed history taken regarding when and where the event occurred, how many assailants were present, whether penetration or ejaculation happened
- A complete narration of history as described by the patient and her escort is noted
- Emotional status of patient is also recorded.

POINTS TO BE NOTED IN EXAMINATION

Carefully and systematically conducted examination would not allow missing on any findings. The examination is conducted in following steps:

Preservation of Clothes

Patient is asked to take out her outer clothes on a big piece of paper. The same is wrapped in the paper and sealed. She is provided with a gown to cover herself. Then her under clothes are collected in a separate piece of paper, wrapped and sealed. The patient is provided with a fresh set of clothes from hospital in which she can go home.

Face, Breast and Whole Body Examined Closely

- Injury marks on body are described and documented clearly. Drawings should be used to describe injuries
- Debris from any site is collected in a separate envelop, labeled and sealed and marked
- Loose debris from finger nails and scrapings collected in envelop, sealed and marked
- Any suspected stains on body are collected by putting distilled water and rolling a swab stick over it. The stick is dried and placed in an envelop.

Examination of Oral Cavity

Swabs are taken from the sides of molar teeth, slides prepared and swabs kept in the tubes

Collection of Pubic Hair

A paper is placed under the buttocks of the patient, patient's public hair combed with the comb and loose hairs collected on the paper are sealed. Patient's pubic hair which appear matted are cut and sealed in another envelop

Local Examination

Vulva is examined for signs of injury and the findings noted down. Condition of the hymen, whether torn or intact, is documented

Per Speculum Examination

This examination may be painful and traumatic to the person who has already suffered. Therefore the procedure should be explained again to the woman and the smallest size of speculum should be chosen. If the survivor denies for its use or the hymen is intact then specimens should be collected by just separating the labia and gently introducing the swab stick into vagina. The reason for omitting speculum examination must be properly documented.

- If she agrees for this examination then swab is collected from the posterior fornix, four slides are prepared, dried and sealed. After drying the swab is put separately in the tube. Two of the four slides prepared are handed over to the accompanying police constable and the other two are sent to the forensic lab
- Swab is also taken from fluid and mucus from the cervix and a smear is prepared on a slide. After drying the swab is placed in a tube and sealed. Another swab is collected from cervix and streaked on chocolate agar plate and the swab is discarded
- Wash the vagina with saline from a preloaded syringe, stir it by the speculum, draw back the fluid with syringe, put it on a slide and examine under a microscope for spermatozoa.

Rectal Examination

Proctoscopy would also be an unpleasant examination for the survivor and should be performed only if the survivor agrees, using smallest size of the instrument. Any injury should be noted; a swab is collected and kept in a tube.

Per Vaginum Examination (Finger Test)

Performing this exam on a survivor of sexual assault is questionable. We do not gain anything by performing this examination and should be omitted as a routine until it is indicated.

INVESTIGATIONS

Samples Collection and Radiological Examination
1. Following body fluids samples are collected after performing the examination:
    - *Blood:* For ABO grouping and Rh typing, HIV, Hepatitis, Syphilis
    - *Urine:* For alcohol intoxication and pregnancy test.

2. *X-ray:* Wrist, pelvis, shoulder and knee for confirmation of age.
3. Sample for gonorrhea was already taken on chocolate agar plate.

Precautions while Handling the Samples

- All the samples should be properly dried (drying is very important otherwise it gets putrefied) and sealed by the nursing staff in presence of doctor conducting the examination.
- All the labels and enclosures must be signed by the doctor and staff nurse across the seal. The requisition form should be properly filled mentioning about the type of samples.
- No specimen should be left alone at any time. All specimens are placed in a yellow bag which is kept in locked refrigerator till the time samples are handed over to the police constable who would take them to the central forensic laboratory. Two swabs from vagina are also sent to the hospital's forensic department.
- The record of all the specimens sent is kept in the register.

Special Tests

If required following test can be performed where indicated:
- Colposcopy—For examining area of microtrauma.
- Toludine blue—It stains microtrauma areas on vulva which can be better visualized. It is then washed with water.
- Woods lamp examination—It help identify seminal stains on body because these stains are fluorescent in ultraviolet light. The florescent area should be swabbed with cotton tipped applicator moistened with sterile water, dried and preserved.
- Bite mark casting can be done by unwaxed dental floss.

TREATMENT

A prophylactic cover against sexually transmitted diseases and tetanus and emergency contraception is provided to the survivor of a sexual attack:
1. *For gonorrhea*
    - Oral azithromycin 1 gm orally single dose
      or
    - Oral cefixime 400 mg orally single dose
2. *For Chlamydia*
    - Oral azythromycin 1 gm single dose
      or
    - Oral doxycycline 100 mg twice daily for 7 days
3. *For HIV* (initiate within 4 hr for maximum benefits), the basic regimen includes:
    - Oral Zidovudine 300 mg twice daily for 4 weeks
      plus
    - Oral Lamivudine 150 mg twice daily for 4 weeks
    If the transmission risk for HIV is perceived to be high (bleeding or the assailant was at high risk of having HIV): Expanded regime to be given which includes:
    - Basic regimen
      plus
    - Indinavir 800 mg thrice daily for 4 weeks or Nelfinavir 750 mg thrice daily for 4 weeks
4. *Tetanus:* Injection tetanus toxoid 0.5 mL subcutaneous
5. *Emergency contraception* is offered
    - Tab Levonorgestrel 75 microgram with in 72 hours and to be repeated after 12 hours
      or
    - Tab mala N2 tab stat followed by 2 tab after 12 hours.
6. Any injury or trauma to the genital tract is dealt with accordingly.

CASE SCENARIO-2

An 11-year-old girl brought by her parents with a history of sexual assault presented at 2 AM to the emergency.

In this case:

- The examination is performed on the request of parents
- Since the survivor is a minor (<16 years) consent of the parents/guardian is taken. If the survivor does not give consent then she and her guardians should be explained about the importance of examination and also the possibility of losing evidences as the time passes
- Steps of examination are the same. However her mother should be allowed to be present at the time of examination
- Since survivor is a child, pediatrician should perform the general physical examination
- The prophylactic doses of drugs for prevention of sexually transmitted disease should be given in pediatric doses
- The child should be attended by a psychologist after the examination and evidence collection and must ensure that the survivor is under safe custody and proper care.

In April 2009, Delhi high court passed a judgment and laid down the guidelines for response to survivors of sexual assault to be followed by different concerned agencies. The honorable court directed all hospitals to identify a place of examination and to use SAFE kit (developed by Mumbai based NGO CEHAT).However the SAFE Kit is not commercially available and either the kit can be generated at hospital level or the evidences can be collected in a systematic order using hospital resources only.

For a model response by health department, protocols must be laid down by the health facilities and it should clearly state the roles and responsibilities of each individual dealing with the survivor. There should be regular training of staff so that they can handle the situation in an efficient and holistic manner.

SAFE (Sexual Assault Care and Forensic Evidence Collection) Kit

SAFE kit is for comprehensive care and collection of evidences in cases of sexual assault. This kit was first adapted from Ontario Provincial Government, Canada. After that it has undergone several reviews depending on feedbacks by forensic experts, gynecologists as well as women's right activists from several parts of country. This kit is scientifically sound, easy to use and helps in examination and collecting the evidences in such a way that no step in examination would be left out. It has following contents:

1. Manual-to-guide doctor—21 pager document to guide the doctor
2. Protocol book containing forms-
   Form 1: Consent
   Form 2: Medical history
   Form 3: Sexual assault history
   Form 4: Forensic examination
   Form 5: General exam and age estimation
   Form 6: Discharge slip
   All forms have 2 copies
3. A box containing envelopes-
   4 envelopes (1A to 1D): Clothes
   11 envelopes (2A to 2K): Body samples
   8 envelopes (3A to 3H): Genital and anal samples
   Step-wise arrangement of all envelops to prevent omissions

Organizations Dealing with the Survivors of Sexual Assault

1. NGOs working for the survivors of sexual assault
   i. CEHAT (Center for Enquiry into Health and allied Themes)
      Aram Society Road
      Vakola, Santa Cruz (E), Mumbai-400055
      Tel-91-22-26673154, 26673571
      Email:cehat@vsnl.com
   ii. SAMA-Resource Group for Women and Health
      2nd floor, B 45, Shivalik Main Road,
      Malviya Nagar, New Delhi-110017
      Tel-91-11-65637632
      Email:sama.womenshealth@gmail.com
2. Legal services
   i. Rape Crisis cell
      Delhi Commission for Women
      C-block, 2nd floor, Vikas Bhawan, I.P.Estate
      New Delhi Tel-23370557
   ii. Delhi Legal Service Authority
      Fab Building, Patiala House Court
      New Delhi
      Tel 12525(toll free)

KEY POINTS

- Every registered medical practitioner must be able to conduct the examination of a female survivor of sexual assault.
- The survivor must always be examined immediately without any delay and should be treated as an emergency.
- The place of examination must be a separate room so as to ensure absolute privacy.
- Examination must be performed keeping certain goals in mind and carried out in a systematic and stepwise manner.
- Proper documentation of the findings and collection of the evidences is extremely important because it makes an important document in the court.

References

1. High Court of Delhi. Delhi Commission for Women v. Delhi Police, W.P (CRL) 696/2008 [Internet]. 2009 Apr 23 [cited 2010 Mar 15]. Available from: http://www.ncw.nic.in.
2. Jagadeesh N. Legal changes towards justice for sexual assault victims. Indian J Med Ethics. 2010;7:108-12.
3. http://www.cehat.org/go/SafeKit/Home as on 15.1.11
4. Avid A. Baram. Sexuality and Sexual Function. In: Jonathan S. Berek, Eli Y. Adashi, Paula A. Hillard (eds). Novak's Gynecology. 12th edn. Baltimore: Williams & Wilkins, 1996. pp. 279-98.

Chapter 33

Emergencies of Gynecologic Oncology

Gauri Gandhi, Manoj Sharma, Neha Singh, Shonali Chandra

INTRODUCTION

Oncological emergencies are acute conditions that are caused by the cancer itself or by the side effects of therapy, which require rapid intervention to avoid death or severe permanent damage.[1]

This can occur in patients with a curable disease like invasive mole, but the majority occur in patients with advanced often incurable disease. Prompt recognition and treatment can lead to improved survival and quality of life.

The important oncological emergencies related to gynecology are:

- Hemorrhage
- Obstructive uropathy
- Malignant ascites and malignant pleural effusion
- Intestinal perforation
- Intestinal obstruction
- Febrile neutropenia.

HEMORRHAGE DUE TO CANCER CERVIX

Predisposing Factors of Hemorrhage in Carcinoma Cervix are:

- Locally advanced cancer
- Thrombocytopenia/pancytopenia from chemotherapy/radiotherapy
- Uremia

CASE SCENARIO-1

Mrs. C, a 52-yr-old lady, postmenopausal for 5 years, presented to the casualty with heavy bleeding per vaginum for 1 day. She had history of slight bleeding off and on for the last 4 months.

> **Comments:** A diagnosis of genital cancer should be considered when a woman presents with post menopausal bleeding. The commonest cause would be cervical cancer.

Differential Diagnosis

- Endometrial cancer
- Rare malignancies like choriocarcinoma and uterine sarcomas

- Benign conditions including endometrial polyps and hyperplasia, but these usually do not cause heavy bleeding.

POINTS TO BE NOTED IN HISTORY

- Parity – multiparity goes in favor of cervical cancer and nulliparity goes in favor of endometrial cancer
- History of postcoital bleeding, which goes in favor of carcinoma cervix
- History of foul smelling discharge, which goes in favor of cervical malignancy
- History of urinary symptoms like hematuria
- History of diabetes, hypertension which favor endometrial cancer.

> **History in this case:** This lady has history of postcoital bleeding and irregular bleeding. She was married at 20 years of age and is P4L4. She also had history of unhealthy vaginal discharge. No history of diabetes or hypertension.

POINTS TO BE NOTED IN EXAMINATION

General Examination

General condition, pulse rate, respiratory rate, blood pressure (BP),temperature, pallor, jaundice, any signs of bleeding diathesis

Cardiovascular and Respiratory System Examination

Abdominal Examination (P/A)

To detect presence of any masses

Pelvic Examination

Per Speculum (P/S) Examination

Any lesion or growth on cervix or vagina

Per Vaginum (P/V) Examination

To detect any pelvic pathology like cervical growth or enlarged uterus. Enlarged uterus may be due to pyometra or due to endometrial growth.

Combined Vaginal and Rectal (P/V/R) Examination

To assess for parametrial involvement.

> **Examination in this case:**
> The general condition was poor. Pulse—120/min, low volume; BP—90/60 mm Hg.
> She looked moderately pale with clinical hemoglobin of 7 gm%.
> P/A : Unremarkable
> P/S : Cervix was replaced by 4*4 cm friable cauliflower growth, which was bleeding.
> P/V/R : Uterus normal size, left parametrium thickened till lateral pelvic wall, rectal mucosa free

Diagnosis

A clinical diagnosis of carcinoma cervix Stage III B was made.

INVESTIGATIONS

- Hemoglobin, hematocrit, complete blood counts
- Blood group
- Kidney and liver function tests, serum electrolytes
- Coagulation profile.

> **Investigations in this case:**
> - Hemoglobin—8 gm% ; hematocrit—24 % ; TLC—12,000/mm³ ; Platelets—2.3 lakh/mm³
> - Blood group: Rhesus type- A +
> - Renal function tests, liver function tests—Normal
> - Bleeding time, clotting time, prothrombin time—Normal

MANAGEMENT

- Venous access should be established immediately and samples sent for complete hemogram, blood group and cross matching, renal function tests, blood sugar. A bedside bleeding time / clotting time/clot retraction time should be done.
- Fluid replacement to be done with crystalloids, while blood is awaited.
- A cervical punch biopsy should be taken to confirm the diagnosis and hasten initiation of treatment.
- For control of bleeding the following methods can be used:[2]
  1. Tight *packing of* cervix and vagina with roller gauze. Monsel's solution (ferric subsulfate) may be put on the portion of the pack abutting the tumor. The patient should be catheterized when packing is done.
  2. *Embolization:* Massive bleeding from a case of advanced cancer cervix may require embolization or ligation of internal iliac arteries. The help of an interventional radiologist can be taken for embolization. The specific bleeding site can be evaluated by injection of contrast and the bleeding vessel is embolized using gelfoam or polyvinyl alcohol particles. Yalvac et al [3] reported selective embolization of uterine arteries in 8 patients of cancer cervix and in all cases bleeding was controlled. The most common side effect was temporary severe pain related to ischemia of tumor.
  3. *Laparoscopic ligation of internal iliac artery* has been used to control massive bleeding in advanced cancer cervix. Sobiczewski et al [4] reported 3 cases in which this was done followed by external radiotherapy. However, in several cases surgical approach may be difficult because the pelvic anatomy is distorted due to the disease itself or due to previous radiotherapy or because the patient is too ill to withstand surgery.
  4. *Hemostatic Radiation:*
     Brachytherapy
     A single low dose rate intracavitory insertion with tandems and colpostats for approximately 6000 mgh (55 Gy to point A) will suffice. If irradiation was delivered previously, lower intracavitory doses should be prescribed (4000 to 5000 mgh).[5] Grigsby et al used two fractions of high dose rate brachytherapy with a ring applicator (once weekly) with control of bleeding in 14 out of 15 patients.[6]
     Teleradiation
     Whole pelvic radiation using a simulator demarcation or a 10 cm X 10 cm field to give 300 c Gy per day for three fractions or 200 cGy for five fractions.
  5. *Hemostatic Chemotherapy:*
     Hemostatic chemotherapy has been found useful in Indian scenario for bleeding advanced stage cancer cervix patients, when radiation therapy or interventional radiology facilities are not immediately available.
     Sharma et al [7] have reported the use of chemotherapy (5 fluorouracil 350 mg D1-5, cisplatin 30 mg D1-4 and bleomycin 10 mg D1&D5) in 60 patients of cancer cervix Stage IIb and beyond. This achieved hemostasis in 90 percent of cases.
- Futher management involves chemoradiation or surgery if it is at an operable stage.

Treatment in this case:
The diagnosis in this case was confirmed by histopathological report of biopsy which came out to be poorly differentiated squamous cell carcinoma. This patient was planned for chemoradiation (Stage IIIb).

URINARY OBSTRUCTION DUE TO CANCER CERVIX

CASE SCENARIO-2

A 40-yr-old lady admitted with complaints of blood stained vaginal discharge for 4 months, vomiting and reduced urinary output for 1 week and anuria for 10 hours

Comment: A diagnosis of locally advanced carcinoma cervix with ureteral obstruction should be considered in view of these two symptoms.

Differential Diagnosis

Other malignancies that can cause ureteral obstruction rarely are:
- Advanced endometrial cancer
- Extrinsic compression by large ovarian malignancies
- Enlarged metastatic lymph nodes.

POINTS TO BE NOTED IN HISTORY

- History of puffiness or edema
- History of altered sensorium or drowsiness (due to uremia)
- History of vomiting (symptom of uremia)

POINTS TO BE NOTED IN EXAMINATION

- General examination:
  General condition and sensorium, pulse rate, BP, pallor, edema and lymphadenopathy
- Cardiovascular and respiratory system examination
- Abdominal examination for any distention or masses
- Pelvic examination
  - Per speculum for any growth on cervix
  - P/V/R to detect cervical growth and stage the patient clinically and to see uterine size and any adnexal mass

History and examination in this case:
There was history of vomiting, but no history of altered sensorium.
The patient was well oriented, with normal sensorium. Her pulse was 100/min and B.P 110/70 mm Hg. There was mild facial puffiness and mild pedal edema. There was no significant lymphadenopathy. On pelvic examination, there was exophytic cervical growth of 4 x5 cm with parametrial involvement upto lateral pelvic wall.

Diagnosis

A clinical diagnosis of carcinoma cervix stage IIIb with anuria was made.

Investigations in this case:
- Hemoglobin—9 gm%
- Blood urea—112 mg% and serum creatinine—12 mg/dL
- Serum electrolytes—normal

Contd...

Contd...

- Arterial blood gas analysis—normal
- Ultrasound abdomen and pelvis showed bilateral hydronephrosis. The uterus was of normal size and there was no pyometra. A cervical growth 4x5 cm was seen. Transvaginal sonography (TVS) did not show bladder involvement. Bilateral ovaries were normal.
- Cervical biopsy—Squamous cell carcinoma.

MANAGEMENT

Ureteral obstruction due to malignancy has poor prognosis and treatment is palliative with some diversion procedure. Treatment aims at providing relief of obstruction till a definite treatment is given. It is important to select patients carefully for curative treatment. Those cases with frozen pelvis and a nonfunctioning kidney are unlikely to show response and are best treated with supportive care. For all other cases treatment aims at providing relief of obstruction till definitive treatment is done.

Initial Management

- Initial management consists of cystoscopy and bilateral ureteral stenting.
- If stenting is not successful, then percutaneous nephrostomy should be done.
- Dialysis may be necessary for some patients till obstruction is relieved and kidney function tests improve. The recovery of kidney functions after relief of obstruction depends on age of the patient and renal cortical thickness. Patient in older age group and those with renal cortical thickness < 13 mm have a poor prognosis.

Cases with complete renal recovery by 4 weeks after diversion have improved survival despite the malignancy.

Elective stenting or nephrostomy may be done in cases showing bilateral hydronephrosis and low creatinine clearance (< 50 mL/min).[8]

Definitive Treatment

Definitive treatment in the form of chemoradiation can be started when renal functions improve. Cisplatin should not be used as a radiosensitizer because it is nephrotoxic. Other drugs like carboplatin and gemcetabine can be used.

In selective younger patients who report early in the course of renal failure, an aggressive initial ureteric diversion followed by chemoradiation may be curative. In cases with frozen pelvis and long-standing renal failure, the prognosis is bad even with diversion procedures.

HEMOPERITONIUM DUE TO INVASIVE MOLE

CASE SCENARIO-3

Mrs A, 29 yrs P2L2 was admitted with history of bleeding per vaginum off and on for 2 months, acute abdominal pain for 1 hour and fainting half an hour back.

Comment: Complications of pregnancy should be considered as the most likely cause in this young woman.

Differential Diagnosis

- Ectopic pregnancy
- Incomplete abortion
- Trophoblastic disease.

POINTS TO BE NOTED IN HISTORY

- History of amenorrhea
- History of passage of products of conception
- History of acute pain
- History of dilatation and evacuation/molar evacuation
- History of urinary or bowel complaints.

History in this case:
Patient had history of molar evacuation of 12 weeks gestation 2 month ago. The histopathological report revealed molar pregnancy.

POINTS TO BE NOTED IN EXAMINATION

- General condition: Pulse, respiratory rate, blood pressure, pallor
- Per abdominal examination: Distention, fluid thrill, guarding and rigidity, or any other palpable mass
- Per speculum examination: Any growth on cervix, vagina, suburethral area (metastasis for choriocarcinoma), bleeding from os
- Per vaginal examination: Uterine size, cervical os open/closed, any adnexal mass/tenderness.

Examination in this case:
Pulse—120/min, low volume; BP- 90/60 mm Hg, Pallor++
P/A : Lower abdomen fullness, fluid thrill present, slight tenderness and guarding
P/S : No growth, bleeding from os present
P/V: Bogginess in fornices present , uterine size 12 weeks.

Investigations in this case:
Hemoglobin—7 gm%
BT—5 min, CT—13 min
Urine pregnancy test—Positive
β-hCG was sent
Ultrasound pelvis: Significant free fluid in abdomen, uterus enlarged to 12 weeks full with mixed echogenic mass in the cavity. Vascularity present in the mass

MANAGEMENT

Emergency Hysterectomy

Emergency hysterectomies have been reported in case of invasive moles or choriocarcinoma causing severe intra-abdominal bleeding or severe vaginal bleeding. Pongsaranantakul S et al[9] reported a series of 18 total abdominal hysterectomies in cases of gestational trophoblastic neoplasia, out of which 4 emergency hysterectomies were done in patients presenting with hemoperitoneum. Hysterectomy in gestational trophoblastic disease can prove very difficult. The uterine vasculature is very prominent, leading to excessive bleeding during dissection, especially in cases where the tumor has gone beyond uterus into the parametrium. If bleeding is difficult to control then ligation of internal iliac arteries will have to be done.

Embolization

In cases which appear wide spread or if the coagulation profile is difficult to correct, embolization of bleeding arteries has to be done to reduce bleeding.

Conservative Myometrial Resection

Conservative myometrial resection combined with uterine reconstruction might be considered in selected patients with invasive moles who are desirous of fertility. Ideally frozen section of margins should be sent. Kanazawa et al [10] evaluated 72 cases with myometrial resection of invasive moles. They recommend that in an elective situation, the patients are selected if:

- Lesions are localized to myometrium, defined by ultrasound, CT or pelvic angiography
- Urinary hCG < 10,000 IU/day
- No evidence of pulmonary involvement
- If metastasis to lungs, it should be controlled by chemotherapy prior to operation

However in an emergency situation, local resection may have to be done without strict compliance to these guidelines.

During hysterectomy or myometrial resection for these indications, ovarian removal is not usually required, because gestational trophoblastic neoplasia rarely metastatizes to the ovaries. These tumor are not hormonally influenced.

Primary Uterine Oversewing

Estrella et al[11] have reported 2 cases of uterine rupture in low-risk GTN managed with primary uterine repair by over-sewing the rupture area with figure of eight sutures. They recommended that cases where uterus is to be conserved and the tumor is large but area of rupture is small, can be managed by simple suturing followed by chemotherapy. This was attempted because removal of large tumor would not leave much of the uterus for future fertility.

> **Treatment in this case:**
> - Paracentesis revealed hemoperitoneum.
> - Fresh frozen plasma and blood transfused rapidly to correct deranged coagulation.
> - Once coagulation was corrected, laparotomy was done.
> - Findings on laparotomy : Friable mass perforating through uterine wall and bleeding into peritoneal cavity (perforating trophoblastic tumor)
> - An emergency hysterectomy was done.
> - This was followed by chemotherapy and serial β-hCG levels.

MALIGNANT ASCITES

Malignant ascitis represents advanced stage of the disease.

CASE SCENARIO-4

A 65-year-old patient presented with abdominal pain, distention which had increased in the last 1 week. She also had complaints of vomiting and dyspnea.

> **Comment:** In a postmenopausal patient with abdominal distention, dyspnea and vomiting, the diagnosis of ovarian malignancy should be considered.

Differential Diagnosis

- Gastrointestinal malignancy
- Abdominal tuberculosis

POINTS TO BE NOTED IN HISTORY

- Parity (nulliparity could favor both ovarian cancer and abdominal Koch)
- History of anorexia and weight loss (more marked in advanced malignancy)

- History of nausea, vomiting, diarrhea or constipation
- Family history or exposure to tuberculosis
- History of fever
- Family history of ovarian, gastrointestinal or breast malignancy

> **History in this case:**
> This lady was P2L2. She had history of anorexia and weight loss for 6 months, vomiting off and on and abdominal distention for 1 month. She did not have history of diarrhea, fever or exposure to tuberculosis.

POINTS TO BE NOTED IN EXAMINATION

- General examination—General condition including BMI of patient, pulse, BP, pallor, pedal edema and lymphadenopathy.
- Cardiovascular and respiratory system examination
- On abdominal examination—Distention, percussion note (dull or resonant), fluid thrill (for ascitis), any mass or hepatosplenomegaly
- Pelvic examination:
  - Per speculum examination for any abnormality visible on cervix and vagina
  - Per vaginal examination for uterine size and any adnexal mass
  - P/V/R for any nodularity in the pouch of Douglas (POD)

> **Examination in this case:**
> The patient was cachexic and general condition was poor. She was dyspneic with respiratory rate of 25/min. Pulse was 96/min and blood pressure was 100/60 mm Hg. She had moderate pallor, no palpable lymph nodes, but had mild pedal edema.
> P/A: Marked distention of abdomen was present. On percussion, there was dull note all over abdomen and fluid was present. A firm mass was palpable in lower abdomen, margins not well delineated
> P/S: Cervix and vagina healthy.
> P/V: Uterus small. Nodular mass tipped through right fornix and extending into abdomen approximately 20x20 cm.
> P/V/R: No nodularity in POD.

Diagnosis

A clinical diagnosis of ovarian tumor with massive ascitis was made.

> **Investigations in this case:**
> Hemoglobin—8 gm%, total leukocyte count—10,000/mm³ and differential count did not show lymphocytosis
> Kidney and liver function tests—normal
> Ultrasound showed significant fluid in abdomen. A large 20 × 22 cm mass seen in pelvis extending from right side to umbilicus. Mixed echogenicity with solid areas.
> Tumor markers CA-125, CEA were sent.

MANAGEMENT

The treatment options are:
1. *Paracentesis:* This provides immediate relief of pain and other symptoms like dyspnea. Usually 500-2000 mL of fluid is drained per procedure although drainage of upto 3 liters of fluid per procedure has been reported to be tolerated. However, the results are short-lived and repeated drainage is required. Also repeated paracentesis can lead to significant protein loss, electrolyte imbalance, hypotension, sepsis and visceral and vascular injury. To minimize these complications, indwelling catheter has been devised, but it can get malpositioned or lead to infection. [12]

2. *Peritoneo-venous shunt:* Shunts can be placed in patients who are in relatively good condition. Commonly used shunts are the LeVeen and Denver shunts (uni-directional shunts) which direct fluid from the abdominal cavity into the vena cava.

   The risks associated with shunt placement are shunt obstruction, sepsis, coagulation dysfunction, spreading of tumor cells from the abdominal cavity.

   Survival and quality of life is not greater than in case of repeated paracentesis.

3. *Diuretics:* Based on studies by Becker et al[13] and Pockros et al,[14] it is recommended that diuretics are helpful only in those cases of malignant ascitis which have evidence of portal hypertension. However, this has not been validated in prospective studies.

4. *Intraperitoneal chemotherapy:* Agents like bleomycin, cisplatin, 5-fluorouracil, thiotepa, cyclophosphamide, doxorubicin, paclitaxel have been tested in small studies but the results are inconsistent.

5. *Immunotherapy:*

   • *Catumaxomab:* It is a tri-functional antibody. It acts by 1) binding to epithelial cell adhesion molecules (EpCAM) of the tumor cells and thus inhibiting these cells and 2) activating T cells and accessory immune cells which destroy the tumor cells.this is most effective in cases of ovarian cancers which contain EpCAM positive tumor cells. Four to five infusions of 5 to 200 µg are given within 9 to 13 days. The side effects include transient fever, nausea, vomiting and most of them are grade 1-2.[15]

   This is the most effective therapy for malignant ascitis reducing the need for paracentesis and prolonging puncture free survival. This is used in addition to systemic chemotherapy and surgery.

   • *Bevacizumab (Avastin):* This is a recombinant humanized monoclonal antibody that blocks the binding of Vascular Endothelial Growth Factor (VEGF) to receptors in the tumor cells leading to decreased vascularization of tumor and reduces ascitis. Numnum et al[16] reported the i.v. application of bevacizumab (15 mg/kg every 3 weeks) to four heavily pretreated patients with end-stage ovarian cancer in order to palliate symptomatic ascites. In all four patients, repeated paracentesis was not required because of dramatically reduced levels of ascites after the initiation of therapy with bevacizumab. Its side effects can be hypertension, proteinuria, thrombosis, delayed wound healing and rarely gut perforation.

OTHER EMERGENCIES

MALIGNANT PLEURAL EFFUSION

Effusion may be an initial sign of cancer or it may signal advanced disease. One-third will be bilateral. Most common are carcinoma of lung, breast, primary unknown, leukemia, lymphoma, genitourinary and gastrointestinal tumors.

Clinical features: Dyspnea, orthopnea, dry non-productive cough, chest pain, heaviness, tachypnea, dull percussion, restricted chest expansion, impaired transmission of breath sounds. Bloody effusion is strongest indicator of malignancy.

Investigations: Chest X-ray, CT scan, diagnostic and therapeutic pleural tap

Management: Observation, therapeutic pleural aspiration, intercostal tube drainage and intrapleural instillation of sclerosant, pleurectomy.

GASTROINTESTINAL OBSTRUCTION

Intestinal obstruction as a presenting symptom of a gynecologic cancer is most commonly caused by advanced ovarian cancer.

History

- Symptoms due to the primary cancer.
- Symptoms pertaining to gastrointestinal obstruction: the common presenting symptoms of small bowel obstruction are abdominal cramps, nausea, vomiting and abdominal distention.
- The time course of symptoms, character of the emesis, and degree of distention provide important historical clues. For example, a rapid course, bilious vomiting, minimal distention points towards a high-grade obstruction. Whereas a more insidious course, nonbilious vomiting and marked abdominal distention suggests a more distal or large bowel obstruction.

Management

Initial therapy involves correction of fluid and electrolytes and nasogastric tube decompression.

Assessment of location and extent of obstruction is done by upper gastrointestinal series with small bowel follow through or a contrast enhanced CT scan.

Severely malnourished patients have to be given total parenteral nutrition (TPN) even before definitive surgery is planned for debulking of tumor and to relieve obstruction. If there is extensive carcinomatosis then neoadjuvant chemotherapy may be a better option than surgical intervention. If this strategy is taken then nasogastric decompression and TPN will be required for several weeks while the neo-adjuvant chemotherapy has the time to result in tumor response. Fortunately many patients with ovarian cancer will regain intestinal function after 2 to 3 cycle of chemotherapy.[2]

COLONIC OBSTRUCTION

It is an acute surgical emergency. It necessitates urgent surgical intervention in order to prevent colonic perforation, peritonitis, sepsis and death. As adequate mechanical bowel preparation is difficult because of malignant colonic obstruction, resection and anastomosis is out of question, and a colostomy must be performed. If the patient has an excellent response to chemotherapy, colostomy takedown in the future is reasonable to consider.

Recent advances in endoscopy have established a role for colonic stenting, either as a palliative measure or as a bridge toward definitive operative management in patients with resectable disease. Stenting carries the risk of perforation, migration and re-obstruction.

THROMBOEMBOLISM

Most women with gynecologic cancers have several risk factors that increase the probability of developing deep venous thrombosis or pulmonary embolism during the course of their therapy. Prophylactic and therapeutic anticoagulation therapy should be instituted.

UNUSUAL ACUTE PRESENTATIONS OF OVARIAN MALIGNANCIES

Ovarian torsion: Takeda et al [17] has seen an ovarian dysgerminoma presenting with acute abdomen due to adnexal torsion in a 17-year-old girl.

Hemoperitoneum: Geisler et al [18] have presented a 40-year-old with acute pain abdomen, nausea and light-headedness. On examination she had severe anemia and hemoperineum. On laparotomy, 1500 cc of blood and a ruptured ovarian mass was found which was reported as malignant mixed mesodermal tumor of ovary.

POSTTREATMENT COMPLICATIONS

NEUTROPENIA

Neutropenia is defined as absolute neutrophil count (ANC) < 2000 (WHO) or ANC <1500 (other sources).
- Mild—ANC between 1000-2000
- Moderate—ANC between 500-1000
- Severe—ANC < 500

Chemotherapy is usually not given if ANC < 1000
NADIR occurs 8 to 10 days after chemotherapy. Some drugs cause prolonged neutropenia.
Recovery occurs in 8 to 89 days
Clinical features: Fever>100.5°F, ANC <1000

Management

- Start antibiotics.
- Maintain hygiene.
- *Neupogen:* This colony stimulating factor or biological response modifiers (BRMs) stimulate the WBC proliferation. Filgrastim or Neupogen is the first of these BRMs.
  Preventive Dose: Start with 5 μg/kg subcutaneous or intravenous <u>daily</u>. Begin 24 hours after end of chemotherapy. Continue past nadir (upto 14 days until ANC >1000)
  If needed in one cycle, they will need support after every subsequent course.
- *Neulasta or Peg Filgrastim:* This is made with a bigger molecule, has a slow release action and only one dose subcutaneous is needed per chemotherapy cycle
  Dose: 6 mg subcutaneous (pre-filled syringe) one time given 24 hours after completion of chemotherapy and not closer than 14 days before next cycle.
  Major side effects of these two drugs are bone pain due to stimulation of bone marrow.

HEMORRHAGIC CYSTITIS

The incidence of severe hemorrhagic cystitis following radiation for cancer cervix is low and can occur many years following treatment. Minor episodes of hematuria are managed by empiric antibiotic therapy until the results of urine cultures are available. Cystoscopy is done in patients with persistent bleeding to rule out clot retention or the possibility of a second primary tumor or recurrent disease. Biopsy or fulgration should be avoided if obvious radiation changes are present. Clot evacuation and continuous bladder irrigation remain the standard treatment for patients with heavy bleeding. Bladder irrigation can be done using 0.5 to 1 percent acetic acid or 1:1000 potassium permanganate solution. As a last resort , bladder may be sclerosed with formaldehyde. In most extreme cases cystectomy and urinary diversion may be required to control bleeding.[2,19]

POSTRADIATION HEMORRHAGIC PROCTITIS

Grade 1-3 rectal bleed can occur in 8 to 12 percent cases undergoing external radiotherapy and high dose brachytherapy. Most develop rectal bleed within 2 years with a median time of 16 months. The risk factors for this complication are- 1) advanced cervical cancer, 2) teleradiation to parametrium >55 Gy and 3) rectal biological equivalent dose >100 Gy.

Management

Steroid Rectal Enema: Six tablets of betnesol to be dissolved in 60 ml of distilled or saline water and to be instilled as high steroid enema. Such six days of once a day enema. Repeat such enema after 7 days if the symptoms are not controlled.

Sucralfate enema for 1 month and/or *coagulation* are effective in grade 1-2 bleeding without formation of stricture or fistula.[20]

POSTRADIATION BOWEL PERFORATION

The incidence of small bowel perforation after radiotherapy has been reported to be 7 to 8 percent.[21] The median time between completion of radiotherapy and perforation was 6 to 13 months (range 2-58 months). The main symptom is acute pain abdomen. There may be signs of generalized peritonitis. This may require small bowel resection and anastomosis or diversion.

KEY POINTS

- Oncological emergencies occur due to cancer itself or due to the side effects of therapy.
- Majority occur in patients with advanced often incurable disease.
- The important oncological emergencies are hemorrhage, obstructive uropathy, malignant effusions, intestinal obstruction and chemotherapy induced, febrile neutropenia.
- Prompt recognition and treatment can lead to improved survival and quality of life.

REFERENCES

1. Cervantes A, Chirivella I. Oncological emergencies. Ann Oncol 2004;15 Suppl 4:iv299-306.
2. Clarke-Pearson DL. Complications of disease and therapy. In: DiSaia PJ, Creasman WT, (eds). Clinical Gynaecologic Oncology. 7th edn. Elsevier Inc; 2007.pp.533-64.
3. Yalvac S, Kayikcioglu F, Boran N, Tulunay G, Kose MF, Bilgic S, et al. Embolization of uterine artery in terminal stage cervical cancers. Cancer Invest 2002;20:754-8.
4. Sobiczewski P, Bidziński M, Derlatka P. Laparoscopic ligature of the hypogastric artery in the case of bleeding in advanced cervical cancer. Gynecol Oncol 2002;84(2):344-8.
5. Perez CA, Kavanagh BD. Uterine cervix. In: Halperin EC, Perez CA, Brady LW,(eds). Perez and Brady's Principles and Practice of Radiation Oncology. 5th edn. Philadelphia: Lippincott William & Wilkins; 2008.pp.1532-609.
6. Grigsby PW, Portelance L, Williamson JF. HDR cervical ring applicator to control bleeding from cervical cancer. Int J Gynecol Oncol 2002;12:18-21.
7. Sharma M, Sharma A, Arora R, A, Sharma K. Haemostatic Chemotherapy in Bleeding Cancer Cervix : Rationale and back ground for necessity of the same . IGCS Asia Pacific conference. 2011.
8. Horan G, McArdle O, Martin J, Collins CD, Faul C. Pelvic radiotherapy in patients with hydronephrosis in stage IIIB cancer of the cervix: renal effects and the optimal timing for urinary diversion? Gynecol Oncol. 2006;101:441-4.
9. Pongsaranantakul S, Kietpeerakool C. Hysterectomy in gestational trophoblastic neoplasia: Chiang Mai University Hospital's experience. Asian Pac J Cancer Prev 2009;10:311-4
10. Kanazawa K, Sasagawa M, Suzuki T. Clinical evaluation of focal excision of myometrial lesion for treatment of invasive hydatiform mole. Acta Obstet Gynecol Scand 1988;67:487-92
11. Estrella JL, Soriano-Estrella AL. Conservative management of uterine rupture in gestational trophoblastic neoplasia: a report of 2 cases. Int J Gynecol Cancer 2009;19:1666-70.
12. DeVita VT, Lawrence TS, Rosenberg SA editors. DeVita, Hellman and Rosenberg's cancer principles and practice of oncology. 8th edn. Philadelphia: Lippincott William & Wilkins; 2008.pp.2427-539.
13. Becker G, Galandi D, Blum HE. Malignant ascites: systematic review and guideline for treatment. Eur J Cancer 2006;42:589.
14. Pockros PJ, Esrason KT, Nguyen C. Mobilization of malignant ascites with diuretics is dependent on ascetic fluid characteristics. Gastroenterology 1992;103:1302.
15. Burges A, Wimberger P, Kümper C, Gorbounova V, Sommer H, Schmalfeldt B. Effective relief of malignant ascites in patients with advanced ovarian cancer by a trifunctional anti-EpCAM x anti-CD3 antibody: a phase I/II study. Clin Cancer Res 2007;13:3899-905.
16. Numnum TM, Rocconi RP, Whitworth J.The use of bevacizumab to palliate symptomatic ascites in patients with refractory ovarian carcinoma. Gynecol Oncol 2006;102:425-28.
17. Takeda A, Mori M, Sakai K, Mitsui T, Nakamura H. Laparoscopic management management of ovarian dysgerminoma presenting with acute abdomen caused by adnexal torsion in a 17-year-old girl. J Pediatr Adolesc Gyecol 2009;22:9-13.
18. Geisler JP, Denman BJ, Cudahy TJ, Lee TH, Geisler HE. Ovarian carcinoma presenting as intra-abdominal hemorrhage. Gynecol Oncol 1994;53:380-1.
19. Levenback C, Eifel PJ, Burke TW, Morris M, Gershenson DM. Hemorrhagic cystitis following radiotherapy for stage Ib cancer of the cervix. Gynecol Oncol 1994;55:206-10.
20. Chun M, Kang S, Kil HJ, Oh YT, Sohn JH, Ryu HS. Rectal bleeding and its management after irradiation for uterine cervical cancer. Int J Radiat Oncol Biol Phys 2004;58:98-105.
21. Yamashita H, Nakagawa K, Tago M, Igaki H, Shiraishi K, Nakamura N, et al. Small bowel perforation without tumor recurrence after radiotherapy for cervical carcinoma: report of seven cases. J Obstet Gynaecol Res 2006;32:235-42.

Chapter 34

Postoperative Complications

Vijay Zutshi, Binni Makkar

INTRODUCTION

The majority of potential postoperative complications associated with gynecological surgery are common to other surgical procedures, and represent the complicated response of the body to the stresses imposed by surgery.

The highest incidence of postoperative complications is between 1 and 3 days after the operation. However, specific complications occur in the following distinct temporal patterns: early postoperative, several days after the operation, throughout the postoperative period, and in the late postoperative period.[1]

Postoperative complications may either be general or specific to the type of surgery undertaken, and should be managed with the patient's history in mind.

- General
- Specific to the type of surgery

General Complications

Immediate—primary hemorrhage, perioperative myocardial infarction
Early complications—Wound infection, secondary hemorrhage, deep vein thrombosis
Late complications—Incisional hernia, bowel adhesions.

Immediate

- Allergic reactions
- Hypotension or arrhythmia due to anesthesia drugs, poor intubation technique or pre-existing cardiac disease
- Primary hemorrhage
- Postoperative anuria (may be due to bladder neck spasm, hypovolemia due to inadequate fluids or blood loss, shock, accidental ligation of both ureters.

Early Complications

- Occur within a few hours to within a week of surgical procedure
- Intraoperative sepsis
- Vomiting

- Postoperative fever—early (days 0-2), late(> day 2) (necrosis, hematoma formation, transfusion reactions)

Late Postoperative Complications

- Fever due to any one of the below written causes
  - Atelectasis
  - Wound infection
  - Superficial phlebitis
  - Secondary to intravenous (IV) injections and infusions
  - Pelvic abscess
  - Deep vein thrombosis
  - Urinary tract infection
- Secondary hemorrhage
- Wound dehiscence in 2 percent of midline incisions usually noted form 5th day onwards
- Fibrous adhesions
- Incisional hernia.

Complications Specific to Gynae Surgery

- Ureteric injury
- Bladder injury
- Bowel injury
- Small bowel adhesions
- Ovarian infections
- Pelvic cellulitis, abscess
- Development of enterocele
- Vault prolapse
- Damage to fallopian tube during myomectomy
- Rupture of uterus postmyomectomy in subsequent pregnancy.

In this chapter major complications like hemorrhage, visceral injury and thromboembolic phenomenon will be discussed. These situations warrant immediate attention to avert mortality and long-term morbidity.

POSTOPERATIVE HEMORRHAGE

Hemorrhage in the postoperative period can broadly be divided into two categories-
1. Reactionary hemorrhage
2. Secondary hemorrhage.

REACTIONARY HEMORRHAGE OR DELAYED PRIMARY HEMORRHAGE

Causes

- Return to normal blood pressure or local vasodilatation
- Vessel not secured properly starts to bleed
- If adrenaline has been added to local anesthetic or to normal saline to render planes of cleavage more prominent while performing vaginal hysterectomy.

Effects of Reactionary Hemorrhage

Small hematoma in abdominal wall or vaginal wound

Signs
- Dark, infected discharge precedes the actual bleeding
- This type of bleeding is seldom self limiting and can be at times profuse to change vital signs

- Pulse and blood pressure may be maintained
- Patient looks ill
- Pallor will be present
- Sometimes mass can be felt locally

Early /Subtle Signs of Hypovolemia

Sometimes the vital signs in the postoperative period may initially remain stable for 12 to 18 hours but if there is a continuous trickle then following signs may ensue like:
- Tachycardia
- Pallor
- Persistent low blood pressure
- Low urine output
- Uncomfortable patient
- Low hemoglobin.

Major Hemorrhage

With major and rapid hemorrhage which is beyond compensatory mechanisms there will be:
- Rapid fall in blood pressure
- Restlessness
- Tachypnea
- Abdominal distension

Diagnosis

- Primarily based on clinical assessment
- Vital signs may be stable for 12 to 18 hours after surgery and then suddenly severe hypotension, tachycardia, tachypnea, restlessness, and abdominal distention may lead to a diagnosis of intraperitoneal hemorrhage
- Sometimes diagnosis may be difficult as peritoneal signs may be subtle and can be masked by incisional pain and analgesia
- As much as 3,000 mL of blood can be hidden in the peritoneal cavity in a person weighing 70 kg with only 1 cm increase in the radius of abdomen
- Abdominal ultrasound scan if diagnosis uncertain
- Rapid low-tech method is to insert a long 18-gauge spinal needle into the abdominal cavity in one of the lower quadrants under local anesthesia
- An abdominal and pelvic CT scan is another good way to identify or rule out intraperitoneal hemorrhage or a hematoma.

CASE SCENARIO-1

A 50-year-old female with fibroid uterus was taken up for total abdominal hysterectomy with bilateral salpingo oophorectomy. The surgery lasted for 2 hours with average blood loss during the surgery. In the immediate postoperative period, patient was stable. After 4 to 5 hours of surgery patient started complaining of dizziness. On examination, she was found to be drowsy. There was marked pallor, pulse was rapid and feeble with blood pressure (BP) of 80/60 mm Hg.

Comment: In such situation possibility of intraperitoneal bleeding has to be kept in mind.

Management

- Arrange whole blood
- Till the blood is cross matched correct hypovolemia by IV infusion of colloids or crystalloids. As per the recent Cochrane review colloids are not better than crystalloids.[2]

- Urgent full blood count
- Coagulation profile
- Arterial blood gases (ABG)
- Decide whether or not the patient should be taken back to theatre for exploration
- Portable ultrasonography (USG) abdomen and pelvis should be done where ever possible
- Decision for laparotomy has to be taken timely before patient enters a state of irreversible shock or develops disseminated intravascular coagulopathy
- Simultaneously other options like arterial embolization have to be kept in mind if facilities are available.

> **Initial management in this case:**
> This patient was rapidly resuscitated with 2 liters of IV fluids
> USG revealed moderate amount of fluid in the abdomen suspected to be blood
> Decision for an immediate laparotomy was taken.

Factors deciding the technique to be chosen for management of intraperitoneal bleeding:
- Unstable patient like rapid pulse, falling blood pressure, and/or low urine output—Relaparotomy
- Interval since surgery is short with unstable patient—Relaparotomy
- Reasonably stable patient—Identify the bleeding artery and embolization by interventional radiological technique

Hemorrhage after Hysterectomy

In patients with signs of hemorrhage and vaginal bleeding after hysterectomy:
- Vault can be reopened
- Bleeder can be identified
- Secure the bleeder with suture
- If hemostasis is achieved vaginal vault can be stitched back
- In all other cases relaparotomy has to be done.

Relaparotomy

- During relaprotomy, all pedicles should be thoroughly inspected.
- More often, the bleeding is due to generalized ooze, and adequate hemostasis is difficult to achieve surgically.
- Recently exploration of postoperative bleeding with laparoscopy has also been reported.[3]
- Sometimes it is difficult to identify the bleeder because it may be venous ooze. In such situation following measures are undertaken-
  - Compression with large packs for few minutes
  - If above not effective then bilateral ligation of internal iliac artery is done
  - Angiographic embolization of bleeding vessel if facility and expertise are available
  - Failure to achieve hemostasis could be due to coagulopathy which needs to be corrected immediately
  - If hemostasis is not possible, bleeding site is kept compressed with surgical packs.

Goals of Postoperative Monitoring

- To determine whether a coagulopathy resulted due to blood therapy
- To determine the success of specific component therapy and identify the need for additional components
- To enable the surgeon to distinguish surgical from nonsurgical bleeding.

Iatrogenic Causes of Abnormal Coagulation Studies

- Low platelet count due to transfusion of only packed red cells or fresh-frozen plasma (FFP).
- Prolonged prothrombin time (PT) and activated partial thromboplastin time (APTT) owing to replacement with packed red cells without fresh-frozen plasma
- Low fibrinogen levels owing to dilution with plasma expanders or concurrent development of disseminated intravascular coagulation.

Further management in this case:
In this case, infundibulopelvic ligament was loose and she was gradually loosing blood and that is why she took time to go into shock. If ligature would have completely slipped, then patient would have gone into shock immediately.
The pedicle was reclamped and doubly ligated, the abdomen was rechecked for adequate hemostatis after which closure was done. Peroperatively 4 units of whole blood and 2 FFP were given. She was shifted to ICU for strict monitoring. Patient had a normal recovery thereafter.

SECONDARY HEMORRHAGE

- The underlying cause is sepsis which erodes blood vessels
- Presents usually between 7th and 10th postoperative day
- Can also occur after day 14 of surgery.

Signs

- Dark, infected discharge precedes the actual bleeding
- This type of bleeding is seldom self limiting and can be at times profuse and affect vital signs
- Pulse and BP may be maintained
- Patient looks ill
- Pallor will be present
- Sometimes mass can be felt locally due to hematoma formation.

CASE SCENARIO-2

A 35-year-old lady underwent Manchester repair with bilateral laparoscopic ligation for second degree uterovaginal prolapse. She was doing well till day 4 of the surgery. On day 5 she complained of bleeding per vaginum.
On examination vital signs were stable; she was afebrile and had mild pallor.
Uterus was just palpable abdominally.
Vaginal bleeding—Continuous trickle with small clots.

Comment: In this situation one must think of hematoma at the repair site or secondary hemorrhage.

Vault Hematoma

Incidence of vault hematomas: 20 to 30 percent of patients.

Various Sites of Pelvic Hematomas

- Above the vaginal vault
- Along the pelvic side wall
- In the paravesical space
- In the abdominal wall
- Ischiorectal fossa and
- Vulva

Presentation

- Most cases asymptomatic
- Lower abdominal pain
- Low-grade temperature
- Vaginal discharge/bleeding.

Diagnosis

- Pelvic ultrasound scan, or
- Computerized tomography (CT) scan.

Management

- Majority are managed conservatively
- Drainage can be done under anesthesia via vaginal approach
- If interrupted sutures have been used, removal of one or two may be sufficient to introduce a finger into the gap
- One can even use bimanual compression to expel the clot
- A small penrose drain can be inserted through the drainage tract and left in place for a day or so
- If drainage cannot be achieved in this simple way, drainage under CT guidance or through an abdominal incision may be necessary.

> **Management in this case:**
> This patient had a hematoma at the anterior colporrhaphy site, which was diagnosed by pelvic USG. Two stitches from the anterior colporrhaphy repair site were removed in OT under sedation. Clots got expelled and gradually bleeding stopped.
> She was given antibiotics and hemostatic agents for control of bleeding.

Hemorrhage after Cervical Conization

Another very frequent cause of reactionary or secondary hemorrhage is after cervical conization which occurs in first 24 hours or 7 to 14 days later.
- If the patient is bleeding at any time after conization, cervix should be inspected.
- Measures to control the bleeding include:
  - Tight packing
  - Resuturing
  - Cautery
  - Monsel's solution

THROMBOEMBOLIC PHENOMENON

Clinical Presentation of Patients with Venous Thromboembolism[4]

- Asymptomatic—30 percent
- Symptomatic—8 percent
- Symptomatic non fatal Pulmonary embolism—1-2 percent
- Fatal pulmonary embolism—0.5 percent

Diagnosis of Phlebothrombosis

- On history:
  - Swelling of leg
  - Erythema
  - Pain over the calf muscles
- On examination:
  - Low-grade pyrexia
  - Calf muscles can be swollen, tender and warm
  - Positive Homans' sign.

CASE SCENARIO-3

A 50-year-old female weighing 85 Kg, a known case of type 2 diabetes mellitus (controlled on oral hypoglycemic) was taken up for extrafascial hysterectomy in view of endometrial cancer. The surgery lasted for 3 hours and she was given 2 units of packed cell transfusion per operatively. She remained stable for first two days postoperatively. On day 3 patient developed pain and swelling in the left leg. On examination, the left leg was found to be slightly swollen and there was erythema of the overlying skin and calf tenderness.

Comment: Since this patient did not receive thromboprophylaxis, there should be a high index of suspicion for venous thromboembolism.

Investigations

Doppler ultrasound of leg veins. USG has sensitivity and specificity of 97 percent for detection of proximal DVT.

Investigations in this case:
In this patient an urgent Doppler ultrasound revealed a thrombus in popliteal vein of the left lower limb thus confirming the diagnosis of deep venous thrombosis.

Treatment

Anticoagulant treatment of venous thrombosis and pulmonary embolism:
• Unfractionated heparin:
  – It is given in the initial bolus dose of 80 U/kg followed by maintenance dose of 18U/kg/hr. Adequate anticoagulation is achieved by monitoring the APTT to maintain INR of at least two and a half to three time.
    OR
  – Intravenous infusion, 10,000 units six hourly
    OR
  – Intravenous injection in doses of 10,000 to 15,000 units, four to six hourly.
• Alternatively low molecular weight heparin may be started in the dose of 2 mg/kg. Its administration does not require monitoring with APTT values.
Antidote for heparin overdose is injection of 1 percent solution of protamine sulfate.
To counter act action of 10,000 units of heparin 4 to 5 mL of latter will be required.

Treatment in this case:
The patient was immediately started on unfractionated heparin with initial bolus dose of 80 U/kg followed by maintenance dose of 18 U/kg/hr. Simultaneously warfarin was started in the dose of 2.5 mg daily. Symptomatic treatment in the form of nonsteroidal anti-inflammatory drug (Ibuprofen) was administered for relieving her pain.
The heparin was discontinued after 5 days after adequate anticoagulant effect was achieved with warfarin which was further continued for 6 months.

PULMONARY EMBOLISM

One should think of pulmonary embolism if the above mentioned case had following symptoms:
• Abrupt onset chest pain
• Hemoptysis
• Dyspnea

Screening for Pulmonary Embolism

• Positive D dimer with signs and symptoms of pulmonary embolism. In such cases, diagnostic imaging is indicated
• ECG (abnormal in 20% cases) may show tachycardia, nonspecific ST wave abnormalities, peaked P wave, right axis deviation, right bundle branch block, atrial fibrillation
• Chest X-ray : To rule out other causes like pneumonia, pneumothorax.

Table 34.1: Clinical Presentation of Pulmonary Embolism		
Classical presentation	*Nonspecific symptoms*	*Signs of Pulmonary embolism*
Abrupt onset of pleuritic chest pain	Shoulder pain	Tachypnea
Shortness of breath and hypoxia	Upper abdominal pain	Tachycardia
Less frequent symptoms	Syncope	Low-grade fever
Hemoptysis	Painful respiration	Rales
Dyspnea	High-grade fever	Accentuated S2 heart sound
	Productive cough	
	Hiccups	
	Wheezing	

Clinical Presentation of Pulmonary Embolism (Table 34.1)

Investigations

- Contrast angiography
- Spiral CT
- Ventilation/perfusion scan.

Management

- Propped up position
- Oxygen by positive pressure, 2 to 12 liters/minute.
- Thrombolytic therapy—Tissue plasminogin activator (TPA) 0.9 unit/kg to be given over a period of 10 to 30 minutes followed by full heparinization same as in any thrombotic phenomenon.
- ICU care
- Thrombus fragmentation/surgical embolectomy where ever indicated.

URETERIC INJURY

The ureter is injured in 0.5 to 2.5 percent of gynecological procedures. The risk is lower for vaginal versus abdominal hysterectomy and lower still for major laparoscopic surgery.[5]

Surgical details should be elicited like:
- Whether adhesions were present or not
- Whether anatomy was distorted
- Any slippage of ligature
- Difficulty during stitching of vault
- Hemostasis at vault.

Risk of ureteric injury during gynecological surgeries is at four sites
- Pelvic brim
- Lateral to ovarian fossa
- As it passes under uterine artery
- Where it runs into the bladder.

CASE SCENARIO-4

Mrs A underwent total abdominal hysterectomy for fibroid uterus. Surgery was uneventful. Indwelling catheter revealed hematuria which did not clear after 24 hours. Urinary leak was observed.

Comment:
In this situation one should suspect injury to the urinary tract—bladder injury and ureteric injury

Diagnosis of Ureteric Injury

- Three swab test with methylene blue to differentiate from bladder injury
- The bladder is filled with 200 mL of saline stained with 1 to 3 cc of methylene blue
- If blue fluid leaks, it confirms bladder injury
- Inject 5 mL of indigo carmine intravenously. If the watery discharge from vagina stains blue, a ureteral fistula is present
- Urography
- CT scan with contrast provided serum creatinine is normal (Intravenous contrast can cause renal damage if serum creatinine is elevated).

Indications for Postoperative Excretory Urography

- Loin tenderness
- Unexplained hematuria (like in the case mentioned above)
- Unexplained or persistent fever, with or without chills
- Persistent abdominal distension
- Escape of watery fluid through the vagina (like in the case mentioned above)
- Appearance of lower abdominal or pelvic mass after operation
- Oliguria or elevated serum creatinine levels
- Any surgery for extensive pelvic disease that distorts the ureters
- Any question of ureteral integrity.

> **Investigations in this case:**
> In this patient, methylene blue test was done; no leakage of dye was seen. Ureteric injury was suspected. Cystoscopy was done in which blood stained urine was seen coming through the left ureteric opening, bladder walls were normal.

Management

Management depends on the type of ureteral injury (Table 34.2):

> **Management in this case:**
> In this case immediate stenting was done, following which leakage of urine stopped and hematuria started to get clear
> She was further managed by antibiotics
> Alternate day urine culture and sensitivity for one week
> Patient was called back after 6 weeks for follow up and removal of stent
> Retrograde pyelogram was done to check the integrity of the ureter.

Thus, in this case:
- Timely suspicion of ureteric injury could save patient from developing ureterovaginal fistula later.
- Simple measure like stenting could avert second surgery which patient would have to undergo had diagnosis been delayed at first go.

Table 34.2: Guidelines for management of ureteral injuries	
Type of injury	*Corrective procedure*
Ligation	Deligation, stent placement
Partial transaction	Primary repair over stent
Total transaction:	
Upper & middle third	Ureteroureterostomy over stent
Lower third	Ureteroneocystostomy with psoas hitch over ureteral stent

GASTROINTESTINAL COMPLICATIONS

PARALYTIC ILEUS

Definition

Gut ileus persisting beyond three days following surgery.
Normal functions of gastrointestinal tract after abdominal gynecological surgery:[6]
- Small bowel regains function within hours
- Stomach regains activity in 1 to 2 days
- Colon regains activity in 3 to 5 days.

Symptoms

- Abdominal distention
- Nausea/vomiting
- Delayed passage of flatus or feces.

Signs

- Absent or hypoactive bowel sounds
- Distention of abdomen.

Diagnosis

- X-ray abdomen revealing dilated bowel loops.

CASE SCENARIO-5

Mrs Y, a 36-year-old lady with the diagnosis of tubo-ovarian mass was posted for diagnostic laparoscopy. Per operatively visualization was difficult due to dense adhesions and thus laparotomy was done. TAH with BSO was done in view of endometriosis. First 2 days, patient was stable but not comfortable. She had not passed flatus. On 3rd postoperative day patient started complaining of pain in upper abdomen. On examination, abdomen was nontense, nontender, there was slight distension and bowel sounds were absent.

> **Comment:**
> In this situation one should rule out paralytic ileus.

Investigations

- Complete blood counts
- Serum electrolytes
- Serum calcium.

Management

Conservative treatment like
- Nil per oral
- Nasogastric tube drainage
- IV fluids
- Correction of electrolyte imbalance
- Severe protein depletion to be corrected

- Ambulation
- Occasionally localized intestinal stimulation by rectal suppositories may be helpful.

> **Management in this case:**
> In this patient, X- ray abdomen showed multiple gas fluid levels.
> Surgical consultation was taken. She was managed as a case of paralytic ileus.
> But patient did not improve and bowel sounds continued to be absent. Tachycardia worsened and abdominal distension increased. Possibility of bowel leak was considered. Decision for laprotomy was taken which revealed small bowel leak.

BOWEL INJURY

Incidence of bowel injury is 0.3 to 0.8 percent during benign gynecological surgery.

Presentation after Surgery

- Bowel injury due to direct trauma and missed intraoperatively—Leak will present 48 to 72 hours later.
- Thermal damage/necrosis due to devascularization—May manifest as late as 6 to 8 days after surgery.

Small Bowel Leak

Symptoms

- Abdominal distention
- Pain abdomen
- Vomiting.

Signs

- Initially bowel sounds may be present
- Later symptoms will worsen with localized signs of tenderness and development of a pelvic mass.

Severity of Physiological Disturbance

- Fistula of stomach, duodenum, or high jejunum may be devastating
- Distal ileal or colonic fistulas may be well tolerated.

Diagnosis

- May be difficult if opening is very small
- CT with contrast may be required if in doubt
- X-ray abdomen may be helpful sometimes.

Management

- More proximal the fistula, the more urgent is the need for closure
- Performing enterostomy distal to fistula
- Total parental nutrition
- Most fistulas close in 4 to 6 weeks
- Closure of enterostomy after 4 to 6 weeks and may be even later if required.

Large Bowel Leak

Symptoms

- Abdominal pain
- Distention
- Nausea/vomiting.

Signs

- Guarding of abdomen
- Absent bowel sounds
- Deterioration of patients general well being
- Swinging temperature if localized abscess formation and not responding to antibiotics.

Diagnosis

- Distended bowel loops on X-ray abdomen
- Gas under diaphragm.

Management

- Laparotomy after correction of electrolyte imbalance
- Repair of fistula
- End colostomy.

ELECTROLYTE IMBALANCE

All types of electrolyte imbalance may occur in a postoperative case. They are discussed in detailed in Chapter 40 and are summarized below.

Correction of Hypokalemia

20 mEq of K in 100 mL normal saline (NS) over 1 hr. Maximum rate of infusion is 20 mEq/hr
Ideally KCL should be mixed in NS since dextrose solution may initially exacerbate hypokalemia due to insulin mediated movement of potassium into the cells.[7]
KCL 1 vial = 10 mL, concentration is 2 mEq/mL = 20 mEq = 1.5 g
Magnesium depletion promotes urinary potassium losses and can cause refractory hypokalemia.[8]

Correction of Hypocalcemia

Special attention for correction of hypocalcemia
1 vial = 10 mL (containing 10% cal gluconate and 0.931 % of elemental calcium =1 g of calcium gluconate= 9 mg/mL of elemental calcium)
Treatment for symptomatic hypocalcemia: levels like 4 mg/dL
Bolus 200 mg of elemental Ca (22 ml of 10% calcium gluconate) in 100 mL NS over 10 min followed by continuous infusion of 1 to 2 mg elemental calcium/kg/hr for 6 to 12 hours.[9]

Correction of Hypomagnesemia

1 vial= 2mL (50%) = 1g =8 mEq (4mmol) of elemental magnesium
Ringer Lactate (RL) is not used as diluents because calcium in RL will counteract the actions of infused magnesium.
Intravenous replacement if symptomatic.
Levels = 1.0-1.8 mEq/dL

Magnesium sulfate 0.5 mEq/kg in NS 250 mL IV over 24 hours for 3 days.
Recheck levels in 3 days.
Levels < 1.0: Magnesium sulfate 1 mEq/kg in NS 250 mL IV over 24 hr for 1 day
Followed by 0.5 mEq/kg in NS 250 mL over 24 hr for 2 days. Recheck levels in 3 days.

KEY POINTS

- If postoperative complications occur, it is the responsibility of the operating gynecologist to liaise with the appropriate specialty and ensure that the patient is investigated and treated promptly.
- Gynecology patients are relatively young and fit before surgery, and thus may not reveal signs of internal hemorrhage until the late stages and then quickly decompensate.
- Pelvic hematomas are common after hysterectomy and may be the cause of postoperative pyrexia or unexpected anemia.
- There is significant risk of DVT after major gynecological procedures, and each patient must be given appropriate prophylaxis relevant to risk status.
- The majority of DVT's which precede pulmonary embolism are not recognized clinically, so be vigilant to detect potential DVT's.
- Early recognition of bowel and urinary tract damage reduces the risk of serious morbidity.
- Damage to bowel and urinary tract should only be repaired by experienced specialist.
- Local audit will identify areas of concern in surgical technique and infection control.

REFERENCES

1. Thompson JS, Baxter BT, Allison JG, Johnson FE, Lee KK, Park WY. Temporal patterns of postoperative complications. Arch Surg 2003;138:596-603.
2. Perel P, Roberts I. Colloids versus crystalloids for fluid resuscitation in critically ill patients. Cochrane Database Syst Rev. 2011;3:CD000567.
3. Sobolev VE, Dudanov IP, Alontseva NN, Bogdanova VS. The role of laparoscopy in the diagnosis and treatment of early postoperative complications. Vestn Khir Im I I Grek 2005;164:95-9.
4. Scottish Intercollegiate Guidelines Network. Prophylaxis of venous thromboembolism. Edinburgh: SIGN, 2002. http://www.sign.ac.uk/guidelines/fulltext/62/index.html.
5. Amer S. Postoperative care. In: Shaw R, Luesley D, Monga AK (eds). Gynaecology. 4th edn. Churchill Livingstone Elsevier, 2010. pp. 116-27.
6. Cameron JL (ed.), Current Surgical Therapy.7th edn. St. Louis: Mosby, 2001.
7. Kruse JA, Carlson RW. Rapid correction of hypokalemia using concentrated intravenous potassium chloride infusions. Arch Intern Med 1990;150:613-7.
8. Whang R, Flink EB, Dyckner T, Wester PO, Aikawa JK, Ryan MP. Magnesium depletion as a cause of refractory potassium repletion. Arch Intern Med 1985;145:1686-9.
9. Marino PL. The ICU Book.3rd edn. Philadelphia: Lippincott Williams & Wilkins, 2007.

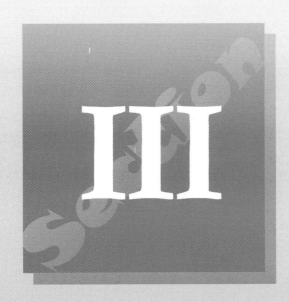

Emergencies Common to
Obstetrics and Gynecology

Chapter **35**

Acute Urinary Retention

Saritha Shamsunder, Parul Rathore

INTRODUCTION

Acute urinary retention (AUR) is a sudden inability to empty the bladder. This is associated with severe discomfort and is a medical emergency. The incidence of AUR in women is estimated to be 7 per 100,000 population per year; being 13 times more common in males.[1]

Physiologically, voiding requires a coordinated bladder contraction and outlet relaxation, with sustained detrusor contraction achieving complete bladder emptying.

Urinary retention occurs as a consequence of one or more of reduced bladder contractility, poorly sustained detrusor contraction, lack of an adequate anatomical outlet, deficient outlet relaxation, or impaired neurological coordination of the voiding process.[2]

Urinary retention (UR) is a severe impairment of voiding, which can be defined as inability to achieve complete bladder emptying by voluntary micturition.

Acute urinary retention (AUR) is painful bladder distension, which usually presents as an emergency.

Incomplete bladder emptying signifies the presence of a postvoid residual (PVR).

Agreement as to what constitutes a clinically significant PVR has not been achieved, with absolute volumes, proportion of bladder capacity, or presence of relevant symptoms all included in some contexts.

Cause of Acute Urinary Retention

There can be several causes of acute urinary retention (Tables 35.1 to 35.3).

Approach to Diagnosis and Management of Acute Urinary Retention

- Detailed history, abdominal and pelvic examination should be carried out to make a diagnosis. Neurological examination may be rarely needed
- Immediate management of AUR requires bladder decompression with catheterization, either indwelling or intermittent catheterization (IC). IC not only avoids potential morbidity with an indwelling catheter but also allows monitoring of return of voiding function, which is usually preceded by a reduction in PVR
- Any urinary tract infection should be treated with appropriate antimicrobial therapy. Other reversible causes such as prolapse should be identified and rectified

Table 35.1: Obstetric and Gynecological causes of acute urinary retention	
Obstetric Causes	*Gynecological causes*
Early pregnancy • Incarcerated retroverted gravid uterus • Impacted pelvic tumors *During labour* • In coordinate uterine action • Obstructed labor *During puerperium* • Diminished bladder tone • Reflex from pain due to vulval injuries • Bruising from edema of bladder neck • Hematomas	• Pelvic organ prolapse • Uterine fibroid • Pelvic tumor • Poorly fitting pessary • Post incontinence procedure

Table 35.2: Urological causes of acute urinary retention	
Urethral causes • Stricture • Meatal stenosis • Thrombosed urethral caruncle • Diverticulum • Skene's gland abscess or cyst	**Bladder** • Stone • Tumor • Ureterocele
Impaired detruser contractility • Senile bladder changes • Diabetes mellitus • Neurological disease (lower motor neuron lesions)	**Functional (impaired coordination)** • Fowler's syndrome • Neurological (upper motor neuron lesions)

Table 35.3: Other causes of acute urinary retention		
Perioperative	*Infective/inflammatory*	*Pharmacological*
• Pain • Analgesia or anesthetic, e.g. epidural	• Urinary tract infection • Acute vulvovaginitis • Lichen planus/sclerosis • Genital herpes	• Opiates • Antipsychotics • Antidepressants • Antimuscarinic • α- adrenergic agonist

• Further radiological and pressure-flow investigation may be required in some patients. Pelvic ultrasound occasionally reveals relevant findings that may contribute to the symptoms in women with urinary retention. Gynecological causes, such as large uterine fibroids, are unusual but they must be considered among the underlying causes of urinary retention.

• Flexible cystoscopy under local anesthesia can provide additional anatomical information. In patients with primary bladder neck obstruction, reported in 9 to 16 percent of women with bladder outlet obstruction, bladder neck incision or transurethral resection can improve voiding.[3,4,5] In some women, α-blockers can lower the resting urethral pressure.[6]

RETROVERTED GRAVIS UTERUS AND URINARY RETENTION

Retroversion of the first trimester uterus occurs in 6 to 19 percent of all pregnancies and usually does not cause problems. The cause of urinary retention associated with retroverted gravid uterus has been reported to be mechanical compression of the lower bladder by the anteriorly and superiorly displaced uterine cervix.[7] The urethra itself is not compressed or distorted. It occurs most commonly between 10 and 16 weeks' gestation. These patients may present in extreme distress. There may be recurrence in subsequent pregnancy.[8]

CASE SCENARIO-1

A 23-yr-old primigravida with three months amenorrhea came to the casualty with complaints of inability to pass urine and severe lower abdominal pain.

> **Comments:** Life threatening conditions like ectopic pregnancy should be ruled out first in any case with severe lower abdominal pain in early pregnancy. Urinary retention due to retroverted, gravid uterus though an uncommon disorder should be considered in differential diagnosis. These patients may present in extreme distress

Differential Diagnosis

- Pregnancy with urinary tract infection
- Chronic ectopic pregnancy with a pelvic hematocele
- Renal calculus impacted in the urethra.

POINTS TO BE NOTED IN HISTORY

- Prior history of urinary symptoms/abdominal pain
- History of vaginal bleeding/fainting attacks (suggests a chronic ectopic pregnancy)
- History of interference (suggests septic abortion with renal failure)
- Past gynecological history.

> **History in this case:** She was about 13 weeks pregnant with no preceding history of urinary problems, abdominal pain or vaginal bleeding.

POINTS TO BE NOTED IN EXAMINATION

General Examination

- General condition
- Pallor
- Temperature, pulse rate
- Respiratory rate and blood pressure (BP)

Cardiovascular and Respiratory System Examination

Abdominal Examination

- Location and severity of pain
- Guarding, rigidity, rebound tenderness, renal angle tenderness
- Suprapubic swelling suggestive of bladder enlargement

Pelvic Examination

Per Speculum (P/S) Examination

Location of the os, as it may be displaced forwards behind the pubic symphysis.

Per Vaginum (P/V) Examination

Uterine size, position, tenderness and any adnexal mass (suggestive of tubo-ovarian mass, pelvic hematocele)

Examination in this case:
- 23-yr-old lady, anxious, doubled up in pain
- Pulse 120/min, temperature 98.4°F, respiratory rate—20/min
- General examination—unremarkable
- Abdominal examination—Abdomen soft, no guarding/rigidity noted, supra-pubic cystic swelling corresponding to 20 weeks gestational size
- P/V examination—Cervix visualized with difficulty, vaginal healthy
- P/V examination—Cervix pointing forwards, cervix long, os closed, midline cystic swelling felt arising from the pelvis up to umbilicus. Uterine size not clearly made out.
- On catheterization, 2 liters of urine was drained and cystic swelling disappeared. On repeat examination uterus was retroverted 12 weeks size, non-tender, no adnexal mass/tenderness noted

Diagnosis

Retroverted gravid uterus with retention of urine

INVESTIGATIONS

- Hemogram
- Blood group
- Urine routine and microscopy
- Urine culture
- Pelvic ultrasonography (USG)

Investigations in this case:
- Hemogram-Hb—10.5 g%, PCV—32%, TLC—11,000 P74L20M2E2
- Blood group—O positive
- Urine routine and microscopy—Albumin/sugar-nil; pus cells—5 to 6/hpf
- Urine culture—Sterile
- Transabdominal ultrasonography (USG)—Retroverted uterus with a single live fetus of 13 weeks gestation. No free fluid in pouch of Douglas, both ovaries normal
- USG whole abdomen—Normal

MANAGEMENT

Principles

Continuous bladder drainage and await spontaneous correction or retroversion and antibiotic cover.
- She is asked to lie in a prone position to facilitate anteversion
- Bladder is kept empty by continuous bladder drainage until the uterus ascends out of the pelvis
- Urine samples are sent for culture and sensitivity
- Urinary antiseptics (ampicillin 500 mg 8 hourly) are started empirically.

Rarely Attempted Techniques

Other treatments are described though, these are rarely used.
- Manual correction by pushing the uterus digitally through the posterior fornix. This procedure is done with the patient in Sims' or knee-chest position. After successful repositioning, the patient is generally advised to sleep in the prone position.
- In obstinate cases, the above method may fail due to intraperitoneal adhesions, and laparotomy may be necessary
- In diagnosed cases of anterior sacculation of the uterus, delivery by cesarean section is the method of choice.[10]

Prevention

In early pregnancy, she is advised to empty her bladder frequently and lie in a prone position.

Postpartum Urinary Retention

CASE SCENARIO-2

A 23-yr-old primigravida delivers a healthy male baby weighing 3.2 kg after prolonged labor and forceps application for 2nd stage fetal distress. There was an extension of the episiotomy wound with difficult repair. Few hours later, she complained of severe abdominal pain with perineal discomfort. On examination, she was tachycardic, BP was normal. Abdominal examination revealed a cystic suprapubic swelling up to the umbilicus. The episiotomy wound was edematous; pelvirectal examination was normal.

On catheterization, 2 liters of urine was drained with disappearance of the cystic abdominal mass.

Comment: Excessive perineal trauma with pain could be the cause of urinary retention.

Differential Diagnosis

Pudendal neuropathy (due to overstretching of the perineum during delivery)

Management

The indwelling catheter is left for a few days till the edema subsides. After catheter removal, she is asked to void 3 hourly as over distension of a traumatized bladder can result in long-term voiding dysfunction. If the condition persists, self-catheterization may be the only option.

Prevention

Adequate pain relief should be given after operative vaginal delivery. With extensive perineal injuries, an indwelling catheter may be left prophylactically for 48 to 72 hours.

Acute Urinary Retention due to Gynecological Causes

Various gynecological causes of AUR are listed in Table 36.1. Some of the common clinical presentations are discussed below.

Urinary Retention due to Fibroid Uterus

CASE SCENARIO-3

A 38-yr-old P2L2 presented to the emergency with inability to pass urine and severe lower abdominal pain for 6 hours; she revealed a history of difficulty in micturition for the last 15 days. There was no past history of urinary symptoms. Her past menstrual cycles were regular with excessive blood flow and dysmenorrhea.

Comment: The history is suggestive of a gynaecological cause for her symptoms; possibly a fibroid uterus.

Differential Diagnosis

- Urinary tract infection
- Renal calculus impacted in the urethra

Examination in this case:
- General examination was unremarkable.
- Abdominal examination revealed a soft abdomen, bowel sounds were present with no guarding/rigidity, a suprapubic bulge was seen due to full bladder
- Bladder was catheterized and 2000 mL of clear urine was drained
- Pelvic examination revealed a splayed out posterior cervical lip with a large anterior cervical fibroid about 7x8 cm, with the uterus of normal size on top of the cervical fibroid.

Diagnosis

Anterior cervical fibroid with retention of urine

Investigations in this case:
- Transabdominal USG revealed a heterogenous mass of 7x8 cm in the cervical region with a normal sized uterus
- USG whole abdomen—Normal
- Hemogram—Hb-8.5 g%, PCV-28%
- Intravenous pyelogram—Both renal pelvis and ureters normal
- Urine routine and microscopy—Normal
- Urine culture—Sterile

Management in this case:
In view of her fibroid causing urinary retention, considering her parity, hysterectomy was advised.

POSTOPERATIVE URINARY RETENTION

Contributing factors include traumatic instrumentation, bladder over-distension, reduced contractility of bladder, increased outlet resistance, nociceptive inhibitory effect, pharmaceutical influences, pre-existing outlet pathology and decreased micturition reflex activity. Various studies have shown that specific types of anesthesia and analgesia can increase the risk of postoperative urinary retention, e.g. epidural anaesthesia. In a review of more than 3000 obstetric deliveries Olofsson and colleagues demonstrated that patients who received epidural anesthesia had an increased risk of UR.[11]

CASE SCENARIO-4

A 58-yr-old diabetic woman had type III radical hysterectomy with pelvic lymphadenectomy performed for stage 1B cervical cancer. Her postoperative period was uneventful. After 1 week of catheterization, her catheter was removed. A few hours later, she complained of inability to pass urine with severe abdominal discomfort. On examination the abdomen was distended with a cystic swelling in the suprapubic region. On catheterization, 1 liter of urine was drained.

Comment: Urinary retention is common after radical hysterectomy due to denervation.

Differential Diagnosis

- Urinary tract infection
- Hypotonic/atonic bladder due to autonomic neuropathy.

Prevention and Management

A radical hysterectomy substantially denervates the bladder and upper urethra as the parasympathetic and sympathetic nerve fibres to and from the bladder and urethra are removed along with the paracervical, paravaginal, cardinal ligament and pelvic lymph nodes.

- The indwelling catheter is left for up to 2 weeks and taken out only if the residual urine is <50 mL (as assessed on ultrasonography) with the advice to empty her bladder frequently
- If >50 mL of residual urine is found, she should be recatheterized and discharged only when the residual urine is <50 mL.
- She should be given bladder training and asked to pass urine frequently with the help of suprapubic pressure.

CASE SCENARIO-5

A 65-yr-old diabetic P3L3 had vaginal hysterectomy with Kelly's repair under epidural anesthesia for stress urinary incontinence. She was catheterized for 5 days with good urine output. However, following removal of the catheter on the 6th day, she complained of inability to pass urine with severe lower abdominal pain. On examination, she was afebrile, lower abdomen was distended with a cystic swelling suggestive of an over-distended bladder. On catheterization, 2 l of cloudy urine was drained.

Comment: Overzealous repair or tissue edema could be the cause of urinary retention.

Differential Diagnosis

- Urinary tract infection
- Bladder hypotony due to autonomic neuropathy or secondary to anesthesia.

Management

- Send urine culture and give appropriate antibiotics
- Recatheterization to relieve tissue edema
- Bladder training in refractory cases.

FOWLER'S SYNDROME

Fowler's syndrome is an uncommon condition which affects young women after menarche, who develop painless urinary retention. There is an unconnected precipitating event, such as minor surgery. Most of the women will not report any prior urinary tract problems. It is estimated that around 40 percent of women affected have polycystic ovary syndrome.[6] It is important to exclude occult or undiagnosed neurological problems as a cause. It is hypothesized that changes in the ion channels of the skeletal muscles of the urinary sphincter may be affected by the hormonal environment of the menarche ("hormonal channelopathy") leading to abnormal communication directly between muscle cells. As a consequence, the sphincter becomes overactive and hypertrophic, and reacts excessively to direct stimulation.

Diagnostic Criteria: UR of at least 1 litre on at least one occasion; exclusion of other causative factors; raised maximum urethral closure pressure on urethral pressure profilometry; increased sphincter volume on ultrasound or MRI assessment; and a characteristic urethral sphincter EMG. The most specific diagnostic test for Fowler's syndrome is a urethral sphincter EMG (USEMG).

Management of Fowler's syndrome: A sympathetic approach is essential with exclusion of psychological factors. Intermittent catheterization, percutaneous sacral nerve stimulation, botulinum injections into the urethral sphincter and continent diversion are the options available for these patients.

CONCLUSION

Acute urinary retention could be a mode of presentation of a gynecological pathology previously undiagnosed in a woman. Careful examination and evaluation alone can help in arriving at a diagnosis. Urodynamics is needed in only a small percentage of women.

KEY POINTS

- Acute urinary retention is associated with severe discomfort and is a medical emergency.
- AUR could be the mode of presentation of a gynecological pathology previously undiagnosed in a woman.
- Retroverted gravid uterus is a common cause.
- Gynecological causes are unusual, however should be considered in undertaking a complete evaluation.
- A distended bladder should always be considered in the differential diagnosis of a cystic abdominal mass, catheterization should be the first step prior to the battery of investigations.

REFERENCES

1. Klarskov P, Andersen JT, Asmussen CF, Brenoe J, Jensen SK, Jensen IL, et al. Acute urinary retention in women: A prospective study of 18 consecutive cases. Scand J Urol Nephrol 1987;21:29-31.
2. Abrams P. Bladder outlet obstruction index, bladder contractility index and bladder voiding efficiency: Three simple indices to define bladder voiding function. BJU Int 1999;84:14-5.
3. Blaivas JG, Flisser AJ, Tash JA. Treatment of primary bladder neck obstruction in women with transurethral resection of the bladder neck. J Urol 2004;171:1172-5.
4. Kumar A, Mandhani A, Gogoi S, Srivastava A. Management of functional bladder neck obstruction in women: Use of alpha-blockers and paediatric resectoscope for bladder neck incision. J Urol 1999;162:2061-5.
5. Peng CH, Kuo HC. Transurethral incision of bladder neck in treatment of bladder neck obstruction in women. Urology 2005;65:275-8.
6. Fowler CJ, Kirby RS. Abnormal electromyographic activity (decelerating burst and complex repetitive discharges) in the striated muscle of the urethral sphincter in 5 women with persisting urinary retention. Br J Urol 1985;57:67-70.
7. Yang JM, Huang WC. Sonographic findings in acute urinary retention secondary to retroverted gravid uterus: pathophysiology and preventive measures. Ultrasound Obstet Gynecol 2004;23:490-95.
8. Suzuki S, Ono S, Satomi M. Recurrence of urinary retention secondary to retroverted gravid uterus. North Am J Med Sci 2009;1:54-7
9. Misra R. Local Abnormalities. In: Misra R (ed). Ian Donald's Practical Obstetric Problems. 6th edn. BI Publications, 2007.pp. 261-79.
10. Hoenigl W Asymptomatic urinary retroversion at 32 weeks gestation: sonographic features. J Ultrasound Med 1999;18:795-8.
11. Olofsson CI, Ekblom AO, Ekman-Ordeberg GE, Irestedt LE. Post-partum urinary retention: A comparison between two methods of epidural analgesia. Eur J Obstet Gynecol Reprod Biol 1997;71:31-4.

Chapter 36

Nonobstetric Trauma to the Genital Tract

Deepti Goswami

Introduction

Injuries of the genital tract occur in patients with trauma to the lower abdominal and pelvic region or penetrating injuries of a sexual or nonsexual nature. Many injuries are minor and do not require hospitalization; however, serious coitus related and accidental injuries require appropriate evaluation and management.

Indians studies have documented that nonobstetric injuries of the female genital tract constitute 0.8 percent of all gynecological admissions.[1] One third of women with nonobstetric lower genital tract injuries in rural India presented with coital trauma while two third sustained noncoital injuries. Many women have multiple injuries and require blood transfusion.[2]

Coital Injuries to the Female Genital Tract

Coital injuries are usually in the form of vaginal lacerations. These injuries may be abuse related and may present late. It has been postulated that vigorous intercourse increases intra-abdominal pressure in women causing tensing of the culdesac, decreasing the elasticity of the posterior fornix, resulting in vaginal laceration.[3]

Predisposing Factors for Coital Injuries

- First experience of coitus
- Coitus after a long abstinence
- Congenital anomalies of the vagina[4]
- Coital positions that permit deep penetration
- Substance abuse (alcohol or drugs), brutality, violence
- Insertion of foreign objects
- Also reported- In women with thrombocytopenia, Ehler's Danlos syndrome, after radical hysterectomy.[5-7]

Clinical Presentation

- The vaginal vault, especially the right and posterior fornices have been reported to be the frequent sites of coital injury for parous women. Lower vaginal and introital injuries result following first acts of coitus.[8]

- Women with coital injuries may develop shock, requiring rapid resuscitation and operative repair.[9]
- Hemoperitoneum has been reported after coital injury even without associated vaginal injury. The causes reported are ruptured ovarian/corpus luteum cysts and laceration of ovary and round ligament. In one of the reported cases hemoperitoneum occurred from a liver laceration produced by the disruption of an adhesion between the colon and liver during coitus.[10]

Noncoital Injuries to the Female Genital Tract

Noncoital injuries are usually accidental in nature. Blunt traumas due to vehicular accidents and falling from a height are the most common causes of these injuries. Other causes include straddle injuries, cattle horn injury, burns, high pressure liquid injection (as in water sports, water slides) and vaginal foreign bodies.[2]

Concomitant Injuries in Cases with Accidental Pelvic Trauma

Most of these patients have multiple severe injuries and require operative intervention and a multidisciplinary approach for management.[11]

- *Pelvic fractures*—Most serious presentation is the one with open pelvic fracture where there is a direct communication between a skin, rectal, or vaginal wound and the fracture. The mortality in such cases may be as high as 30 to 50 percent. These high energy injuries are usually due to motor vehicle accidents and may be associated with extrusion of the pelvic contents. Resultant boney spicules may lacerate the urethra, vagina and bladder.
- *Urinary tract injuries:*
  Urethral injuries—are rare in females. All patients should be carefully examined. A Foley catheter is passed to check for any hematuria (indicating injury to genital tract) and to monitor urinary output.
  Urinary bladder—Rarely, traumatic fracture of the pelvis may lead to urethral injury, bladder rupture and fistulization into the vagina. Rupture of the urinary bladder, either intra- or extraperitoneal, may go undiagnosed initially and must be properly identified during the emergency gynecology and urology examination.[12]
  Ureteral injuries—are relatively rare in blunt injuries.
- *Anorectal lacerations*

CASE SCENARIO-1

A 19-year-old lady, P1L1, was referred to our hospital in April 2009, four hours after a road traffic accident which resulted in a pelvic fracture and perineal trauma.

> **Comments:** Vehicular accidents cause high energy injuries and may result in open fractures of pelvis, often associated with extrusion of the pelvic contents. Early assessment and resuscitation is vital.

Points to be Noted in History

In cases with genital tract injuries which are due to vehicular accidents or fall from height:
- Nature of accident
- Time elapsed since the accident
- Estimated blood loss so far as noted by the attendants
- Any care provided so far
- History of loss of consciousness, vomiting, headache, seizures, inability to move, incontinence of bladder or bowel
- Ask whether she is pregnant
- In a pregnant woman ask regarding abdominal pain, bleeding or leaking per vaginum and fetal movements.

In all the cases also check for the following:
- Check whether the history provided is compatible with the injuries found on examination
- In children, sexual abuse should always be considered when genital injury is identified, especially when history is vague. History from the child provides the single most important information when diagnosing child sexual abuse
- Individuals with developmental delay and disabilities are an at-risk group for sexual abuse.

History in this case:
Patient had a vehicular accident 4 hours back. There was a history of direct trauma to the perineum by a motorcycle wheel.
She complained of severe pelvic pain.
History of significant bleeding from perineal wound.
There was no history of loss of consciousness, vomiting, headache, seizures or incontinence of bladder or bowel.
She was not pregnant and had a 1-year-old child.

POINTS TO BE NOTED IN EXAMINATION

General Examination

Assessment of vital signs, airway, breathing, circulation
- General condition
- Pulse, blood pressure (BP), respiratory rate (RR) and temperature
- Other associated injuries which may require immediate attention
- Pallor
- Urinary output.

Cardiovascular and Respiratory System Examination

Abdominal Examination

- Tenderness, guarding, rigidity and rebound tenderness
- Presence of free fluid in peritoneal cavity
- Bowel sounds
- Whether the uterus is palpable per abdomen.

Pelvic Examination

In genital trauma note the severity of the injury and the amount of bleeding:
- If the injury is not severe, the patient may be examined in the clinic or emergency department without sedation
- General anesthesia may be required for cases of severe genital injury and for children. It helps in a better examination, assessment and repair.

Local Examination

Assess for perineal injuries, involvement of urethra, bladder, anal sphincter.

Per Speculum (P/S) Examination

Check vagina and cervix

Per Vaginum (P/V) Examination

Size of the uterus, any hematoma

Per Rectal (P/R) Examination

Check for any anorectal lacerations

The examination in a case of suspected sexual abuse is discussed in a separate chapter. In these cases the genital examination may provide some supportive evidence or may be normal or non-specific. A normal genital examination does not rule out the possibility of sexual abuse.

Examination in this case:

Patient was conscious, oriented, pulse -106/min, blood pressure (BP) 94/70 mm Hg significant pallor. There was no involvement of the spine or lower limbs.

Cardio-respiratory examination—Unremarkable.

Abdominal examination—Soft on palpation, no guarding or rigidity.

Local examination—Revealed an open pelvic fracture with a large laceration extending from the perineum to the pubic symphysis, which was split wide apart with bladder lying exposed between the symphyseal edges. The perineal tear extended posteriorly to involve the anal sphincter and the sphincteric tone was completely lost. Right vaginal wall was avulsed from its lateral attachment and pulled to the left side leaving a gaping defect medial to the right labia minora.

Urethra could not be located. Bladder was aspirated by a sterile needle; there was no hematuria. Further pelvic examination was not feasible due to local pain.

Diagnosis

Pelvic fracture with vaginal avulsion, complete perineal tear and extensive trauma to the external genitalia.

INVESTIGATIONS

- Hemoglobin, hematocrit
- Blood group, Rh testing
- Complete blood count
- Coagulation profile in cases with excessive hemorrhage
- Blood urea, serum creatinine, liver function tests—particularly in cases requiring exploration under general anesthesia
- Urine—albumin, sugar and microscopy
- Anteroposterior and lateral pelvic X-ray in cases with vehicular accidents and fall from height
- Ultrasonography (USG)—Useful to detect free fluid in abdominal cavity and to check condition of the fetus in a pregnant woman
- Investigations required for other concomitant injuries
- Investigations required in a suspected case of sexual abuse are discussed in a separate chapter.

Investigations in this case:

Hemoglobin—7 gm/dL, complete blood counts—normal.

Renal and liver function tests, serum electrolytes—Normal

Coagulation profile—Normal

Urine albumin, sugar and microscopy—Normal

Pelvic X-ray—Symphyseal diastasis with bilateral superior pubic rami fracture and vertical shear injury of the left sacro-iliac joint (type C pelvic fracture).

TREATMENT

Early assessment and resuscitation is vital. Life-threatening injuries, including hemorrhage and unstable pelvic fracture are addressed first.

1. The principles of management in cases with high-impact injuries causing pelvic fracture and extensive genital tract/perineal injuries:

- Pelvic fracture stabilization
- Wound debridement
- Repair of the genital and urinary/anorectal injuries if wound is not infected
- Selective diverting colostomy is carried out in patients with rectal or perineal lacerations to avoid sepsis due to contamination from fecal matter
- Colostomy takedown (6weeks~3months).

2. Urethral catheterization is attempted carefully in such cases, if passage is not easy, a urological consultation is required.
3. Coital injuries require primary definitive surgical repair.
4. Management of a survivor of sexual assault is discussed in detail in a separate chapter. The main aspects of management are:[13]
   - Medicolegal examination with documentation for law enforcement authorities
   - Care of injuries
   - Prevention of venereal disease
   - Prevention of pregnancy
   - Prevention/alleviation of psychological damage

> **Treatment in this case:**
> Pelvic fracture was stabilized with an external fixator.
> The broken ends of the pubic bone were brought together by an orthopedic wire.
> The detached vaginal wall and torn anal sphincter were surgically repaired after making a diverting colostomy. The postoperative period was uneventful.
> Colostomy was reversed after 3 months.

PROGNOSIS

The commonest posttraumatic symptoms are related to lower urinary tract, bowel, and sexual life.[14] Pelvic trauma is a known factor predisposing to pelvic floor disorders. Apart from direct pelvic floor disruption, indirect damage to the muscle, connective tissue, nerve and blood supply can result in neuropathy and pelvic floor dysfunction.[15] However, the general incidence of pelvic floor dysfunction following pelvic trauma remains unclear.

Late sequelae are minimal after both coital and noncoital injuries, and even severe injuries do not preclude normal pregnancy and sexual function.[11]

> **Obstetric and gynecological outcome in this case:**
> Postoperatively patient developed a cystocele, dyspareunia and vaginal pain
> She conceived spontaneously and was planned for an elective cesarean at 37 weeks gestation in view of pubic symphyseal injuries; however, she presented in labor at 36 weeks and had a normal vaginal delivery in January 2011.

TRAUMA IN PREGNANCY

The most common causes of genital tract trauma in pregnancy include vehicular accidents, falls, violent assaults, and burn injuries.[16,17]

Blunt trauma most often occurs as a result of motor vehicle accidents which account for two-thirds of all trauma events during pregnancy.[18] Blunt trauma to the abdomen increases the risk for placental abruption, where as penetrating trauma is more likely to cause direct fetal injury.

Potential Complications of Trauma in Pregnancy Include

- Maternal injury or death
- Shock
- Internal hemorrhage

- Intrauterine fetal demise
- Direct fetal injury
- Abruptio placentae
- Uterine rupture

Role of Obstetrician[19]

- Managing genital tract injuries
- Consultative role if nonobstetric surgical care is required
- To intervene if trauma care is compromised by the pregnancy
- Perimortem cesarean delivery may be required in most seriously injured women.

CASE SCENARIO-2

A 37-year-old lady, G5P4L4 with 7 months gestation presented to our hospital in April 2011, ten hours after a fall from height. She complained of excessive vaginal bleeding and lower abdominal pain.

> **Comments:** The patient is pregnant and has presented late after the trauma. Fetal prognosis is of concern.

The history, examination and investigations are carried out as described earlier in the chapter. Fetal well being needs to be checked closely.

> **History in this case:**
> Patient had a fall, 10 hours back, from a first floor terrace over an iron beam sustaining blunt trauma over lower abdomen and perineum.
> History of significant bleeding from perineal wound, lower abdominal pain and inability to pass urine (there was no urge).
> No history of loss of consciousness, vomiting, headache, seizures or incontinence.
> She could not inform about the fetal movements.

> **Examination in this case:**
> Patient was conscious, oriented, Pulse–116/min, BP–100/70 mm Hg
> Significant pallor. There was no involvement of the spine or lower limbs.
> Cardio-respiratory examination–unremarkable.
> Abdominal examination–soft on palpation, no guarding or rigidity. Uterus 26 weeks size, uterine tone was increased, fetal heart sound could not be localized on auscultation.
> *Local examination*–multiple perineal and vaginal lacerations. External urethral meatus was located and Foley catheter was inserted, the tip of the catheter emerged out in between the traumatized vaginal tissue indicating bladder rupture and fistulization in vagina.
> *P/S examination*–was not feasible due to local pain.
> *P/V examination*–cervix -2 cm, 30% effaced, membranes intact, cephalic at -3 station.
> *P/R examination*–no anorectal lacerations

Diagnosis

Pelvic trauma with vaginal and perineal lacerations, traumatic vesicovaginal fistula and abruptio placentae.

> **Investigations in this case:**
> Hemoglobin—7 g/dL, complete blood counts—Normal
> Renal and liver function tests, serum electrolytes—Normal
> Coagulation profile—Normal
> Urine albumin, sugar and microscopy—Normal
> USG abdomen—Single fetus, cephalic, no cardiac activity, small retroplacental clot present.
> Pelvic X-ray—Fracture left suprapubic rami

MANAGEMENT

- The management of pregnant trauma victims requires a multidisciplinary approach involving the anesthesiologist, the obstetrician and the trauma surgeon
- While managing these cases it is important to consider the unique changes in anatomy and physiology that take place during pregnancy.[20]
- Initial evaluation and resuscitation should always be maternally directed. Expeditious maternal resuscitation is the most effective method of fetal resuscitation.
- Once maternal stability is established, vigilant evaluation of fetal well-being, including continuous cardiotocographic (CTG) monitoring, should be initiated as soon as possible. Patients with viable gestations require at least 4 hours of monitoring after even minor trauma.[21]
- Imaging studies should not be delayed because of concerns of fetal radiation exposure, because the risk is minimal with usual imaging procedures, especially in mid-to-late pregnancy
- Early ultrasonographic evaluation can identify free intraperitoneal fluid and assess fetal health
- *Abruptio placentae:* For early diagnosis of abruptio placentae after blunt trauma to the abdomen, continuous monitoring of the fetal heart rate and uterine contractions is required. Monitoring should be continued for at least 4 hours, and whenever the frequency of uterine contractions exceeds one per 15 min or tenderness of the abdomen or vaginal bleeding is present, the pregnant trauma patient should be carefully monitored under hospital conditions for at least 24 hours.[18]
- Open peritoneal lavage, and/or exploratory laparotomy may be indicated in most severe cases of trauma as in suspected uterine rupture
- It is essential to maintain documentation of the chronology of events, the maternal and fetal assessment, and the management and outcome of the pregnancy.

Treatment in this case:
Patient was taken up for urgent exploration and repair of injuries under general anesthesia after arranging 2 units of blood. Surgeon was called in view of extensive bladder injury.
Per operative-
Urinary bladder was torn transversely with both ureteral openings lying close to the edges of the laceration. Bladder was repaired after stenting the ureters taking care not to include the ureters in the stitch line.
Suprapubic urinary catheter was inserted to ensure bladder drainage
Vaginal lacerations and perineal tears were repaired with good hemostatsis.
Postoperative-
Broad spectrum antibiotics were given
Hourly urine output record was maintained to ensure adequate bladder drainage
Perineal care was given
Pelvic traction was applied for the pelvic fracture.

PROGNOSIS

The severity of the trauma is an important prognostic factor for survival of both mother and fetus. Fetal injury can be caused even by apparently mild forms of maternal trauma. In cases with delayed presentation after trauma, infection is likely to set in and jeopardize the outcome of primary repair.

Obstetric and gynecological outcome in this case:
Postoperatively patient had fever and infection of the perineal stitches
She developed labor pains and had a preterm still birth on 3rd postoperative day
She developed urinary leakage per vaginum on 5th postoperative day suggesting failed bladder repair
Ureteric stents were removed after 2 weeks cystoscopically
Suprapubic and urethral catheters were removed after 3 weeks
Patient was planned for repair of the urinary fistula after 3 months.

BURNS IN PREGNANCY

Burn injuries during pregnancy are relatively rare and the exact incidence is not known. Burns may be caused by scalding or as a result of flames. Most burns are minor, and erythema usually subsides within 24 hours during the outpatient therapy. Severe burns during pregnancy though rare, are alarming events. Maternal and perinatal mortality increases significantly when > 50% of the total body surface area (BSA), is burnt. The genitals are generally well protected by the thighs unless burns are extensive (> 30 to 50% of the total BSA).

Most chemical burns are work-related, and occur as a result of accidental contact with a chemical agent. They usually appear on the face, hands, and upper limbs. The respiratory system can be affected by inhalation of the agent. Chemically induced genital and perianal burns have been reported from caustic substances used for douching, abortifacients, and vaginal foreign objects. The severity of the chemical injury generally depends on the concentration of the agent and the duration of exposure.

MANAGEMENT

- Acute management of thermal injuries in pregnancy is essential for maternal and fetal well-being. Therapy should be directed to saving the mother
- Care should be provided at a regional facility with expert burn care and fetal monitoring
  - Attempts should be undertaken during maternal transport to avoid hypovolemia, hypotension, and hypoxia
  - The wound should be covered with sterile dressings to prevent further contamination
- Complications to be considered during the emergent and acute phases of recovery include:
  - Fluid and electrolyte imbalance
  - Respiratory difficulties
  - Systemic and wound infection
  - Inadequate nutrition
  - Emotional disturbances
- Periodic ultrasonographic and biophysical testing of the fetus is recommended
- Obstetrical management should be individualized
- If conditions are considered unfavorable to meet fetal circulatory and oxygen demands, prompt delivery during the third trimesters has been advocated if the mother's burn covers 50 percent or more of the BSA.

PROGNOSIS

Multiple factors influence morbidity and mortality resulting from burn injuries during pregnancy:[23]
- Depth and size (BSA involved)of the burn
- Woman's underlying health and age
- Estimated gestational age of the fetus
- Associated inhalation injury and
- Development of other significant secondary complications

There is a direct correlation between the extent of the burns and survival of the fetus.
- If the patient has recovered satisfactorily and there has been no evidence of fetal jeopardy or premature labor within the first week following the burn injury, the eventual delivery of a healthy-appearing, term-sized fetus is quite likely.[24]
- In all burns above 30 % BSA, abortion, premature labour and intrauterine fetal death are potential complications and fetal mortality exceeds 50%. Nearly all these complications occur during the first week after the burn
- For patients in the third trimester of pregnancy with burns above 50 percent BSA the fetal survival is uncommon unless the pregnancy is terminated within 24 to 48 hours after the burn.[25]

KEY POINTS

- Varied presentations of the coital injuries demand careful evaluation and timely management.
- Noncoital genital tract injuries are usually accidental in nature. Most of the patients have multiple severe injuries, often associated with pelvic fractures. Early assessment and resuscitation is vital. Life-threatening injuries, including hemorrhage and unstable pelvic fracture are addressed first.
- Initial evaluation and resuscitation of pregnant trauma victims should always be maternally directed. Once maternal stability is established, fetus is closely monitored.
- For early diagnosis of abruptio placentae after blunt trauma to the abdomen, continuous monitoring of the fetal heart rate and uterine contractions is required.
- Patients with viable gestations require at least 4 hours of monitoring after even minor trauma.
- Acute management of thermal injuries in pregnancy is directed to saving the mother.
- Maternal and perinatal mortality increases significantly when >50% of the total body surface area is burnt.

REFERENCES

1. Sau AK, Dhar KK, Dhall GI. Nonobstetric lower genital tract trauma. Aust N Z J Obstet Gynaecol 1993;33:433-5.
2. Jana N, Santra D, Das D, Das AK, Dasgupta S. Nonobstetric lower genital tract injuries in rural India. Int J Gynaecol Obstet 2008;103:26-9.
3. Sivalingam N, Rajesvaran D. Coital injury requiring internal iliac artery ligation. Singapore Med J 1996;37:547-8.
4. Kriplani A, Agarwal N, Garg P, Sharma M. Transvaginal repair of post-coital rectovaginal fistula in patients of vaginal agenesis. J Obstet Gynaecol 2007;27:209-10.
5. Rabinerson D, Fradin Z, Zeidman A, Horowitz E. Vulvar hematoma after cunnilingus in a teenager with essential thrombocythemia: a case report. J Reprod Med 2007;52:458-9.
6. Howard JM, Diaz MC, Soler ME. Hemorrhagic shock resulting from post-coital vaginal bleeding in an adolescent with Ehlers-Danlos type IV. Pediatr Emerg Care 2009;25:397-8.
7. Elbiss H, Jain Y, Watts JF. Post-coital vaginal vault rupture following radical hysterectomy. J Obstet Gynaecol 2005;25:522-3.
8. Ahmed E, Syed SA, Parveen N. Female consensual coital injuries. J Coll Physicians Surg Pak 2006;16:333-5.
9. Jeng CJ, Wang LR. Vaginal laceration and hemorrhagic shock during consensual sexual intercourse. J Sex Marital Ther 2007;33:249-53.
10. McColgin SW, Williams LM, Sorrells TL, Morrison JC. Hemoperitoneum as a result of coital injury without associated vaginal injury. Am J Obstet Gynecol 1990;163:1503-5.
11. Fallat ME, Weaver JM, Hertweck SP, Miller FB. Late follow-up and functional outcome after traumatic reproductive tract injuries in women. Am Surg 1998;64:858-61.
12. Bittard H, Bernardini S, Khenifar E, Lévy T, Pradines M, Vichard P. Ureterovesival rupture with vaginal fistula following pelvic fracture. Value of early diagnosis and emergency surgery. J Urol (Paris) 1995;101:159-62.
13. Massey JB, García CR, Emich JP Jr. Management of sexually assaulted females. Obstet Gynecol 1971;38:29-36.
14. Mikos T, Papanicolaou A, Tsalikis T, Ioannidis E. Uterine prolapse after pelvic trauma: case report and literature review. Int Urogynecol J 2008;20:881-84.
15. Baessler K, Bircher MD, Stanton SL. Pelvic floor dysfunction in women after pelvic trauma. BJOG 2004;111:499-502.
16. Mirza FG, Devine PC, Gaddipati S. Trauma in pregnancy: a systematic approach. Am J Perinatol 2010;27:579-86.
17. Weiss HB. Pregnancy-associated injury hospitalizations in Pennsylvania, 1995. Ann Emerg Med 1999;34:626-36.
18. Schneider H. Trauma and pregnancy. Arch Gynecol Obstet 1993;253:S4-14.
19. Brown HL. Trauma in pregnancy. Obstet Gynecol 2009;114:147-60.
20. Kuczkowski KM. Trauma during pregnancy: a situation pregnant with danger. Acta Anaesthesiol Belg 2005;5:13-8.
21. Shah AJ, Kilcline BA. Trauma in pregnancy. Emerg Med Clin North Am 2003;21:615-29.
22. Smith BK, Rayburn WF, Feller I. Burns and pregnancy. Clin Perinatol 1983;10:383-98.
23. Kennedy BB, Baird SM, Troiano NH. Burn injuries and pregnancy. J Perinat Neonatal Nurs 2008;22:21-30.
24. Polko LE, McMahon MJ. Burns in pregnancy. Obstet Gynecol Surv 1998;53:50-6.
25. Srivastava S, Bang RL. Burns during pregnancy. Burns Incl Therm Inj 1988;14:228-32.

Chapter 37

Postexposure Prophylaxis to HIV and Hepatitis B

Shakun Tyagi, Shalini Jaluthria

INTRODUCTION

The term postexposure prophylaxis (PEP) denotes the medical response given to prevent the transmission of blood-borne pathogens following a potential exposure to the causative agent.[1] This term is most commonly used for Human Immunodeficiency virus (HIV) and Hepatitis B virus (HBV). Avoiding exposure to substances contaminated with these viruses is the primary way to prevent transmission. Once exposure has occurred PEP plays an important role in preventing the development of the infection. Initially PEP was described only following occupational exposure but later exposure following sexual assault, isolated or episodic needle-sharing among injectable drug users and consensual unprotected sexual exposure were also included in this category.

In prospective studies of Health Care Personnel (HCP), the average risk of HIV transmission after a percutaneous exposure to HIV-infected blood has been estimated to be approximately 0.3 percent[2] and after a mucous membrane exposure the risk is approximately 0.09 percent.[3]

The risk of HBV infection is primarily related to the degree of contact with blood and to the hepatitis B e antigen (HBeAg) status of the source person. In studies of HCP who sustained injuries from needles contaminated with blood containing HBV, the risk of developing clinical hepatitis if the blood was both hepatitis B surface antigen (HBsAg) and HBeAg-positive was 22 to 31 percent; the risk of developing serologic evidence of HBV infection was 37 to 62 percent. The risk of developing clinical hepatitis from a needle contaminated with HBsAg-positive, HBeAg-negative blood was 1 to 6 percent, and the risk of developing serologic evidence of HBV infection, 23 to 37 percent.[4] As compared to HIV which is a relatively fragile virus HBV has been demonstrated to survive in dried blood at room temperature on environmental surfaces for at least 1 week.[5]

CASE SCENARIO-1

A surgeon accidently pricks herself while performing emergency cesarean section. The double gloves which she wore were punctured and there was superficial puncture wound of the skin. There was slight ooze of blood underneath the gloves.

Comments: Universal precautions (Annexure-1) prevent exposure to infected biological material but if exposure occurs in spite of these, the procedure should be interrupted and first aid should be undertaken. This is followed by further precautions in a stepwise approach.

FIRST AID

First aid is a term describing the set of actions that should be taken immediately after potential exposure occurs. The aim of first aid is to reduce contact time with the source person's blood, body fluids or tissues and to clean and decontaminate the site of the exposure.

- Do not squeeze or rub the injury site
- Wash the site immediately using soap or a mild disinfectant solution that will not irritate the skin. WHO recommends the use of a chlorhexidine gluconate solution
- Same actions need to be taken in case of a splash to unbroken skin
- If running water is not available, clean the site with a gel or other hand-cleaning solution, whatever is available
- Do not use strong solutions, such as bleach or iodine, to clean the site as these may irritate the wound and make the injury worse.

First aid in this case: The surgeon washed her hands with soap and water and continued with surgery after scrubbing again. She went to the HIV counseling center 1 hour after the exposure with the blood sample of the source person.

DECIDING WHETHER PEP SHOULD BE INITIATED OR NOT

While assessing for PEP the *exposed person* is the person who has been potentially at risk of acquiring HIV infection through exposure to blood or body fluids. The *source person* is the person who is the possible source of infection through blood or body fluid. If the sero-status of the source person is unknown, he or she should be asked to provide informed consent for HIV testing before the sample is taken.

WHO recommends following eligibility criteria for postexposure prophylaxis in occupational settings:[1]

- Less than 72 hours have elapsed since exposure;
- The exposed individual is not known to be HIV infected;
- The person who is the source of exposure is living with HIV or has unknown HIV status;
- Exposure was to blood, body tissues, visibly blood-stained fluid, concentrated virus, cerebrospinal fluid, synovial fluid, pleural fluid, peritoneal fluid, pericardial fluid or amniotic fluid;
- Exposure penetrated the skin with spontaneous bleeding or there was a deep puncture or splash of significant amount of fluid to mucous membrane or prolonged contact with nonintact skin.

Further management in this case:
The HIV test for the exposed person was negative.
HIV test of the source person was positive by three Rapid tests. The source person did not have any clinical features of AIDS and was asymptomatic (WHO Classification for AIDS: Annexure 2).

INVESTIGATIONS

- HIV pretest counseling should be provided to the exposed and the source persons prior to conducting HIV test if HIV status is not already known
- Tridot test for both the source and the exposed person are performed which provide the status for HIV, Hepatitis B and Hepatitis C. HIV post-test counseling should be provided after the HIV test.
- Hemoglobin estimation may be needed, especially when zidovudine is used for postexposure prophylaxis in areas where anemia is common
- Liver and kidney function tests (LFT, KFT) should be done as Nonnucleoside Reverse Transcriptase Inhibitor (NRTI) drugs can cause hepatitis.

Table 37.1: Categories of exposure according to NACO[6]

Category	Definition and example
Mild exposure	Mucous membrane/non intact skin with small volumes. E.g. a superficial wound (erosion of the epidermis) with a plain or low caliber needle, OR contact with the eyes or the mucous membrane, subcutaneous injections following small-bore needles
Moderate exposure	Percutaneous superficial exposure with solid needle, e.g. a cut or needle stick injury penetrating gloves
Severe exposure	Percutaneous with large volume e.g.: • An accident with a high caliber needle(>18G) visibly contaminated with blood • A deep wound (hemorrhagic wound and/or very painful) • Transmission of a significant volume of blood • An accident with the material that has previously been used intravenously or intra-arterially. The wearing of gloves during any of these accidents constitutes a protective factor

BASIC REGIMEN VERSUS EXPANDED REGIMEN

Risk assessment needs to be performed to decide whether basic regimen or the expanded regimen needs to be provided and for counseling the exposed person.

Basic regimen comprising two nucleoside—analogue reverse—transcriptase inhibitors is recommended.

Expanded regimen comprises of two nucleoside—analogue reverse—transcriptase inhibitors plus a boosted protease inhibitor.

Following factors need to be considered in risk assessment

Type of Exposure or Source Factor

Table 37.1 describes the various categories of exposure according to NACO.
- *Sharps injury:*[8] To describe the exposure by a sharp needle or blade, the following points need to be taken into consideration-
  - The type (solid or hollow bore) and size of the needle or sharp object
  - What the needle or sharp object had been used for
  - The severity of the injury
  - Whether the penetration site bled
  - Whether the injury was through gloves or clothing
  - How recently the sharp object had been used
- *Splash:* It is described in following terms.
  - The type of body fluids to which the person was exposed
  - Whether the fluid to which the person was exposed contained blood
  - The amount of blood or body substance to which the person was exposed
  - Whether non-intact skin or mucous membrane was exposed
  - When the exposure occurred.

Source of the Blood, Body Fluids or Tissue

- Identity of the source person (known or unknown) (Table 37.2)
- HIV status (if known)

Table 37.2: Categories of situations depending on laboratory and clinical results of the source suggested by NACO[6]

Source: HIV Status	*Definition of risk in source*
HIV negative	Source is not HIV infected but consider HBV and HCV
Low-risk	HIV positive and clinically asymptomatic
High-risk	HIV positive and clinically symptomatic (see WHO clinical staging) Annexure:2
Unknown	Status of the patient is unknown, and neither the patient nor his/her blood is available for testing (e.g. injury during medical waste management the source might be unknown). The risk assessment will be based only upon the exposure(HIV prevalence in the locality can be considered)

- Stage of HIV infection (if known)
- HIV RNA viral load (if known)
- Antiretroviral therapy history of the source person (if known)
- Estimated population prevalence of HIV and the prevalence of resistance in that population, including geographical region and country prevalence
- Prevalence within the cultural, ethnic or behavioral group

Starting the Required PEP for HIV to the Eligible Exposed Person

PEP after exposure to HIV is short-term 28 day antiretroviral treatment to reduce the likelihood of HIV infection. The efficacy of PEP has been reported in a case control study.[7]

- The first dose of PEP should always be offered as soon as possible after exposure (preferably within 2 hours, without waiting for HIV testing and counseling or for the HIV test results of the source person unless rapid testing, which provides results within one hour, is available) and in cases of sexual assault. Basic two drug regimen should be started as soon as possible.
- The exposed person should be provided counseling prior to starting PEP which should include information about the risk of transmission, the possibility of side effects of the regimen and advice about the importance of adherence to PEP.
- WHO (2010)[1] recommends that either the basic regimen or the expanded regimen is started (Annexure 3) according to the type of exposure, the HIV status of the source person and the prevalence of resistance to antiretroviral drugs. It recommends expanded regimen (three drug regimen) only in severe per cutaneous exposure in following situations:
  - The source person is HIV positive, taking antiretroviral therapy and is known to have signs or personal history of or proven antiretroviral therapy resistance; OR
  - The source person's HIV status is unknown and the background prevalence of resistance to antiretroviral therapy in the community exceeds 15 percent (where this is known).
- National AIDS Control Organization (NACO) recommends that the basic regimen or the expanded regimen should be started (Table 37.3 to 37.5) according to the type of exposure and the HIV status of the source person and whether symptoms of AIDS are present or not (according to the WHO classification).

Follow-up

The exposed person should be monitored for drug toxicity by testing at baseline and again 2 weeks after starting PEP. Lab monitoring for toxicity should include a complete blood count and renal

Table 37.3 : HIV Post-exposure Prophylaxis evaluation and decision regarding the PEP regimen (NACO)[6]

Exposure	HIV+ and asymptomatic	HIV+ and Clinically symptomatic	HIV status unknown
mild	Consider 2-drug PEP	Start 2-drug PEP	Usually no PEP or consider 2-drug PEP
moderate	Start 2-drug PEP	Start 3-drug PEP	Usually no PEP or consider 2-drug PEP
severe	Start 3-drug PEP	Start 3-drug PEP	Usually no PEP or consider 2-drug PEP

Table 37.4: The Recommended two-drug combination therapies for HIV post-exposure Prophylaxis[1]

Preferred regimens
Zidovudine 300 mg BD + Lamivudine 150 mg BD

Alternative regimens[a]
Tenofovir 300 mg OD+ Lamivudine 150 mg BD/Lamivudine 300 mg OD
Stavudine 30 mg BD + Lamivudine 150 mg BD

[a] Tenofovir is available for antiretroviral therapy as an alternative drug. Emtricitabine is an acceptable alternative to Lamivudine where it is available. Abacavir and Didanosine are discouraged due to their relatively higher potentially serious side effects of fatty liver and pancreatitis.

Table 37.5: Recommended triple drug combination for PEP

Zidovudine + lamivudine plus lopinavir with a ritonavir boost
Alternate Regimens
• NRTI: Lamivudine
• + NRTI: Zidovudine/Tinofovir/Stavudine
• + boosted protease inhibitor: Atazanavir with a ritonavir boost/Saquinavir with a Ritonavir boost/ Fos-Amprenavir with a Ritonavir boost
The recommended duration of PEP for HIV infection is 28 days.

and hepatic function tests. Monitoring for evidence of hyperglycemia should be included if regimens include any Protease inhibitor. It is recommended that HIV testing in the exposed person should be performed 3 months and 6 months after exposure.

Every health care delivery place should have following systems in place for providing timely PEP:
• A written algorithm for risk assessment
• Prompt access to and clear protocols for delivering the first dose of PEP
• Adequate availability of PEP medication
• HIV testing and counseling services
• Protocols governing counseling services which would cover risk reduction, side effects of PEP medication and the importance of adherence and HIV testing.

> **PEP and follow-up in this case:** Considering that category of exposure was moderate (as the surgeon had pricked her gloves with a solid needle resulting in blood collecting under her gloves) and the source person was low-risk (as patient was asymptomatic), the exposed person was started on a combination of Zidovudine 300 mg and Lamivudine 150 mg twice a day after counseling and consent. Baseline LFT and hemoglobin were done and she was asked to follow-up after 2 weeks for clinical evaluation. HIV test was done after 3 months and six months which was found to be negative.

CASE SCENARIO-2

An intern accidently pricks himself while taking the blood sample of HBsAg positive patient. The patient is HIV negative. He thoroughly washes his hand. The intern had received only two doses of hepatitis B vaccine one year back.

Comments: First aid in the form of washing of the injured part needs to be provided. It is important to know the vaccination status of the exposed person. If the person has not been vaccinated earlier, full course of Hepatitis B vaccination should be given.

The response of the person to the vaccine needs to be evaluated by measuring anti-HBsAg levels in order to decide whether the patient requires passive immunization with hepatitis B immune Globulins (HBIG) or not. Table 37.6 summarizes the post exposure prophylaxis for hepatitis B.

- If the exposed person has been immunized against hepatitis B earlier and has adequate immune status revealed by anti-HBsAg levels of more than 10 mIU/mL then no treatment is required.
- If the exposed person has been immunized against hepatitis B earlier and shows inadequate response, i.e. value of anti-HBsAg < 10 mIU/mL then the exposed person requires both active immunization by hepatitis B vaccine as well as passive immunization in the form of intra muscular injection of hepatitis B immunoglobulins in the dose of 0.06 mL/kg.
- If immune status against hepatitis is not known then hepatitis B vaccine is administered and anti-HBsAg levels are done. If the levels of anti-HBsAg are less than 10 mIU/mL then HBIG is indicated. When both HBIG and hepatitis B vaccine are indicated, they should be administered as soon as possible after exposure (preferably within 24 hours). When both these drugs are to be administered simultaneously, vaccine should always be administered in the deltoid muscle and the HBIG should be administered at separate site.

Management in this case: The serum anti-HBsAg levels were 6 mIU/mL which is less than required level. Passive immunization with hepatitis B immune globulin at the dose of 0.06 mL/Kg intravenously was given to the exposed person.

Table 37.6: Recommended postexposure prophylaxis to hepatitis B exposure[8]

Vaccination and antibody response status of exposed workers*	Treatment Source HBsAg[1] positive	Source Unknown or not available for testing
Unvaccinated	HBIG X 1 and initiate HB vaccine series[1]	Initiate HB vaccine series
Previously vaccinated Known responder *Antibody to HBsAg>10mIU/ml*	No treatment	No treatment
Known nonresponder *Antibody to HBsAg<10mIU/ml*	HBIG X 1 and initiate revaccination or HBIG X 2	If known high-risk source treat as if source were HBsAg positive
Antibody response unknown	Test exposed person for anti-HBsAg 1. If adequate, no treatment is necessary 2. If inadequate, administer HBIG X 1 and vaccine booster	Test exposed person for anti-HBsAg 1. If adequate, no treatment is necessary 2. If inadequate vaccine booster and recheck titer in 1 to 2 months

KEY POINTS

- Universal precautions should be observed by HCP irrespective of the HIV status of any patient
- First aid and the first dose of PEP should be provided as soon as possible in case of exposure according to the risk category
- Counseling prior to starting PEP and support to the exposed person prevents default in taking PEP.
- Hepatitis B PEP is provided according to the immune status of the exposed person to hepatitis B surface antigen measured by anti-HbsAg levels.

REFERENCES

1. Post-exposure prophylaxis to prevent HIV infection : joint WHO/ILO guidelines on post-exposure prophylaxis (PEP) to prevent HIV infection (/http://whqlibdoc.who.int/publications/2007/9789241596374_eng.pdf)
2. Bell DM. Occupational risk of human immunodeficiency virus infection in healthcare workers: An Overview. Am J Med 1997;102(5B):9-15.
3. Ippolito G, Puro V, De Carli G, Italian Study Group on Occupational Risk of HIV Infection. The risk of occupational human immunodeficiency virus in health care workers. Arch Int Med 1993;153:1451-8.
4. Werner BG, Grady GF. Accidental hepatitis-B-surface-antigen-positive inoculations: use of e antigen to estimate infectivity. Ann Intern Med 1982;97:367-9.
5. Bond WW, Favero MS, Petersen NJ, Gravelle CR, Ebert JW, Maynard JE. Survival of hepatitis B virus after drying and storage for one week. Lancet 1981;1:550-1.
6. Antiretroviral Therapy Guidelines for HIV-Infected Adults and Adolescents Including Post-exposure Prophylaxis downloaded from http://www.nacoonline.org/upload/Policies% 20&%20Guidelines/1. %20Antiretroviral %20Therapy%20Guidelines%20for%20HIV-Infected%20Adults%20and%20Adolescents%20Including%20Post-exposure.pdf
7. Cardo DM, Culver DH, Ciesielski CA, et al. A case-control study of HIV seroconversion in health care workers after percutaneous exposure. Centers for Disease Control and Prevention Needlestick Surveillance Group. N Engl J Med. 1997;337:1485-90.
8. Updated U.S. Public Health Service Guidelines for the Management of Occupational Exposures to HBV, HCV, and HIV and Recommendations for Postexposure Prophylaxis, June 29, 2001/50(RR11);1-42. http://www.cdc.gov/mmwr/preview/mmwrhtml/rr5011a1.htm

Annexure-1

Universal precautions are intended to prevent the exposure of health-care workers and patients to blood borne pathogens. These must be practiced in regard to the blood and body fluids of all patients, regardless of their infection status.

Universal Precautions[6] Include:

- Hand-washing before and after all medical procedures
- Safe handling and immediate safe disposal of sharps:
  - Not recapping needles;
  - Using special containers for sharp disposals;
  - Using needle cutter/destroyers;
  - Using forceps instead of fingers for guiding sutures;
  - Using vacutainers where possible for safe decontamination of instruments;
- Use of protective barriers whenever indicated to prevent direct contact with blood and body fluid such as gloves, masks, goggles, aprons, and boots.
- A HCP who has a cut or abrasion should cover the wound before providing care
- Safe disposal of contaminated waste

Annexure-2

WHO recommendations for deciding the regimen for PEP regimen (2007).[1]

Exposure type	HIV positive	Unknown HIV status
Percutaneous: More severe e.g. a large hollow-bore needle, a deep puncture and contact with visible blood on a device or a needle used in artery or vein	Offer a **basic regimen** (two-drug regimen). **Offer expanded regimen (three drug regimen):** If an HIV-positive source has known or suspected resistance to antiretroviral therapy **or** if the background prevalence of antiretroviral therapy resistance in the community is more than 15%.	Consider population or subgroup prevalence
Percutaneous: Less severe e.g. a small-bore or solid needle and a superficial injury	Offer a two-drug regimen	Do not offer PEP
Sexual	Offer a two-drug regimen	Consider population or subgroup prevalence
Splash: Includes exposure to non-genital mucous membranes or to non-intact skin **More severe:** E.g. include exposure to a large volume of blood or semen	Offer a two-drug regimen	Consider population or subgroup prevalence
Splash: **Less severe**	PEP is not recommended, but a two-drug regimen may be offered on request	Do not offer PEP

Annexure-3

WHO Clinical Staging of HIV/AIDS for Adults and Adolescents[1]

Primary HIV Infection

- Asymptomatic
- Acute retroviral syndrome.

Clinical Stage 1

- Asymptomatic
- Persistent generalized lymphadenopathy.

Clinical Stage 2

- Moderate unexplained weight loss (<10% of presumed or measured body weight)
- Recurrent respiratory infections (sinusitis, tonsillitis, otitis media and pharyngitis)
- Herpes zoster
- Angular cheilitis
- Recurrent oral ulceration
- Papular pruritic eruptions
- Seborrheic dermatitis
- Fungal nail infections.

Clinical Stage 3

- Unexplained severe weight loss (>10% of presumed or measured body weight)
- Unexplained chronic diarrhea for >1 month
- Unexplained persistent fever for >1 month (>37.6°C, intermittent or constant)
- Persistent oral candidiasis (thrush)
- Oral hairy leukoplakia
- Pulmonary tuberculosis (current)
- Severe presumed bacterial infections (e.g., pneumonia, empyema, pyomyositis, bone or joint infection, meningitis, bacteremia)
- Acute necrotizing ulcerative stomatitis, gingivitis, or periodontitis
- Unexplained anemia (hemoglobin <8 g/dL)
- Neutropenia (neutrophils <500 cells/μL)
- Chronic thrombocytopenia (platelets <50,000 cells/μL).

Clinical Stage 4

- HIV wasting syndrome, as defined by the CDC (see Table 37.3, above)
- *Pneumocystis* pneumonia
- Recurrent severe bacterial pneumonia
- Chronic herpes simplex infection (orolabial, genital, or anorectal site for >1 month or visceral herpes at any site)
- Esophageal candidiasis (or candidiasis of trachea, bronchi, or lungs)
- Extrapulmonary tuberculosis
- Kaposi sarcoma
- Cytomegalovirus infection (retinitis or infection of other organs)
- Central nervous system toxoplasmosis
- HIV encephalopathy
- Cryptococcosis, extrapulmonary (including meningitis)
- Disseminated nontuberculosis *Mycobacteria* infection

- Progressive multifocal leukoencephalopathy
- Candida of the trachea, bronchi, or lungs
- Chronic cryptosporidiosis (with diarrhea)
- Chronic isosporiasis
- Disseminated mycosis (e.g., histoplasmosis, coccidioidomycosis, penicilliosis)
- Recurrent nontyphoidal *Salmonella* bacteremia
- Lymphoma (cerebral or B-cell non-Hodgkin)
- Invasive cervical carcinoma
- Atypical disseminated leishmaniasis
- Symptomatic HIV-associated nephropathy
- Symptomatic HIV-associated cardiomyopathy
- Reactivation of American trypanosomiasis (meningoencephalitis or myocarditis)

Annexure-4

Summary of Steps for PEP[6]

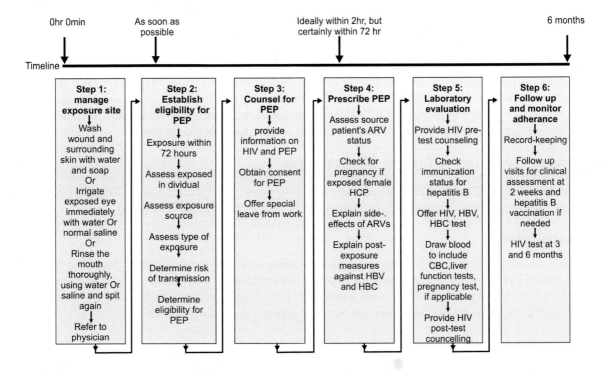

Chapter 38

Endotoxic Shock

Devender Kumar

Severe sepsis and septic shock persist as major health problems and mortality ranges from 30 to 60 percent despite aggressive medical care.[1,2] In 1914, Schottmueller wrote, "Septicemia is a state of microbial invasion from a portal of entry into the blood stream which causes signs of illness." Sepsis occurs when micro-organisms or their toxins break into tissue barrier and the host immune system responds to these microbial molecules and the toxins released by them.[2]

DEFINING SEPSIS AND ITS CLINICAL MANIFESTATIONS

The American College of Chest Physicians (ACCP)/Society of Critical Care Medicine (SCCM) consensus conference[3] defined sepsis, severe sepsis, and septic shock (Table 38.1).

Endotoxic Shock

Endotoxic shock is caused by gram negative bacteria or endotoxins absorbed from the gut or peritoneal cavity in cases of intestinal obstruction, strangulation, perforation, mucosal shut down due to hypovolemic shock or abscess formation. Pneumonia, urinary tract infection, burns or invasive procedure leading to sepsis can be other sources. It has two phases.[4]

Endotoxic Shock Phase 1

In this hyperdynamic phase cardiac output is increased, peripheral resistance decreased, blood pressure is normal or slightly reduced and skin is warm and dry. Tachycardia, hyperventilation, and pyrexia are common. Urine output is satisfactory and patient may not have typical shock syndrome. If patient is not treated within 2 to 12 hours then phase 2 begins.

Endotoxic Shock Phase 2

In this hypotensive phase, cardiac output is decreased, peripheral resistance increased; the patient is hypotensive and oliguric with cold pale cyanotic skin. The features are of typical shock syndrome.

Septic Focus

Usually there is some invasive procedure and it is the job of physician to provide the evidence. Sepsis conference recommended "PIRO" concept.[1,2,3]

Table 38.1: Definition of terms associated with infection	
Bacteremia	Presence of bacteria in blood (blood culture)
Septicemia	Presence of microbes and their toxins in blood
Systemic inflammatory response syndrome (SIRS)	Two of the following conditions
	Fever (>38°C) or hypothermia (<36°C)
	• Tachycardia
	• Tachypnea
	• Leukocytosis (>1200/µL) or leukopenia (<4000/µL) or >10% bands
Sepsis	SIRS with proven suspected microbial etiology
Severe Sepsis	Sepsis associated with hyotension, hypoperfusion and organ dysfunction
	• Systolic BP ≤90 mm Hg or mean arterial blood pressure ≤ 70 mm Hg that responds to iv fluid therapy
	• Urine output ≤0.5 ml/kg per hour for 1 hour despite adequate fluid resuscitation
	• PaO$_2$/FiO$_2$ ≤250 or if lung is the only dysfunctional organ ≤200
	• Platelet counts < 80,000/µL or 50% decrease in platelets from highest recoded over previous 3 days
	• pH ≤7.3 or a base deficit ≥5mEq/L and a plasma lactate levels > 1.5 times upper limit of normal for reporting lab
	• Pulmonary artery wedge pressure ≥12 mm Hg or CVP ≥8 mm Hg
Septic shock	Sepsis with hypotension for at least 1 hour despite adequate fluid resuscitation or need of vasopressors to maintain BP
Multiple organ dysfunction syndrome (MODS)	Dysfunction of more than one organ, requiring interventions

P = Predisposing Factors

Genetic factors, AIDS, life style diseases can aggravate the condition. Patient's age and gender are also important factors.

I = Infectious Insult

Bacterial (gram positive or negative, MRSA) infections are common in severe sepsis. Tuberculosis has chronic course. Fungal infections are seen in AIDS. Viral infections are associated with cancer. The source of sepsis and degree of spread also influence severity of sepsis and response to therapy.

R = Host Response

Host response to infection varies as each patient mounts a different response. The response is assessed by signs and symptoms largely.

O = Organ Dysfunction

This refers to the degree of organ dysfunction related to the sepsis. The evaluation can be done using Sequential Organ Failure Assessment (SOFA) score.

Table 38.2: Sequential Organ Failure Assessment (SOFA)

Sofa score		0	1	2	3	4
Respiration[a]	PaO$_2$/FIO$_2$ SaO$_2$/FIO$_2$ (mm Hg)	>400	<400 221–301	<300 142–220	<2006 7–141	<100 <67
Coagulation	Platelets (10^3/mm^3)	>150	<150	<100	<50	<20
Liver	Bilirubin (mg/dL)	<1.2	1.2 – 1.9	2.0 – 5.9	6.0 – 11.9	>12
Cardiovascular[b]	Hypotension	No hypotension	MAP <70	Dopamine </=5 or dobutamine (any)	Dopamine >5 norepine-phrine </=0.1	Dopamine >15 or norepine-phrine >0.1
CNS	Glasgow Coma Score	15	13 – 14	10 – 12	6 – 9	<6
Renal	Creatinine (mg/dL) or urine output (mL/d)	<1.2	1.2–1.9	2.0–3.4	3.5–4.9 or <500	>5.0 or <200

MAP—Mean arterial pressure; CNS—Central nervous system;
SaO$_2$—Peripheral arterial oxygen saturation
[a]PaO$_2$/FIO$_2$ ratio was used preferentially. If not available, the SaO$_2$/FIO$_2$ ratio was used
[b]vasoactive agents administered for at least 1 hr (dopamine and norepinephrine-µg/kg/min)

Sequential Organ Failure Assessment (SOFA) Score[2,5,6,7]

The SOFA system was created in a consensus meeting of the European Society of Intensive Care Medicine in 1994 and further revised in 1996 (Table 38.2). The SOFA is a six-organ dysfunction/failure score measuring multiple organ failure daily. Each organ is graded from 0 (normal) to 4 (the most abnormal), providing a daily score of 0 to 24 points. The objective to create a simple, reliable, and continuous score, easily obtained in every institution.

Mechanism of Sepsis Leading to Organ Injury (Figure 38.1)

- Bacterial groups such as *Streptococci, Staphylococci, Clostridia* and *Corynebacteria* produce soluble *exotoxins* which initiate inflammatory response.
- Gram negative bacteria such as *E. coli, Klebsiella, Proteus, Pseudomonas,* and *Salmonella* produce *endotoxins*, which are part of cell wall lipopolysaccharide.[2,4,5] When these microbes are killed in bloodstream by the complement or bactericidal drugs, endotoxins are released in the system.
- In phase 1, endotoxin causes fever, increase heart rate and stroke volume. Arteriolar dilatation causes increased vis a tergo and venous return.[4] This leads to increased heart rate by the Bainbridge reflex and increased stroke volume by Starling's law. Blood flow to most vascular beds is raised. Endotoxins cause noncomplement mediated necrosis of endothelium of blood vessels which triggers nitric oxide synthesis. Nitric oxide causes widespread vasodilatation leading to decreased peripheral resistance. These vascular changes lead to hyperdynamic circulation.
- Monocytes/macrophages and neutrophils release inflammatory mediators like cytokines (IL 1, IL 6, IL 12, IL 15, TNF etc.), chemokine, lipid mediators and oxygen radicals, which can activate other cells.
- There is expression of adhesion molecule on the vascular endothelium and circulating cells (platelets, neutrophils and monocytes) allowing adhesion of leukocytes and their migration to subendothelial tissue.

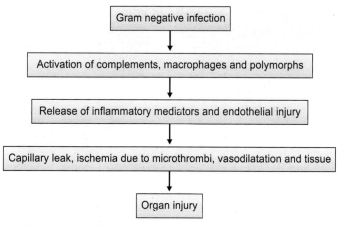

Figure 38.1: Algorithm of Sepsis leading to Organ injury

- Alteration in intercellular endothelial junctions causes increased capillary permeability and generalized edema.
- The inflammatory response activates tissue factor on the surface of endothelial cells and monocytes etc. In addition the inflammatory response leads to reduction in natural anticoagulants like protein C, protein S and antithrombin that ultimately create procoagulant state.
- The products of DIC and platelet aggregation aggravate bleeding tendency & obstruct microcirculation. The decreased blood flow to organs causes hypoxia, lactic acidosis, and organ dysfunction/failure.

"Two Hit" Theory

First "Hit" is tissue injury or ischemia due to trauma, surgery or shock. Second "Hit" is amplified inflammatory response due to infectious insult. But in actual practice it's difficult to differentiate. The enormous inflammatory response generated can affect cardiovascular, respiratory and other organs.

Multiple Organ Dysfunctions (MODs)[2,4,5,8]

The septic and thrombus emboli affect multiple organs on different days by affecting their blood supply (Figure 38.2). The infection itself can occur in multiple organs.

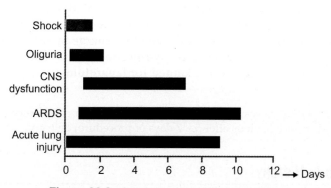

Figure 38.2: Organ damage following sepsis

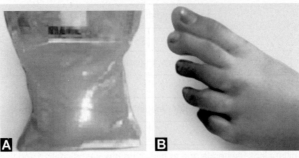

Figures 38.3A and B: Organs affected due to sepsis A) Pyuria, B) Gangrene of toes
(*For color version, see Plate 1*)

Organ Dysfunction

- Cardiovascular system (CVS)
  - Systolic BP ≤ 90 mm Hg or MAP ≤ 70 mm Hg for at least 1 hour despite adequate volume resuscitation, or the use of vasopressors to achieve the same goals.
- Renal
  - Urine output < 0.5 mL/kg/hr, or acute renal failure, Pyuria (Figure 38.3A)
- Pulmonary
  - PaO_2/FiO_2 ≤ 250 if other organ dysfunction present or ≤ 200 if the lung is the only dysfunctional organ.
- Hepatic dysfunction
  - hyperbilirubinemia, raised liver enzymes
- Central nervous system
  - Acute alteration in mental status (e.g. delirium).
- Hematologic
  - Platelet count <80,000/mm³ or decreased by 50 percent over three days, or disseminated intravascular coagulation.
- Metabolic
  - pH ≤ 7.30 or base deficit >5.0 mmol/L and plasma lactate >1.5 x upper limit of normal.
- In severe cases of puerperal sepsis case there may be gangrene of toes. (Figure 38.3B).

CASE SCENARIO

32 years P4 L4 A3 was brought to casualty with complain of pain abdomen for 8 days which had aggravated since 3 days, distension of abdomen 2 days, vomiting, constipation and discharge per vagina 1 day. She had dilatation and evacuation for 2 months amenorrhea in a private clinic 10 days back. She was febrile, pale, tachypenic (30/min) and with tachycardia (102/min). Her BP was 92/62 mm Hg. On examination abdomen was distended, free fluid present and no mass palpable. Her genital examination revealed purulent discharge mixed with blood from cervix. She was diagnosed as septic abortion with pyo-peritonium. Broad spectrum intravenous antibiotic were initiated and patient was planned for laparotomy.

> **Comments:**
> Septic abortion and puerperal sepsis occur when uterine evacuation or delivery is conducted in septic conditions. The sepsis becomes obvious after 5 – 7 days of procedure/delivery.

POINTS TO BE NOTED IN HISTORY

- History of invasive procedure (often by untrained person)
- Patient susceptibility to infection due to recurrent invasive procedure, anemia, diabetes or AIDS
- Place of intervention and experience of person who conducted the procedure

- Onset and duration of symptoms in chronological order and associated complaints of bladder (urine output should be >30 ml per hour or >600 ml in 24 hours) and bowel (constipation/obstipation/altered bowel habits)
- Past history of pelvic inflammatrory disease/blood transfusion/surgery.

> **History in this case:**
> The presenting case had dilatation and evacuation 10 day back probably under septic condition. She developed presenting complaints 2 days after that and symptoms were aggravating

POINTS TO BE NOTED IN EXAMINATION

History followed by examination help make a diagnosis of sepsis. The holistic approach (including investigations) will help in deciding for the conservative approach or surgical intervention.

General Examination

- Consciousness status and orientation of the patient
- Temperature, pulse, respiratory rate & blood pressure
- Pallor, icterus, cyanosis, lymphadenopathy.

Cardiovascular and Respiratory System Examination

- Tachycardia/heart sounds/murmurs/cardiomegaly
- Position of trachea/breath sounds (vesicular/bronchial or absent)/pleural effusion.

Abdominal Examination

- *Inspection:* Distension/movement along with respiration/visible mass or veins or peristalsis/any other abnormality like cough impulse
- *Palpation:* Tenderness/guarding/organomegaly or palpable mass
- *Percussion:* Any free fluid in abdominal cavity
- *Auscultation:* Presence or absence of bowel sounds.

Pelvic Examination

Local Examination

- External genitalia
- Any swelling or congestion

Per Speculum (P/S) Examination

- Vestibule, vagina and cervix are inspected for position/any lesion/discharge/injury
- Cervical os should be inspected (open or close)
- Swab (for microscopy & culture) from cervix or vagina should be kept ready.

Per Vaginum (P/V) Examination

- Cervical tenderness, consistency, dilatation should be noted
- Uterus tenderness, position, size should be observed carefully
- Palpation through fornices should note tenderness, mass, fibrosis, bogginess due to collection.

Per Rectal Examination

- Any collection in the pouch of Douglas (POD).

> **Examination in this case:**
> The presenting case had typical signs of septic shock in examination. She had pyoperitoneun and purulent discharge per vaginum. The infection had spread to peritoneal cavity involving the abdominal organs.

INVESTIGATIONS AND MONITORING

The role of investigations is both diagnostic as well as prognostic. The base line investigations should be done as soon as possible after admission and preferably before initiation of treatment. Following investigations are done but should be chosen judiciously.

- Hemoglobin, packed cell volume, platelets count, total & differential leukocyte counts
- Urine albumin, sugar, microscopic examination and culture
- Liver function tests (bilirubin, AST, ALT, proteins and GGT)
- HIV/HBs Ag
- X-ray chest with both domes of diaphragm – PA view
- X-ray abdomen – AP view (erect)
- Blood sugar, electrolytes, urea and creatinine
- Blood culture and sensitivity
- Specimen (sputum, pus, tissue)/swab/fluid from suspected sites, aspiration or punctures
- Coagulation profile (BT, CT, aPTT, PT)
- Plasma fibrinogen levels
- Fibrin degradation products (FDP)
- Serum cortisol, lactate levels are not obligatory.

Monitor the following Parameters

- Consciousness level
- Pulse oxygen saturation
- Pulse rate, heart rate, BP (NIBP or invasive), temperature and respiration- initially hourly till patient is stabilized, thereafter four hourly
- Urine output—Initially hourly till patient is stabilized, thereafter four hourly
- Central venous pressure (CVP) to be maintained 8 – 12 cm of water column
- Pulmonary wedge pressure[2,5,9] (using Swan-Ganz catheter) to be maintained 15 mm Hg (Table 38.3).
- Arterial blood gas analysis is done if patient undergoes surgery or is critically ill.
- Repeat blood investigations at regular (clinically suitable) interval to note the trend of organ functions.

Rationale for using Swan-Ganz Catheter

Clinical observation is subjective/inadequate in critically ill subjects. It allows measurements of determinants and consequences of cardiac performance thereby helping in the management of perfusion and ventilation of vital organs.

Table 38.3: Normal resting pressure obtained during right heart catheterization		
Cardiac Chamber		*Pressure (mm Hg)*
Right atrium	Range	0 – 6
	Mean	3
Right Ventricle	Systolic	15 – 30
	Diastolic	3 – 8
Pulmonary artery	Systolic	15 – 30
	Diastolic	4 – 12
	Mean	10 – 18
Pulmonary wedge pressure		2 – 15

- Assessment of Shock
  - Cardiogenic, hypovolemic
  - Septic, pulmonary embolism
- Assessment of Respiratory Distress
  - Cardiogenic vs Non-Cardiogenic
- Management of Complicated myocardial infarction
  - Hypovolemia vs Cardiogenic Shock
  - VSD vs MR
  - Severe LVF

TREATMENT OF SEPSIS AND ENDOTOXIC SHOCK[2,5,8,9,10]

Rapid assessment and diagnosis are essential for management of cases with endotoxic shock as these cases are critically ill. It involves:
1. Resuscitation of patient
2. Prediction/identification/removal of pathogens and antibiotics sensitivity
3. Organ specific support
4. Identifying the need for surgical intervention

Resuscitation to Establish Hemodynamic Stability (VIP)

- Ventilation (V)
- Infusion (I) of fluids
- Pumping of circulation with vasoactive agents (P).

Fluid Therapy

- Fluid resuscitation may consist of natural or artificial colloids or crystalloids. There is no evidence-based support for one type of fluid over another. The infusion volume is calculated with simple formula (2 ml/kg per hour + urine output per hour) otherwise fluid infusion depends on CVP or pulmonary wedge pressure.
- Fluid challenge in patients with suspected hypovolemia (suspected inadequate arterial circulation) may be given at a rate of 500–1000 mL of crystalloids or 300–500 mL of colloids over 30 minutes and repeated based on response (increase in blood pressure and urine output) and tolerance (evidence of intravascular volume overload).

Vasopressor Therapy (Table 38.4)

According to the Cochrane review [11], vasopressor therapy is an important part of hemodynamic support in patients with shock. Several randomized controlled trials have compared the effects of various vasopressors. Presently there is not sufficient evidence to prove that any of the vasopressors are superior over others in terms of mortality. Dopamine appears to increase the risk for arrhythmia.

Table 38.4: Different vasoactive drugs and their doses		
Mode of action	*Drugs*	*Doses*
Inotropic agents	Dobutamine	2 – 20 µg/kg/min
	Dopamine (low doses)	5 – 10 µg/kg/min
	Epinephrine	0.06 – 0.20 µg/kg/min
Vasoconstrictors and Inotropic agents	Dopamine (high doses)	>10 µg/kg/min
	Epinephrine (high doses)	0.21 – 0.25 µg/kg/min
Vasoconstrictor	Phenylephrine	0.2 – 2.5 µg/kg/min
	Vasopressin	0.04 – 0.1 units/min
Vasodilators	Milrinone	0.4 – 0.6 µg/kg/min
	Dopamine (Very low dose)	1 – 4 µg/kg/min

The choice of the specific vasopressor may therefore be individualized. Factors like experience, physiological effects (for example heart rate, intrinsic inotropic effects, and splanchnic perfusion), drug interaction with other therapeutics, availability, and cost should be considered.

Corticosteroids

- Intravenous corticosteroids (hydrocortisone 200–300 mg/day, for 7 days in three or four divided doses or by continuous infusion) are recommended in patients with septic shock who, despite adequate fluid replacement, require vasopressors to maintain adequate blood pressure.
- In the absence of shock, corticosteroids should not be administered for the treatment of sepsis. There is, however, no contraindication to continuing maintenance steroid therapy or to using stress dose steroids if the patient's history of corticosteroid administration or the patient's endocrine history warrants.

Treatment of Infection

- *Antimicrobial agents should be initiated as soon as samples of blood and other relevant culture specimens are taken.* Early administration of antimicrobials is important for better outcome. Empirical broad spectrum antibiotics in maximum recommended doses are administered intravenous if culture reports are pending. When culture reports are available then therapy should be simplified as single antimicrobial agent. Meta-analysis have concluded (except one) that combination therapy is not superior to monotherapy for treating gram negative bacteremia.
  - Imipenem-cilastin—0.5g every 6 hr
  - Meropenem—1.0g every 8 hr
  - Piperacillin-tazobactam—3.375g every 4 hr or 4.5 g every 6 hr
  - Cefepime1—2 every 8 hr
  - Gatifloxacin—400 mg IV every day
  - Ceftriaxone—2.0 g every 24 hr
  - Levofloxacin—500mg every day
- Add clindamycin 600 mg every 8 hr
- Removal or drainage of a focal source of infection is essential.

Organ Specific Support

a. *Blood and blood products* –Blood transfusion helps in improving RBCs, platelets, and clotting factors (fibrinogens etc). Packed cells should be transfused to improve hemoglobin (>10 gm %). Plasma transfusion may complicate the condition due to incompatibility and unnecessary immunoglobulins.

b. *Role of FDP* – FDP levels help in diagnosing DIC, but its interpretation should be done carefully with the knowledge of desirable levels to be maintained (fibrinogen >150 mg % and platelets >1 lac/mm³. Fresh frozen plasma or platelets are transfused when fribrinogen or platelets are low.

c. *Renal damage*—In case of renal damage, diuretics should be considered to maintain urine output. Fluid infusion has to be maintained for adequate perfusion.

d. *Hepatic damage* requires conservative management, with high carbohydrate and low protein diet. Once the regeneration of liver cells begins, functions will improve.

e. *CNS involvement* has more long-term complications and neurologist should be involved to restrict the damage.

f. *Stress ulcer prophylaxis* should be given to all patients with severe sepsis. Proton pump inhibitors are very effective.

g. *Deep vein thrombosis (DVT) prophylaxis* is provided to patients having severe sepsis using either low-dose unfractionated heparin or low-molecular weight heparin. If there is a contraindication for heparin use (i.e. thrombocytopenia, severe coagulopathy, active bleeding, recent intracerebral hemorrhage), the use of a mechanical prophylactic device (graduated compression stockings or intermittent compression device) is recommended (unless contraindicated by the presence of peripheral vascular disease).

h. *Bicarbonate therapy* for the purpose of improving hemodynamics or reducing vasopressor requirements is not recommended for treatment of hypoperfusion induced lactic acidemia with pH >7.15. The effect of bicarbonate administration on hemodynamics and vasopressor requirement at lower pH as well as the effect on clinical outcome at any pH has not been studied.

i. *Mechanical Ventilation* in sepsis-induced Acute Lung Injury (ALI)/ARDS should be done under expert supervision.

j. *Nutrition of the patient*- In severe cases parentral nutrition should be considered. Oral nutrition (balanced diet) should begin once patient is able to tolerate and in convalescent state.

Identifying the Need for Surgical Intervention[12]

Surgery has specific role in cases of sepsis. ***When not to operate is more important than performing surgery.***

- The removal of pus or septic foci (abscess or gangrenous uterus) and bowel injury are the main indications for laparotomies.
- Another area of clinical importance is tuberculosis. Antitubercular therapy (ATT) is the mainstay treatment and surgery is limited to tubo-ovarian masses not responding to ATT (4 to 6 months of therapy), or doubtful diagnosis.
- Laparoscopy should be considered if diagnosis is doubtful. Cultures obtained will identify the organism. It may be helpful in identifying endometriosis/ovarian tumors.
- *Posterior colpotomy*- Its use is limited to following three conditions:
  - The abscess must be midline approximately
  - The abscess should be in POD and preferably extending to recto-vaginal septum
  - The abscess should be cystic

> **Treatment in this case:**
> In this case, laparotomy findings were as follows:
> - Pus (400 mL) drained from peritoneal cavity
> - Flakes of pus were present on bowel
> - Posterior wall of uterus was gangrenous
> - Subtotal hysterectomy was done
> - Bowel explored for any injury
> - Peritoneal lavage was done and a drain was kept in POD
>
> *Postoperatively:* Patient had persistent fever, renal output did not improve (350 ml/24hour) and she developed ARDS on fourth post- op day. PT was prolonged despite sufficient amount of fresh frozen plasma transfusion and she had cardiac arrest on post op day 7 which responded to CPR (subsequently patient was put on ventilator).

PREVENTION

- Aseptic techniques with universal precaution are essential to prevent infection
- Immunizations against tetanus, hepatitis B, chicken pox etc
- Nutrition and correction of anemia can improve the host resistance
- Broad spectrum antibiotics prophylaxes covering the most probable organism are essential in susceptible case with diabetes, AIDS etc.

CONCLUSION[13,14]

In 2005, WHO had a theme "every mother counts"! Pregnancy and childbirth claim the lives of an estimated 514,000 women each year globally. This translates to one woman dying every minute.

The overwhelming majority of these deaths (98 per cent) occur in the developing world. Sepsis is the third leading cause of maternal mortality and major cause of morbidity. If we have answer to "why they are so prone to become septic?" we can think of elimination of cause(s). We should stress more on aseptic techniques instead of expanding the spectrum and misuse of antibiotics.

KEY POINTS

- History and examination establish the clinical diagnosis of sepsis. Early diagnosis and treatment (with broad spectrum antibiotics) can improve the condition of patient
- Investigations are important to confirm diagnosis and judicious use at particular interval will give the prognosis.
- Isolation of organism and sensitivity pattern will help in exact treatment.
- The insult due to infection can become worse soon after initiation of antimicrobial treatment to destruction of organism and release of endotoxins, so perfusion of tissue and ventilation of patient require intensive care.
- Maintain the circulatory volume, clotting factors, hemoglobin and nutrition of the patient for better results.
- Swan-Ganz catheter (pulmonary wedge pressure) is required in severe sepsis or septic shock.
- FDP help in evaluation of fibrinogen and platelets. DIC cases may need low-dose anticoagulant and clotting factors. Correction of DIC and clotting factors is mandatory before any surgical intervention
- The knowledge of pathophysiology (organism/endotoxin) and intensive care can prevent/ restrict damage to lungs, liver, kidneys, heart, CNS and other organs

---

REFERENCES

1. Levy MM, Fink MP, Marshall JC, et al. 2001 SCCM / ESICM / ACCP / ATS / SIS International sepsis definition conference. Crit Care Med 2003;31:1250-56.
2. Jean-Louis Vincent. Septic shock. In: Fink MP, Abraham E, Vincent JL, Kochanek PM (eds). Text book of critical care. 5th edn. Elsevier Saunders, 2005. pp. 1259-65.
3. R C Bone, R A Balk, F B Cerra, et al. Definitions for sepsis and organ failure and guidelines for the use of innovative therapies in sepsis. The ACCP/SCCM consensus conference committee. American college of chest physicians/ society of critical care medicine. Chest 1992;101:1644-55.
4. Wright MO. Shock. In: Glasby MA, Huang CLH (eds). Applied physiology for surgery and critical care. Butterworth-Heinemann Ltd, Oxford, 1995.pp. 677-87.
5. Robert S M. Severe sepsis and septic shock. In: Fauci AS, Braunwald E, Kasper DL, Hauser SL, Longo DL, Jameson JL, Loscalzo J (eds). Harrison's principles of internal medicine.17th edition. Mc Graw Hills, 2008. pp.1699-1782.
6. Acharya SP, Pradhan B, Marhatta MN. Application of "the Sequential Organ Failure Assessment (SOFA) score" in predicting outcome in ICU patients with SIRS. Kathmandu Univ Med J 2007;5:475-83.
7. Williams L, Gannon J. Use of the SOFA score in pandemic influenza — a prospective study. JICS, 2009;10:3,179-82.
8. Matthew RM, Scott TM, Marin H, et al. The Management of Severe Sepsis and Septic Shock. Infect Dis Clin N Am 2009;23:485-501.
9. Elizabeth J. Bridges, Susan D. Cardiovascular Aspects of Septic Shock: Pathophysiology, Monitoring and treatment. Crit Care Nurse 2005;25:14-40.
10. Mariana B, Batista, Augusto C, et al. Pressor response to fluid resuscitation in endotoxic shock: Involvement of vasopressin. Crit Care Med 2009;37:2968-72.
11. Havel C, Arrich J, Losert H, Gamper G, Müllner M, Herkner H. Vasopressors for hypotensive shock. Cochrane Database Syst Rev 2011;5:CD003709.
12. Mark GM. Pelvic inflammatory disease. In: John AR, Howard WJ (eds). Te Linde's Operative Gynecology 10th edn, Lippincott Williams & Wilkins, 2008. pp.660-86.
13. WHO, UNICEF, UNFPA World bank. Maternal mortality in 2005. Estimates developed by WHO, UNICEF, UNFPA, and the World Bank. WHO Geneva 2007.
14. MOH & FW report. Estimates of maternal mortality ratios in India and its states – A pilot study. ICMR, July 2003.

Chapter **39**

Management of Hyperglycemic and Normoglycemic Ketoacidosis in Diabetes Mellitus

Dinesh K Dhanwal, Sanjay Kumar

INTRODUCTION

Diabetic ketoacidosis (DKA) is a hyperglycemic emergency. It is commonly seen in Type 1 DM but may occur in Type 2 DM subjects as well. It is characterized by hyperglycemia (glucose > 250 mg/dL), acidosis (pH < 7.35), low serum bicarbonate, high anion gap and ketonuria. DKA is the result of absolute or relative deficiency of insulin and increase in the level of counter regulatory hormones. This leads to reduced cellular glucose uptake, an increased degree of lipolysis and proteolysis, the end-result being hyperglycemia, volume depletion and metabolic acidosis.

Gestational diabetes mellitus (GDM) is an increasingly recognized abnormality of glucose metabolism during pregnancy, which affects fetal development and leads to peripartum complications.[1-4] The prevalence of DKA in pregnant type 1 and type 2 diabetics was reported to be 9.3 percent.[5] The development DKA in pregnancy is an emergency, requiring treatment in an intensive care setting. Both the mother and the fetus are at risk for significant morbidity and mortality.[6] Occasionally ketosis or ketoacidosis during pregnancy can occur in setting of GDM or pre-existing diabetes with normal or not so high blood glucose. This condition has been recognized as euglycemic ketoacidosis.[7] This condition is seen commonly in type 1 diabetic patients.

Clinical Presentation

- In DKA, metabolic decompensation usually develops over a period of hours to a few days. Patients with DKA classically present with lethargy and a characteristic hyperventilation pattern with deep slow breaths (Kussmaul respirations) associated with the fruity odor of acetone.
- These patients often complain of nausea and vomiting, and abdominal pain is somewhat less frequent.
- The abdominal pain, when present, can be quite severe and may be associated with distention, ileus, and tenderness without rebound but usually resolves relatively quickly with therapy unless there is underlying abdominal pathology.
- Most patients are normotensive, tachycardic, and tachypneic and have signs of mild-to-moderate volume depletion.
- Hypothermia has been described in DKA, and patients with underlying infection might not manifest fever.
- Cerebral edema may occur occasionally during treatment of DKA.

- Patients with DKA can have stupor and obvious profound dehydration, and they often demonstrate focal neurologic deficits such as Babinski reflexes, asymmetrical reflexes, cranial nerve findings, paresis, fasciculations, and aphasia.
- The clinical presentation of diabetic ketoacidosis in pregnancy is similar to that of non-pregnant diabetics. Infection may or may not be apparent.

Laboratory Findings in DKA

Laboratory findings include acidemia, hyperglycemia, a raised anion gap, ketonemia, ketonuria, and renal dysfunction. However, a substantial minority may have glucose level less than 12 mmol/L. Fifteen percent of DKA patients present with blood glucose levels below 300 mg/dL.[8] Various reasons noted for this discrepancy include insulin pump use, administration of insulin on the way to the hospital, pregnancy, prolonged fasting and alcohol consumption. *Euglycemia does not rule out DKA and a high index of suspicion is required in the appropriate clinical setting.* Most of the euglycemic DKA patients are young well hydrated on insulin and facing an intercurrent illness. The exact cause of euglycemic ketoacidosis is unknown, but it is important to recognize the condition.

Precipitating Factors

The usual precipitating factors include:
- Intercurrent illness
- Infections especially of the urinary tract
- Emesis and dehydration
- Non-compliance, insulin pump failure
- Undiagnosed pregnancy
- Unrecognized new onset diabetes—Accounts for 30 percent of the cases of diabetic ketoacidosis.

In Indian context missing insulin dose or reducing insulin dose in type 1 DM may be responsible for ketoacidosis. A retrospective survey conducted by Rodgers and Rodgers to identify the precipitant of diabetic ketoacidosis in pregnant women, revealed non-compliance to be the cause in 17 percent and a contributory factor in a further 25 percent.[9]

Factors Contributing to Increased Risk of Diabetic Ketoacidosis in Pregnancy

Pregnancy in particular can predispose a patient to ketoacidosis in several ways.
- In the fasting state, the increased use of glucose by both the fetal and maternal units can lead relatively quickly to conversion to a catabolic metabolism.[10] This condition of accelerated starvation is further characterized by hypoinsulinemia, hypoglycemia and more importantly hyperketonemia and protein catabolism[11]
- Pregnancy-associated nausea and vomiting can contribute as well
- Relative respiratory alkalosis associated with increased alveolar minute-ventilation causes a compensatory increase in renal bicarbonate excretion. As a consequence, a deficit in buffering capacity develops, which becomes especially important in the presence of an acid load, as is the case in ketonemia.
- The production of diabetogenic hormones, such as human placental lactogen, prolactin and cortisol, increases over the course of gestation, thereby predisposing the patient to ketoacidosis.[12]
- During pregnancy, miscellaneous conditions, such as infection, beta-sympathomimetic therapy, and labor can increase endogenous catecholamine release, thereby contributing to the onset of diabetic ketoacidosis. β_2-agonists, used to suppress premature uterine contractions, cause an increase in blood glucose, free fatty acids and ketones through stimulation of gluconeogenesis, glycogenolysis, and activation of lipolysis leading to hyperglycemia and ketosis. Similarly, the use of corticosteroids in diabetic pregnancy for fetal lung maturation may worsen hyperglycemia and insulin resistance leading to ketosis.[13-14]

- In addition, it has been demonstrated that, during pregnancy, diabetic ketoacidosis can occur at glucose levels as low as 200 mg/dl.[15]

Effects of Diabetic Ketoacidosis on the Fetus

The precise effects of diabetic ketoacidosis on the fetus are unknown, although abnormal heart-rate patterns consistent with fetal acidosis have been reported. In severe cases of ketoacidosis, especially those associated with maternal coma, fetal demise is common.[16] Most series report good outcomes for the fetus, if it is alive upon presentation to the hospital and prompt, appropriate, maternal interventions are initiated.[17] The importance of continuous fetal heart-rate monitoring in this setting cannot be overemphasized. In cases of maternal diabetic ketoacidosis, a number of factors contribute to the development of fetal acidosis. Maternal hypovolemia and catecholamine excess may result in decreased uterine blood flow.[17] Fetal hyperinsulinemia, resulting from hyperglycemic conditions, will increase fetal oxygen demand. Maternal phosphate deficiency may deplete erythrocytes of 2,3-diphosphoglycerate, thereby impairing oxygen delivery to the fetus. Hyperglycemia has been shown to decrease myocardial contractility in animal models. Finally, maternal metabolic acidosis and electrolyte disturbances will be directly reflected in the fetal compartment. For example, fetal cardiac arrest has been reported in connection with severe, maternal hypokalemia.[18]

CASE SCENARIOS

Case Scenario-1
A 35-year-old fourth gravida is admitted to the labor room in early labor. She is a known case of gestational diabetes controlled on insulin mixtard 20 units in morning and 16 units at night. Her blood glucose level as tested by glucometer is 120 mg/dL and bed side test for urinary ketones with ketostix showed "large ketones". Examination revealed mild dehydration. There was no acidosis.

Case Scenario-2
A 50-year-old known Type 2 DM patient undergoes hysterectomy for endometrial cancer. Preoperatively her glycemic control was good on oral hypoglycemic agents. On second postoperative day her blood glucose level as tested by glucometer is 320 mg/dL and bed side test for urinary ketones with ketostix showed "moderate ketones". She had a low pH with hypokalemic and hyponatremia.

Differential Diagnosis

Not all patients with hyperglycemia and an anion gap metabolic acidosis have DKA, and other causes of metabolic acidosis must be considered in these patients, particularly if the serum or urine ketone measurements are not elevated. These are lactic acidosis, starvation ketosis, alcoholic ketoacidosis, uremic acidosis, and toxic ingestions especially salicylate intoxication, methanol and ethylene glycol.

INVESTIGATIONS

The first thing to get is the usual laboratory parameters like blood urea, creatinine, serum sodium, potassium, and chloride, blood sugar random, urinary ketones and arterial blood gas analysis. The key feature of DKA is acidosis, and the serum HCO_3 concentration is usually less than 10 mEq/L.

Next thing to calculate is the anion gap which is the index of unmeasured anions in the blood (normal <14 mEq/L)

Anion gap = sodium - (chloride + bicarbonate)

Most patients with DKA present with an anion gap greater than 20 mEq/L, and some present with a gap greater than 40 mEq/L.

Patients with DKA almost invariably have large amounts of ketones in their urine. The serum glucose in DKA is usually around 500 mg/dL. However, an entity known as euglycemic DKA as described earlier occurs, particularly in the presence of decreased oral intake or in pregnancy, in which the serum glucose is normal or near normal. These patient require insulin therapy for the clearance of ketoacidosis.[19] The arterial pH is commonly less than 7.3 and can be as low as 6.5.

MANAGEMENT

Diabetic ketoacidosis is an emergency that demands prompt and vigorous treatment in a high dependency unit under combined medical and obstetric care to reduce the maternal and fetal mortality. Treatment includes aggressive volume replacement, insulin infusion, careful attention to electrolytes, and a search for and correction of precipitating factors.[21] The initial fluid deficit is higher than that of nonpregnant diabetic ketoacidosis. Acidosis occurs at lower glucose levels than in nonpregnant patients. This necessitate simultaneous dextrose infusion to enable insulin treatment.

Fluid Replacement

After initial evaluations and investigations one must quickly assess the hydration status and calculate the amount of fluid required by the patient. When there is physical evidence of dehydration—that is, hypotension, decreased skin turgor, or dry mucous membranes—generally administer 1 L of normal saline over the first hour and 200 to 500 mL/hour in subsequent hours until hypotension resolves and adequate circulation is maintained. If hypotension is severe, there is clinical evidence of hypoperfusion, and hypotension does not respond to crystalloid, therapy with colloid is considered, often in combination with invasive hemodynamic monitoring. If there is no hypotension and no concern about renal failure, administer 1 L of half-normal saline over the first hour.

Remember that glucose is osmotically active and there is free water clearance from the kidneys and thus the measured sodium is erroneously low and needs to be corrected by the below formula before the exact water deficit is calculated.

Corrected sodium concentration = measured sodium + 0.016 × (glucose - 100)

Water deficit in liters = 0.6 x weight in kg × [(sodium/140) - 1]

Hence an 80 kg pregnant woman with a serum sodium of 140mEq/L and glucose concentration of 600 mg/dL will have a water deficit of 2.74L. When the serum glucose reaches 250 - 400 mg/dL, all fluids should contain 5 percent dextrose and therapy should be aimed at maintaining the serum glucose in that range for 24 hours to allow slow equilibration of osmotically active substances across cell membranes.

While cerebral edema is a theoretical risk of diabetic ketoacidosis, especially in children, its association with aggressive fluid replacement has not been consistently proven.[20,21] It has been found to happen in children who have received sodium bicarbonate for acidosis.

Insulin

- When starting insulin, give a priming dose of 5-10-U of intravenous (IV) insulin to saturate the insulin receptors fully before beginning continuous therapy and to avoid the lag time necessary to achieve steady-state insulin levels.
- The continuous therapy should begin with a low-dose insulin infusion (0.1 U/kg or 0.05 U/kg per hour). Prepare the infusate by adding 50-U of regular insulin in 500 ml of normal saline. With this low dose continuous infusion one expects to lower the glucose by 10 to 15 percent or 50 to 100 mg/dL in an hour.
- If it does not fall at this rate then increase the rate by 50 percent to 100 percent and a second bolus of intravenous insulin should be administered. If the fall is more than 100 mg/dL then decrease the rate by 50 to 100 percent. After the glucose reaches approximately 250 mg/dL, it is prudent to decrease the insulin infusion rate and administer dextrose from the other intravenous site while continuing the insulin infusion.

- Further titration of insulin infusion is done based upon the hourly blood glucose monitoring as given in the protocol (see below).
- Insulin infusion must be continued for an additional 12 to 24 hours to clear ketones from the circulation after the hyperglycemia is controlled. With resolution of ketosis, the rate of infusion approaches the physiologic range of 0.3 to 0.5 U/kg per day.
- When the decision is made to feed the patient, the patient should be switched from intravenous or intramuscular therapy to subcutaneous therapy. Subcutaneous insulin should be administered before a meal and the insulin drip discontinued approximately 30 minutes later. The glucose should be checked in 2 hours and at least every 4 hours subsequently until a relatively stable insulin regimen is determined. Early conversion to oral feeding and subcutaneous insulin therapy is associated with a shorter hospital stay.

Potassium

- Once the fluid and insulin is given the potassium levels go down in blood as it is driven back into the cells. Hence the initially high serum potassium will fall dramatically if not replaced immediately with intravenous supplement. It is necessary to anticipate this and start potassium replacement as soon as possible. It has been observed that the potassium losses in DKA is quite high (3-10 mEq/kg). If the serum potassium is less than 5.5 mEq/L, give potassium chloride 1 ampoule (which contains 20 mEq of potassium) in one of the ongoing normal saline over 1 to 2 hours.
- If the patient is oliguric, do not administer potassium unless the serum concentration is less than 4 mEq/L, and even then potassium is administered with extreme caution.
- *Remember not to give replacement very fast as it may lead to arrhythmias.*
- There is a limit to the amount one can replace through a peripheral IV line, i.e. not more than 10 to 20 mEq/hr, however higher replacement can be given via a central line, i.e. 40 to 60 mEq/hr.
- Measure serum potassium every 2 hours initially then every 6 hourly and then decide the rate of replacement.

Bicarbonate

The serum bicarbonate will always be low in DKA, but the use of bicarbonate for treatment is very controversial. When treatment is started for DKA the ketoacids and lactate anions are metabolized to bicarbonate, hence no need to give bicarbonate from outside. However in severe acidosis (pH < 6.9), or patients with hemodynamic instability if the pH is less than 7.1, or patient with hyperkalemia, one can give bicarbonate. About 1 mEq/kg of bicarbonate is administered as a rapid infusion over 10 to 15 minutes, and further therapy is based on repeated arterial blood gases every 30 to 120 minutes. Potassium therapy should be considered before treatment with bicarbonate because transient hypokalemia is not an uncommon complication of the administration of alkali.

Identify the Precipitating Factor

Always search for the underlying cause, although pregnancy itself may precipitate DKA. Careful history and physical examination is very crucial in making strategy of further diagnosis and treatment. Most common cause of DKA is noncompliance with insulin therapy, while the second most common cause is infection of which viral syndromes, urinary tract infection, pelvic inflammatory disease, and pneumonia predominate. One must actively look for infection in the body since the usual signs and symptoms and even the laboratory data are misleading. Fever may be absent, while the total leukocyte count may well be within normal levels. As a result cultures should be performed for most patients and empiric antibiotic coverage should be considered pending reports.

Patients with altered sensorium needs special attention since it may be due to DKA itself or meningitis, or meningoencephalitis. One should have very low threshold for doing a lumbar puncture in these patients. Pneumonia is difficult to diagnose as X-ray may be normal initially because of dehydration and lack of alveolar edema. Serum amylase level will be misleadingly elevated in DKA and one should rely on serum lipase level to diagnose pancreatitis.

Monitoring and Complications

Initial evaluation should contain basic laboratory parameters like serum glucose, electrolytes, BUN, creatinine, ketones, lactate, creatine phosphokinase, and liver function tests as well as urinalysis, ECG, upright chest radiograph with abdominal shield, complete blood count, and arterial blood gases. Initially blood glucose is monitored every hour and once stable, then every two hours. Electrolytes and acid base gas analysis is done atleast once in 6 hours and more frequently if situation demands. Urine ketones are checked every 4–6 hours.

Fetal Monitoring

Continuous fetal monitoring is mandatory to assess fetal wellbeing. A non-reactive fetal heart tracing, repetitive late decelerations, or a non-reassuring biophysical profile may be present indicating some degree of fetal compromise in the ketoacidotic patient but they are not necessarily indications for immediate delivery. *Subjecting a patient in diabetic ketoacidosis to emergency caesarean section could cause further maternal deterioration while offering minimal, if any, benefit to the fetus.* Interestingly, once hyperglycemia and acidosis is reversed and maternal stabilization achieved, fetal compromise may no longer be evident. If preterm labor occurs, magnesium sulfate is the tocolytic of choice and β_2-agonists are relatively contraindicated. In essence, an approach that incorporates in utero resuscitation with maternal stabilization, hydration, and reversal of hyperglycemia and metabolic acidosis under combined medical and obstetric supervision is the cornerstone of management of this condition.

Treatment in the given cases:

In the case histories given above Case-1 has euglycemic ketosis and Case-2 has hyperglycemia with ketoacidosis The management of euglycemic ketoacidosis is on similar lines except that these patients will need glucose insulin infusion at lower doses. These patients have less dehydration and acidosis as compared to hyperglycemic DKA.

The protocol used in our institution is based upon Staged Diabetes Management. In our experience we find this protocol as an effective tool to treat subjects with diabetic ketoacidosis and hyperglycemic emergencies.[22,23]

Both the case scenarios listed above can be treated using this protocol in ICU setting. All these patients should be treated with insulin infusion as per protocol with hourly blood glucose monitoring in beginning but once blood glucose is in target range then one can monitor blood glucose once in 2 to 3 hours. These subjects should also have frequent (at least every 6 hourly) electrolyte monitoring.

PROTOCOL FOR MANAGING DIABETIC KETOACIDOSIS

START IV INSULIN THERAPY

Step 1: Prepare IV Insulin

- 100 units regular insulin/100 mL normal saline or 50 units in 520 mL saline
- Flush all tubing with IV insulin solution

Step 2: Determine Starting Insulin Infusion Rate and Basal Insulin Dose

- 0.05 units/kg/hr for BG 200-600 mg/dL
- 0.1 units/kg/hr if BG >600 mg/dL (and for DKA or HHS)

For patients on insulin regimen prior to admission:
- Hold usual regular or rapid acting insulin doses
- Calculate basal insulin dose to be given subcutaneously in addition to insulin infusion based on basal insulin dose prior to admission

For patients using detemir/glargine:
- Administer 100 percent of current detemir/glargine dose subcutaneously every AM or PM

For patients using two injections of NPH:
- Administer 50 percent of current NPH AM dose and 100 percent of current NPH PM dose every AM and bedtime respectively.

Step 3: Monitor Blood Glucose and Adjust Insulin Infusion Rate as Required

- Target BG 70-140 mg/dL and adjust insulin infusion rate accordingly
- Monitor BG hourly until insulin infusion unchanged for 2 readings, thereafter monitor every 2 hrs.
- If BG decreases <100 mg/dL since last reading, reduce the rate of insulin infusion to half.

Blood Glucose	Action
<70 mg/dL	Give 1 ampoule 50% dextrose IV, reduce the rate of insulin infusion to half, recheck BG in 30 min
70-100 mg/dL	No change in infusion unless BG decreases by > 10 mg/dL since last reading, then decrease infusion 1 unit/hr
101-140 mg/dL	No change in infusion unless BG decreases by > 10 mg/dL since last reading, then decrease infusion by 0.5 unit/hr
141-200 mg/dL	Increase infusion 0.5 units/hr unless BG decreases > 10-20 mg/dL since last reading, then hold increase in infusion rate; if BG decreases > 20mg/dL since last reading, decrease infusion 0.5 units/hr
201-300 mg/dL	Increase infusion 1 unit/hr unless BG decreases >20-40 mg/dL since last reading, then hold increase in infusion; if BG decreases by > 40 mg/dL since last reading decrease infusion 1 unit/hr
>300 mg/dL	Increase infusion 2 units/hr unless BG decreases >40 mg/dL since last reading, then hold increase in infusion.

CONCLUSION

Hyperglycemic emergency whether associated with ketoacidosis or without is a frequent emergency encountered in obstetrics and gynecology. This condition should be treated in ICU setting as a team comprising of obstetrician/gynecologist, physician/diabetologist and dietician. It is important to follow an individualized protocol to treat this condition to reduce associated morbidity and mortality.

KEY POINTS

- DKA is a hyperglycemic emergency characterized by hyperglycemia, acidosis, low serum bicarbonate, high anion gap and ketonuria.
- Occasionally ketoacidosis during pregnancy in gestational diabetics or pre-existing diabetics may occur with normal or not so high blood glucose levels (euglycemic ketoacidosis).
- Important precipitating factors in pregnancy are non-compliance to insulin therapy, infection, administration of beta sympathomimetic agents and corticosteroids for fetal lung maturity.
- Treatment of DKA includes aggressive fluid replacement, insulin infusion, electrolyte correction and correction of the precipitating factors.

REFERENCES

1. Kitabchi AE, Umpierrez GE, Fisher JN, Murphy MB, Stentz FB. Thirty years of personal experience in hyperglycemic crises: diabetic ketoacidosis and hyperglycemic hyperosmolar state. J Clin Endocrinol Metab 2008;93:1541-52.
2. Kitabchi AE, Umpierrez GE, Murphy MB, et al. Management of hyperglycemic crises in patients with diabetes. Diabetes Care 2004;27:S94-102.
3. Maislos M, Harman-Bohem I, Weitzman S. Diabetic ketoacidosis. A rare complication of gestational diabetes. Diabetes Care 1992;15:968-70.
4. Carroll MA, Yeomans ER. Diabetic ketoacidosis in pregnancy. Crit Care Med 2005;33:S347-53.
5. Cousins L. Pregnancy complications among diabetic women: review 1965-1985. Obstet Gynecol Surv 1987;42:140-9.
6. Handisurya A, Bancher-Todesca D, Schober E, Klein K, Tobler K, Schneider B, et al. Risk factor profile and pregnancy outcome in women with type 1 and type 2 diabetes mellitus. J Women's Health 2011;20:263-71.
7. Chico M, Levine SN, Lewis DF. Normoglycemic diabetic ketoacidosis in pregnancy. J Perinatol 2008;28:310-2.
8. Cook CB, Elias B, Kongable GL, Potter DJ, Shepherd KM, McMahon D. Diabetes and hyperglycemia quality improvement efforts in hospitals in the United States: current status, practice variation, and barriers to implementation. Endocr Pract 2010;16:219-30.
9. Rodgers BD, Rodgers DE. Clinical variables associated with diabetic ketoacidosis in pregnancy. J Reprod Med 1991;32:797-800.
10. Metzger BE, Freinkel N. Effects of diabetes mellitus on endocrinologic and metabolic adaptations of gestation. Semin Perinatol 1978;2:309-15.
11. Metzger BE, Vilesis RA, Ravnikar V, et al. "Accelerated starvation" and the skipped breakfast in late normal pregnancy. Lancet 1982;1:588-92.
12. Kallkhoff RK, Kissebah AH, Kim HJ. Carbohydrate and lipid metabolism during normal pregnancy: Relationship to gestational hormone action. Semin Perinatol 1978;2:291-94.
13. Bedalov A, Balasubramanyam A. Glucocorticoid-induced ketoacidosis in gestational diabetes: sequlae of acute treatment of preterm labor. Diabetes Care 1997;20:922-4.
14. Bernstein IM, Catalano PM. Ketoacidosis in pregnancy associated with the parenteral administration of terbutaline and betamethasone: a case report. J Reprod Med 1990;35:818-20.
15. Clark JDA, McConnell A, Hartog M. Normoglycemic ketoacidosis in a woman with gestational diabetes. Diabetic Med 1991;8:388-89.
16. Balsells M, García-Patterson A, Gich I, Corcoy R. Maternal and fetal outcome in women with type 2 versus type 1 diabetes mellitus: a systematic review and metaanalysis. J Clin Endocrinol Metab 2009;94:4284-91.
17. Savage MW. Management of diabetic ketoacidosis. Clin Med 2011;11:154-6.
18. Bard H, Fouron JC, De Muylder X, Ducharme G, Lafond JS. Myocardial function and hemoglobin oxygen affinity during hyperglycemia in the fetal lamb. J Clin Invest 1986;78:191-5.
19. Hoorn EJ, Zietse R. Cerebral oedema in adult diabetic ketoacidosis: the importance of effective serum osmolality. Neth J Med 2010;68:439.
20. Krane EJ. Diabetic ketoacidosis and cerebral edema. Available at: http://PedsCCM.wustl.edu/FILE-CABINET/Metab/DKA-CEdema.html.
21. Foster DW, McGarry JD. The metabolic derangements and treatment of diabetic ketoacidosis. N Engl J Med 1983;309:159-69.
22. Pearson J, Powers MA. Systematically initiating insulin: the staged diabetes management approach. Diabetes Educ 2006;32:19S-28S.
23. Varroud-Vial M, Simon D, Attali J, Durand-Zaleski I, Bera L, Attali C, Letondeur C, Strauss K, Petit C, Charpentier G. Improving glycaemic control of patients with Type 2 diabetes in a primary care setting: a French application of the Staged Diabetes Management programme. Diabet Med 2004;21:592-8.

Chapter 40

Acid Base Balance and Common Electrolyte Abnormalities

Anju Bhalotra, Gunjan Manchanda, Raktima Anand

INTRODUCTION

As a consequence of underlying diseases and therapeutic manipulations, surgical patients may develop potentially harmful disorders of acid-base equilibrium, intra and extravascular volume and serum electrolytes. Precise perioperative management of acid-base status, fluids, and electrolytes may limit perioperative morbidity and mortality. However, the usefulness of arterial blood gas (ABG) analysis is dependent on the ability to correctly interpret and diagnose the results.

Acidemia/ alkalemia: Refers to H^+ state or pH.
- Acidemia is an ↑ in H^+ and a ↓ in arterial pH
- Alkalemia is a ↓ in H^+ and an ↑ in arterial pH

Acidosis/alkalosis: A pathologic process that tends to accumulate acid or alkali but does not necessarily produce a pH change.

pH: Term used to define the acidity/alkalinity of solutions; is the negative logarithm of H^+ concentration.

All acid-base abnormalities result from alterations in the dissociation of water; only three factors independently affect acid-base balance.[1]
- Pa_{CO_2}
- Strong ion difference (SID)
- Total concentration of weak acids (A_{TOT})

Why do we order an ABG?

- To help establish a diagnosis.
- Guides treatment plans and ventilator management.
- An improvement in acid base status allows optimal functioning of medications.
- Correction of acid base disturbances may help correct dyselectrolytemias.

PROPER SAMPLING AND HANDLING FOR ABG

Proper sampling and handling is essential for obtaining accurate results.
Prior to sampling ensure:
- Proper patient identification.
- Correct type and amount of anticoagulant.

- Adequate stabilization of the patient's respiratory condition.
- Adequate removal of flush solution from arterial line.

During Sampling and Handling

- Mixing with venous blood may lead to errors.
- Avoid air bubbles in sample.
- Ensure sufficient mixing with heparin- mix the sample by inverting the syringe 10 times and rolling between palms.

During Storage

- Correct storage
- Prevent hemolysis— do not cool the sample if it can be analyzed within 30 mins; if analysis is likely to be delayed, store sample using a glass syringe and ice slurry.

For Anticoagulation

- Use heparin coated syringes
- Liquid heparin 0.05 mL/mL blood (dead space of a 5 mL syringe with 22G needle = 0.2 mL sufficient for 4 mL blood). Smaller sample leads to a dilution effect due to relatively larger volume of heparin; values of plasma electrolytes, $PaCO_2$, blood sugar and hematocrit (Hct) decrease linearly with dilution whereas pH and PaO_2 are relatively unaffected.

APPROACH FOR INTERPRETATION OF ABG

Verify Accuracy of the Data[2]

i. Henderson Hasselbach Equation;
   $pH = pK + \log HCO_3^-/H_2CO_3$
   (Bunsen solubility coefficient for CO_2; 0.03 mm/L/mm Hg; $H_2CO_3 = PaCO_2 \times .03$
   If $PaCO_2$ is 40, $H_2CO_3 = 0.03 \times 40 = 1.2$ mmol/L)
   $7.4 = 6.1 + \log (24/1.2) = 6.1+1.3 = 7.4$

ii. Modified Henderson equation;
   $H^+ \times HCO_3^- = 24 \times PaCO_2$
   The H^+ is calculated by subtracting the last two digits of pH from 80; if pH is 7.23, then H^+ is 80-23= 57

Obtain a Relevant Clinical History

Indicates the likely etiology of the acid base disorder (Table 40.1).

Check Oxygenation Status (Table 40.2)

- See PaO_2; normal value- 95-100 mm Hg on room air
  (FiO_2 i.e. fraction of inspired $O_2 = 0.21$)
- Always see PaO_2 in relation to FiO_2 and age of patient.
  $PaO_2 = 5 \times FiO_2$
  $PaO_2 = 100 - 0.3 \times$ age (years) mm Hg
- *Hypoxia* is lack of O_2 availability at the tissue level
- *Hypoxemia* is a lack of O_2 in blood.

Check Ventilation Status

See $PaCO_2$

Table 40.1: Common acid base disturbances	
Clinical state	*Acid base disorder*
Pulmonary embolus	Respiratory alkalosis
Hypotension	Metabolic acidosis
Vomiting	Metabolic alkalosis
Severe diarrhea	Metabolic acidosis
Cirrhosis	Respiratory alkalosis
Diuretic use	Metabolic alkalosis
Sepsis	Respiratory alkalosis, metabolic acidosis
Pregnancy	Respiratory alkalosis
COPD	Respiratory acidosis
Renal failure	Metabolic acidosis

Table 40.2: PaO_2 and oxygenation status		
	PaO_2 (mm Hg)	*Oxyhemoglobin Saturation SaO_2 (%)*
Normal range	> or = 80 mm Hg	> or = 95%
Mild hypoxaemia	60-79 mm Hg	90-94 %
Moderate hypoxaemia	40-59 mm Hg	75-89 %
Severe hypoxaemia	< 40 mm Hg	< 75 %

Assess Acid Base Status

1. See pH to identify primary disorder
   - pH< 7.4 → acidemia
   - pH >7.4 → alkalemia
2. Look at $PaCO_2$ (respiratory acid)
   - >40 mm Hg → respiratory acidosis
   - < 40 mm Hg → respiratory alkalosis.

If this explains the pH change it is a respiratory disorder
Otherwise see HCO_3^- (decreased in acidosis and increased in alkalosis); if it explains pH change it is a metabolic disorder.

Type of Disorder

1. *Simple acid-base disorders:* common clinical disturbances; pH is abnormal, compensation is incomplete
   Examples are -
   - Metabolic acidosis
   - Respiratory acidosis
   - Metabolic alkalosis
   - Respiratory alkalosis

   If pH and $PaCO_2$ move in opposite directions and $PaCO_2$ is abnormal → Respiratory
   If pH and $PaCO_2$ move in same direction (normally should not) → Metabolic

   Primary respiratory disturbances → compensatory metabolic response
   Primary metabolic disturbances → compensatory respiratory response[2]
2. *Mixed acid-base disturbances:* are independently coexisting disorders seen in critically ill patients with extreme changes in pH.[3]
   - If HCO_3 and $PaCO_2$ move in opposite directions (normally should not) – MIXED
   - If trend of change in HCO_3 and $PaCO_2$ is similar check the percent difference from normal. The one with the greater % difference is the dominant disorder.[2]

- e.g. pH- 7.20, HCO^-_3 20, $paCO_2$ - 55 (both respiratory and metabolic acidosis)
  % change from normal for HCO^-_3 = 24-20/24 % = 4/24 x100= 16.66 %
  % change from normal for $PaCO_2$ = 55-40/40 % = 15/40 x 100= 37.5%
  Thus the predominant disorder is respiratory acidosis

  Primary acid- base abnormalities are summarized in Table 40.3.

RESPIRATORY DISORDERS

CAUSES OF RESPIRATORY ACIDOSIS

- *Central:* Drugs (anesthetics, morphine, sedatives), stroke, infection
- *Airway:* Obstruction, asthma
- *Parenchyma:* Emphysema, bronchitis, ARDS, barotrauma
- *Neuromuscular:* Polio, kyphoscolioisis, myasthenia, muscle dystrophy
- *Miscellaneous:* Obesity, hypoventilation, permissive hypercapnia

CAUSES OF RESPIRATORY ALKALOSIS

- *CNS stimulation:* Anxiety, pain, psychosis, fever, CVA, meningitis, tumor, trauma
- *Hypoxia:* High altitude, pneumonia, pulmonary edema, aspiration, severe anemia
- *Drugs or hormones:* Pregnancy, progesterone, salicylates,
- *Stimulation of chest receptors:* Hemothorax, flail chest, pulmonary embolism, cardiac failure
- *Miscellaneous;* mechanical hyperventilation, sepsis, hepatic coma, heat exposure, recovery from metabolic acidosis

If primary disorder is thought to be respiratory, correlate with history and clinical presentation:
1. Is the disorder acute or chronic?
2. What is the alveolar arterial oxygen gradient [(A-a)DO_2]?
3. Is there any compensation?
1. **Assess if disorder is acute or chronic**
2. **(A-a) DO_2 gradient;**
   Normal (A-a) O_2 gradient = 5 to 25 mm Hg
   Alveolar air equation; $P_AO_2 = PiO_2 - PaCO_2/RQ$
   $P_AO_2 = (P_B-P_{H2O}) FiO_2 - PaCO_2/RQ$
   P_{H2O} = 47 mmHg; RQ= respiratory quotient= 0.8
   (PiO_2 = inspired PO_2, P_AO_2 = alveolar PO_2, P_B = barometre pressure)
   In hypoxemic respiratory failure → gradient is normal (10-15 mm Hg) or increased
   If < 20→ extrapulmonary cause of respiratory failure

Table 40.3: Classification of primary acid-base abnormalities[1]

Disorder	Acidosis	Alkalosis
Respiratory	↑ $PaCO_2$	↓ $PaCO_2$
Metabolic		
Abnormal SID		
a. Water excess/deficit	Water excess/dilutional/ ↓ Na^+ (↓ SID)	Water deficit/contraction/ ↑ Na^+ (↑ SID)
b. Electrolytes	↑ Cl^- (↓ SID)	↓ Cl^- (↑ SID)
c. Unmeasured anions (UMA)	↑ Lactate & keto acids ; ↑ UMA^- (↓ SID)	-
Abnormal A_{TOT}		
Albumin [Al]	↑ [Alb] rare)	↓ [Alb]
Phosphate [Pi]	↑ [Pi]	-

Table 40.4: Compensation in Respiratory Disorders		
Acute Respiratory Acidosis	The 1 for 10 Rule	Acute 10 mm Hg ↑ $PaCO_2 \rightarrow$ 1 mmol/L ↑ in HCO_3^-
Chronic Respiratory Acidosis	The 4 for 10 Rule	Chronic 10 mm Hg ↑ $PaCO_2 \rightarrow$ 4 mmol/L ↑ in HCO_3^-
Acute Respiratory Alkalosis	The 2 for 10 Rule	Acute 10 mm Hg ↓ $PaCO_2 \rightarrow$ 2 mmol/L ↓ in HCO_3^-
Chronic Respiratory Alkalosis	The 5 for 10 Rule	Chronic 10 mm Hg ↓ $PaCO_2 \rightarrow$ 5 mmol/L ↓ in HCO_3^-

3. **Compensation for pH changes (Table 40.4):**
   * Depends upon proper functioning of lungs, kidneys and the severity of the acid base disturbance.
   * Acute compensation takes 6-24 hours and chronic compensation takes 1-4 days.
   * Respiratory compensation is faster than metabolic.
   * In clinical practice it is rare to see complete compensation.
   * Usually only a 50-75% return of pH to normal is seen, except in chronic respiratory alkalosis where a complete compensation may be seen.
     a. A **Buffer** is a weak acid which reversibly binds H^+ ions and effectively neutralizes them.
        * A buffer can accept or donate H+ ions and modifies pH changes.
        * Buffering of H^+ ions in blood is rapid (1-3 minutes) but incomplete.
        * It is the first line of defence and includes the HCO_3^-, Hb, protein and PO_4 buffers.
     b. **Ventilatory responses:**
        * Prompt increases or decreases in alveolar ventilation.
        * Respiratory compensation is faster but is often incomplete.
     c. **Renal responses:**
        * Kidneys are the most powerful of the acid base regulatory systems.
        * Renal compensation is slow to act (6-12 hours) but continues until the pH almost returns to 7.4.
        * Respiratory acidosis/alkalosis is compensated for by renal induced changes in serum HCO_3^- that serve to maintain a 20:1 ratio of HCO_3^- to CO_2.
        * Regulate H^+ ion concentration by acidification or alkalinization of urine.
        * Reabsorption of HCO_3^- from glomerular filtrate is essentially complete. Renal excretion of HCO_3^- does not occur until plasma $HCO_3^- > 26$ mEq/L.

METABOLIC DISORDERS

SID is the absolute difference between completely disassociated anions and cations.
$SID = (Na^+ + K^+ + Mg^{2+} + Ca^{2+}) - (Cl^- + A^-) = 40$ to 44 mEq/L
* This represents a net positive charge and is called the **SID apparent**.
* The counterbalancing negative charge is called the **effective SID** ; comes from HCO_3^-, poorly disassociated anions and disassociated weak acids, i.e. albumin, PO_4, SO_4.
* Numerically, this is equal to the traditional **buffer base.**

BUFFER BASE is a measure of the concentration of all the buffers present in either plasma or blood. It is represented by the sum of HCO_3^- and the nonvolatile buffer ions (serum albumin, PO_4, hemoglobin).

Applying the law of electric neutrality, the buffer base is forced to equal the electric charge difference between strong (fully dissociated) ions.

A_{TOT} is the total plasma concentration of weak nonvolatile acids, inorganic PO_4, serum proteins and albumin.

The **ANION GAP** is the contribution to electric neutrality ascribed to weak acids (PO_4 and albumin) and unmeasured anions.

$$AG = Na^+ + K^+ - (Cl^- + HCO_3^-) = 12 \pm 4$$

However most critically ill patients are hypoalbuminemic, and many are also hypophosphatemic. Consequently, the gap may be normal in the presence of unmeasured anions.

"Corrected AG"= calculated AG + 2.5 (normal alb – observed alb)

METABOLIC ACIDOSIS

In metabolic acidosis pH < 7.35 ; hypobicarbonatemia < 21 mEq/L. It occurs due to:
- Accumulation of an acid in the body other than CO_2
- Buffering of endogenous or exogenous acid loads by bicarbonate
- An abnormal external loss of bicarbonate.
- Also anything that decreases the SID acidifies the solution.

Causes of Metabolic Acidosis

1. An ↑ in the endogenous acid production (lactate, ketoacids): addition of H^+
   - Anerobic glycolysis, metabolism of aminoacids in TPN, idiopathic, lactic acidosis, renal acidosis, ketoacidosis
2. Loss of bicarbonate (HCO_3^-)
   - Severe diarrhea
   - Renal tubular acidosis (RTA)
   - Hyperchloremic acidosis (↓ HCO_3^- by ECF volume expansion →Dilutional Acidosis)
     a. Large volumes of crystalloids like 5% dextrose, normal saline (NS), mannitol
     b. Mechanical ventilation → ↑ antinatriuretic hormone (ANH) and antidiuretic hormone (ADH) → increased total body water (TBW).
     c. Carbonic anhydrase (CA) inhibitors
3. Accumulation of endogenous acids (kidneys unable to excrete dietary H^+ load)
   - Renal failure, cirrhosis (decreased conversion of lactate to glucose)

Causes of Increased AG Metabolic Acidosis (MUDPILES)

1. Methanol
2. Uremia
3. Diabetic ketoacidosis (DKA)
4. Paraldehyde
5. Iron
6. INH
7. Lactic acidosis
8. Ethylene glycol
9. Salicylates

Causes of Normal AG Metabolic Acidosis

GIT loss of HCO_3^-: Diarrhea , urinary diversion; Small bowel, pancreatic, or bile drainage; fistulae, surgical drains
Renal loss of HCO_3^- : RTA, recovery phase of ketoacidosis, renal insufficiency
Acidifying Substances- :HCl, NH_4Cl, arginine HCl, lysine HCl
Dilutional acidosis

Compensation in Metabolic Acidosis

Compensatory responses result in a fall in $PaCO_2$, restoration of the HCO_3^-/H_2CO_3 ratio to normal and a ↑ pH (although concentrations of HCO_3^- and H_2CO_3 are lower than normal).

Occurs by the following mechanism:
1. *Extracellular buffering:* Immediately
2. *Respiratory compensation:* Within minutes; results in ↑ alveolar ventilation due to stimulation of carotid bodies by H^+ ions.
   The ventilatory response to a metabolic acidosis will reduce $PaCO_2$ to a level defined by the following equations;
   The One & a Half plus 8 Rule for Metabolic Acidosis
   $$\text{Expected } PaCO_2 = (1.5 \times HCO_3^-) + (8 +/- 2)$$
   OR $\quad\quad\quad \Delta PaCO_2 = 1.3 \, \Delta HCO_3^-$
3. *Intracellular and bone buffering:* Within hours
4. *Renal excretion of the H^+ ion load:* Over hours to days i.e. renal tubular secretion of H^+ ions into urine and retention of HCO_3^-

METABOLIC ALKALOSIS

- Acute metabolic alkalosis is unusual
- There is an alkalemic pH >7.45 and $HCO_3^- > 27.0$ mEq/L.
- Due to loss of H^+ and excess of base.
- Anything that increases the SID alkalinizes the solution
- As the normal kidney can excrete HCO_3^- loads of up to 10 mEq/kg/day, for metabolic alkalosis to persist there must be both a process that elevates its serum levels and a stimulus for renal reabsorption.
- The former is usually acid loss from the stomach or kidney, and the last due to hypovolemia with a Cl⁻ deficit, hypokalemia or an increase in mineralocorticoid activity.
- Maintenance of metabolic alkalosis depends on a continued stimulus, such as renal hypoperfusion, hypokalemia, hypochloremia, or hypovolemia.[4]

The HCO_3^-/H_2CO_3 ratio rises as does the pH, but there is no rise in $PaCO_2$ – this is called uncompensated metabolic alkalosis.

Causes of Metabolic Alkalosis (Table 40.5)

Table 40.5: Causes of Metabolic Alkalosis		
Generation	*Example*	*Maintenance*
I. Loss of acid from ECF		
a. Loss of gastric fluid	Vomiting, NG drainage	↓ effective arterial volume (EAV)
b. Loss of acid in urine	Primary aldosteronism	K⁺ depletion & aldosterone
	Diuretics	excess; ↓ EAV & K⁺ depletion
II. Excessive HCO_3^- loads		
a. Absolute		
1. HCO_3^-	NaHCO₃- administration	↓ EAV
2. Metabolic conversion of salts of organic acid anions to HCO_3^-	Lactate, acetate, citrate administration	
b. Relative		
1. Alkaline loads in renal failure	Alkali administration to pts with renal failure	Renal failure
2. Posthypercapnia	Abrupt correction of chronic hypercapnia	↓ EAV
III. Contraction alkalosis	Profuse sweating, fever, dehydration, oozing tissues, inadequately humidified ventilator, polyuric renal failure, diabetes insipidus	↓ EAV

The "GAP-GAP" or **Delta Anion Gap;** to detect a mixed disorder
- Assess the elevation of the AG relative to the ↓ in HCO_3^-.
- Normal value is 1-1.6
- < 1 indicates the presence of concomitant non anion gap metabolic acidosis.
- > 1.6 indicates the presence of concomitant metabolic alkalosis.

Compensation in Metabolic Alkalosis

- There is increased reabsorption and decreased secretion of H^+ ions by renal tubular cells.
- There is alveolar hypoventilation. However respiratory compensation for pure metabolic alkalosis (in contrast to metabolic acidosis) is never more than 75% complete.
- The Point Seven plus Twenty Rule for a Metabolic Alkalosis
- Expected $PaCO_2 = (0.7 \times HCO_3^-) + (21 +/- 2)$
  OR $\Delta PaCo_2 = 0.75 \, \Delta HCO_3^-$
- A $PaCO_2 > 55$ mm Hg is beyond the normal compensatory mechanism for metabolic alkalosis and reflects concomitant respiratory acidosis.

RULES FOR RAPID ABG INTERPRETATION

LOOK AT pH

1. **If pH acidotic** → see $PaCO_2$ & HCO_3^-
   a. If $PaCO_2$ ↑ →   Primary respiratory acidosis
                    See if acute or chronic
                    Calculate compensation
   b. If HCO_3^- and $PaCO_2$ are both low → primary metabolic acidosis
       Calculate expected $PaCO_2$:
           If $PaCO_2$ < expected $PaCO_2$ → associated respiratory alkalosis
           If $PaCO_2$ > expected $PaCO_2$ → associated respiratory acidosis
   c. If HCO_3^- is low see AG
      i. Normal AG → hyperchloremic metabolic acidosis
      ii. High AG → wide gap MA
      iii. Gap gap ratio
2. **If pH alkalotic** → see $PaCO_2$ and HCO_3^-
   a. If $PaCO_2$ low → Primary respiratory alkalosis
                  See if acute or chronic
                  Calculate compensation
   b. If $PaCO_2$ & HCO_3^- are high → primary metabolic alkalosis
       Calculate expected $PaCO_2$
           If $PaCO_2$ < expected $PaCO_2$ → associated respiratory alkalosis
           If $PaCO_2$ > expected $PaCO_2$ → associated respiratory acidosis
3. **If pH normal** → normal ABG or mixed disorder
   ↑ $PaCO_2$ and ↓ HCO_3^- → mixed respiratory and metabolic acidosis
   ↓ $PaCO_2$ and ↑ HCO_3^- → mixed respiratory and metabolic alkalosis
   Calculate % difference to see which is the dominant disorder.

COMMON ELECTROLYTE ABNORMALITIES

Water is the major component of all fluid compartments. Total body water (TBW) represents about 60% of total body weight or about 42 L. It is divided into intracellular (2/3 TBW) and extracellular (1/3 TBW) fluid compartments separated by water-permeable cell membranes. The major components of the ECF are the plasma (1/4 ECF) and interstitial fluid (3/4 ECF).

SODIUM PHYSIOLOGY

Sodium is the most abundant positive ion of ECF and is critical in determining ECF and ICF osmolality. Normal serum sodium values are 134-145 mmol/L. Sodium is essential for generation of action potentials in neurologic and cardiac tissue. An adult requires about 1.5 mEq /kg/day.

HYPONATREMIA

- Serum Na$^+$ < 134 mmol/L amounts to hyponatremia.
- This is the most common dyselectrolytemia in hospitalized patients.
- In most hyponatremic patients, total body sodium is normal or increased.
- It may be associated with increased mortality due to hyponatremia per se and association with severe systemic disease.
- Hyponatremia has no relation with how the kidneys handle sodium, but how it handles free water.
- Despite a large water intake, hyponatremia is usually prevented by formation of a dilute filtrate in the loop of Henle and inhibition of ADH → urine excretion. Impairment of these two steps predisposes to hyponatremia.

CASE SCENARIO-1

A 30 year-old pregnant woman, is admitted comatose to the emergency. She gives a history of vomiting and diarrhea for past 5-6 days. Blood glucose level is normal but serum Na$^+$ is 112 mmol/L.

> **Comment:** In a comatose patient always check blood glucose level at the bedside before proceeding any further, even if there appears to be another explanation for the coma.
> Untreated hypoglycemia can result in serious neurological sequel and is easily corrected with 25 or 50% dextrose.

Clinical Approach in such a Case

- Ensure safe management of the unconscious patient.
- Then consider the broad differential diagnosis of hyponatremia.

Diagnostic Approach

1. Begin with a targeted history to elicit symptoms of hyponatremia.
   - Signs and symptoms depend on the rate and severity of decrease in plasma Na$^+$.
   - Most patients are asymptomatic.
   - Symptoms usually appear when plasma sodium < 120 mEq/L.
   - Early symptoms are subtle- loss of appetite, nausea, vomiting, cramps, weakness, lethargy, headache, irritability, disorientation, confusion, altered consciousness, coma, seizures.
   - In severe hyponatremia, neurologic and GIT symptoms predominate - severe mental status changes, seizure, coma, and respiratory arrest.
   - Hyponatremic encephalopathy is diagnosed when neurologic manifestations are profound;[5] cerebral edema occurs when Serum Na$^+$ < 123 mEq/L.
   - Cardiac symptoms occur when Serum Na$^+$ is about 100 mEq/L.
2. Consider important causes: Table 40.6
   - Sodium loss- Sweating, vomiting, diarrhea, third space losses, burns, diuretics etc
   - Excess TBW- More common; usually associated with nonphysiologic ADH release and impaired renal diluting capacity.
3. Assess patient's volume status clinically:[6]
   - Hypervolemia- Edema, lung crackles, distended neck veins, third heart sound
   - Hypovolemia - Orthostatic hypotension, tachycardia, oliguria/ anuria

Table 40.6: Causes of hyponatremia	
I. **Pseudohyponatremia**	Artifact in severe hyperlipidemia or hyperproteinemia
II. **True hyponatremia**	
i. **Normal S.Osmolality**	Non-sodium solute (mannitol, glucose), renal failure
ii. **High S. Osmolality**	Non-sodium solute (mannitol, glucose, ethanol, methanol, ethylene glycol), renal failure
iii. **Low S. Osmolality**	a. **High total body Na+;**
	Edematous States (urine Na < 15 mEq/l)
	• CHF, cirrhosis, nephrosis
	• Renal failure (urine Na > 30 mEq/l)
	b. **Low total body Na+;**
	Non renal Na losses
	• GIT, skin, third space losses
	• Dietary Na restriction with excess water intake
	Renal Na losses
	• Diuretics, renal failure, mineralocorticoid deficiency
	c. **Normal total body Na+**
	• SIADH (urine Na > 30mEq/L, Uosm > 300-400 mOsm/kg)
	• Chronic renal failure
	• Water intoxication
	• Potassium deficiency

- Euvolemia - absence of hypervolemia/ hypovolemia
- In hypovolemic/edematous patients, the ratio of BUN to S.Cr should be > 20:1.
4. Appropriate investigations – Renal function tests, serum electrolytes
5. Measure Serum osmolality = 2Na + BUN/2.8 + Glucose/18 (normal 275-290 mOsm/kg H_2O)
6. Measure urine osmolality. (1200 to 30 mOsm/kg)
7. Determine urinary Na^+ levels;
   - Urinary Na^+ <15 mEq/L - edematous states, volume depletion
   - Urinary Na^+ > 20 mEq/L - renal salt wasting, renal failure with water retention.
8. Estimate sodium deficit.

When saline is given to treat hyponatremia, the quantity of sodium required to achieve the desired elevation in the serum sodium concentration can be estimated:

Sodium deficit = TBW x (desired serum Na^+ - actual serum Na^+)

TBW (total body water) = 60% body weight (males), 50% body weight (females)

E.g. Amount of Na^+ needed to raise the Na^+ from 106 to 112 in a 70-kg man can be calculated: 60/100 x 70 (112–106) = 252 mEq

Because there is 513 mEq Na^+ /L in hypertonic saline, roughly 0.5 L of hypertonic saline is needed to raise the Na^+ from 106 to 112 mEq/L.

Treatment of Hyponatremia

- Decide if immediate treatment is required – degree of hyponatremia, acute or chronic, presence of symptoms, and any hypotension.
- Mild asymptomatic hyponatremia (120- 134 mEq/L) - Treat underlying factors.
- Hyponatremia with normal/high serum osmolality:
  - Reduce concentrations of responsible solute, e.g. urea or mannitol
  - Uremic patients - free water restriction /dialysis
- Edematous (hypervolemic) patients
  - Na^+ and water restriction, diuretics
- Hyponatremic hypovolemic patients:
  - 0.9% NaCl, curtail Na^+ + losses

- Neurologic symptoms/ profound hyponatremia (Na$^+$ <115 to 120 mEq/L)
  - Hypertonic (3%) saline 1 to 2 mL/kg/hr, to increase plasma Na$^+$ by 1- 2 mEq/L/hr.
  - Intravenous (IV) furosemide and replacement of uinary Na$^+$ losses with 0.9% or 3.0% saline, can rapidly increase plasma Na$^+$
  - Delayed correction → neurologic injury
  - Too rapid correction → abrupt brain dehydration/ permanent neurologic sequelae (osmotic demyelination syndrome ODS), cerebral hemorrhage or congestive heart failure (CHF).
  - Optimal rate of correction is - 0.6 to 1 mmol/L/hr until S. Na+ is 125 mEq/L, then at slower rate. One half of the deficit can be administered over the first 8 hours, and the next half over 1 to 3 days if symptoms remit.
- Symptoms of ODS vary from mild (transient behavioral disturbances or seizures) to severe (pseudobulbar palsy and quadriparesis).
- 3% hypertonic saline (osmolarity 1000 mOsm/L), must be given through a central line
- Treatment should be interrupted or slowed when symptoms improve
- Frequent determinations of Na$^+$ are important to prevent correction at a rate >1 to 2 mEq/L in any 1 hour and >8 mEq/L in 24 hours.
- Avoid overcorrection of serum Na concentration.
- Detect and manage underlying cause.

Syndrome of Inappropriate Antidiuresis (SIAD)

This is a form of hyponatremia in which there is an increased concentration of ADH inappropriate to any osmotic or volume stimuli that normally affect ADH secretion

Causes

- Pulmonary and cranial disorders
- Neoplasms (oat cell Ca lung)
- Sympathetic activation (postoperative pain)
- Drugs (oral hypoglycemics, tricyclic antidepressants, diuretics)

Diagnosis

- Hypotonic hyponatraemia
- Urine osmolality > plasma osmolality
- Urine sodium excretion > 20 mmol/L
- Normal renal, hepatic, cardiac, pituitary, adrenal, thyroid function
- Absence of hypotension, hypovolaemia, oedema and drugs affecting ADH secretion
- Water restriction → 2-3 kg weight loss, correction of hyponatremia, cessation of salt wasting over 2 to 3 days.

Treatment

- Free water restriction in asymptomatic patients
- Isotonic or hypertonic saline in severely symptomatic patients
- Pharmacotherapy- demeclocycline, AVP-receptor antagonists

HYPERNATREMIA

Hypernatremia is defined as plasma sodium >145 mEq/L. It may be accompanied by low, normal or high total-body sodium content. Hypernatremia inevitably leads to hyperosmolality.

CASE SCENARIO-2

While on restricted oral intake after cesarean delivery, a patient gradually became disoriented and agitated in conjunction with markedly increased urine output disproportional to her intravenous crystalloid fluid intake. Investigations revealed marked hypernatremia of 178 mEq/dL and urine osmolality was low at 248 mOsm/L.

The clinical presentation and electrolyte abnormalities were considered consistent with transient DI of pregnancy. The patient responded well to nasal-spray-administered deamino D arginine vasopressin and increased intravenous fluid intake, with resolution of symptoms and gradual normalization of serum sodium levels.[7]

> **Comment:** Transient diabetes insipidus (DI) of pregnancy should be considered in the differential diagnosis of severe hypernatremia in obstetric patients with restricted oral intake after operative delivery.

Differential Diagnosis

Consider all possible causes of hypernatremia (Table 40.7)

Diagnostic Approach

1. Begin with a targeted history to elicit symptoms of hypernatremia:
   - Major symptom thirst; absence of thirst - impaired thirst mechanism/inability to express thirst/access water.
   - CNS dysfunction due to brain cell shrinkage - confusion, lethargy, restlessness, irritability, hyperreflexia, seizures, coma, cerebrovascular damage with subcortical or subarachnoid hemorrhage and venous thromboses.
   - Chronic hypernatremia - lesser degree of brain cell dehydration and CNS symptoms.
   - Patients with hypotonic losses –signs of hypovolemia, renal insufficiency (occasionally progressing to renal failure), and decreased urinary concentrating ability.
   - Clinical consequences of hypernatremia are most serious at extremes of age and when hypernatremia develops abruptly.
   - Mortality of hypernatremia is 40 to 55%, but it is unclear whether hypernatremia contributes to mortality or is simply a marker of severe associated disease.
2. Assess patient's volume status - CVP, urine output, clinically
3. Obtain urine osmolality, serum glucose level
4. Frequent sodium levels
   - Serum Na > 190 mEq/L - long-term salt ingestion
   - Serum Na >170 mEq/L- indicates DI
   - Serum Na 150-170 mEq/L- dehydration

Table 40.7: Causes of hypernatremia	
Hypovolemic Hypernatremia	*Non Renal water losses* (U_{Na}<10-15mEq/L, U_{osm} > 400 mOsm/kg)
	Adipsic hypernatremia (decreased thirst)
	GIT, skin losses
	Renal losses (U_{Na}< 20 mEq/L, U_{osm}> 300 mOsm/kg)
	Osmotic diuresis (DKA, hyperglycemic nonketotic coma, mannitol)
	Diuretics, postobstructive diuresis, intrinsic renal disease
Euvolemic Hypernatremia	*Non Renal water losses* (U_{Na} variable, U_{osm}> 400 mOsm/kg)
	Respiratory, cutaneous losses
	Renal losses (U_{Na} variable, U_{osm} < 290 mOsm/kg)
	Central & nephrogenic DI
Hypervolemic Hypernatremia	*Iatrogenic*
	Hypertonic saline, sodium bicarbonate, TPN, accidental salt ingestion
	Mineralocorticoid excess (U_{Na} > 20 mEq/L, U_{osm}> 300 mOsm/kg)

5. Is the problem acute or chronic
6. Calculate pure water deficit (i.e. normal TBW- current TBW) and replace
   Current TBW x current plasma Na^+ = normal TBW x normal plasma Na^+

Treatment of Hypernatremia

1. The goal rate of correction should be about 0.5-0.7 mmol/L/hr. Only half of estimated volume deficit is corrected in the first 24 hours.
2. Hypovolemic hypernatremia- Hypovolemia correction (0.9% saline), once hypovolemia is corrected, water can be replaced orally/ IV with hypotonic fluids.
3. Hypervolemic hypernatremia- Enhance sodium removal (loop diuretics, dialysis), Replace water deficit (hypotonic fluids).
4. Euvolemic hypernatremia- Replace water deficit (hypotonic fluids).
5. Conscious patients with no GI dysfunction - oral hydration
   Severe hypernatremia/ patients unable to drink - IV hydration
   Hypernatremia of < 24 hr - correct within 24 hr.
   Chronic hypernatremia - correct over 48 hrs and serum osmolality to be lowered slowly.
6. Serum Na^+ is to be monitored hourly; other electrolytes, including serum K^+, should be monitored and replaced as needed.

DIABETES INSIPIDUS

A urinary osmolality <150 mOsm/kg in the setting of hypertonicity and polyuria is diagnostic of DI.

Central DI (ADH deficiency) may be seen in pituitary surgery, basal skull fracture, and severe head injury.

Nephrogenic DI - inability of kidney to produce a hypertonic medullary interstitium.

Clinical Features

- Large volume of dilute urine
- Profound hypovolemia
- Hypernatremia

Diagnosis

- Urine output > 100 mL/hr
- Hypernatremia
- Urine osmolality < 300 mOsm/L

Treatment

- Central DI- Intranasal DDAVP, subcutaneous vasopressin
- Nephrogenic DI - Treat the cause, restrict sodium and water intake, thiazide diuretics

POTASSIUM PHYSIOLOGY

- Potassium is the most abundant cation in the human body and regulates intracellular enzyme function and neuromuscular (NM) excitability.
- Total body K^+ is about 3500 mmol. Of this about 98% is intracellular and 1-2% is extracellular. The intracellular-extracellular potassium ratio (Ki/Ke) largely determines NM tissue excitability.
- Serum K^+ is normally maintained between 3.5- 5.5 mEq/L, whereas that inside the cell is 150 mEq/L.
- Potassium requirements vary with age and growth. An adult needs 1- 1.5 mEq /kg/day.

- Potassium homeostasis:
  - Short-term potassium homeostasis occurs via transcellular potassium shifts influenced by insulin, pH, β-adrenergic agonists, bicarbonate concentration.
  - Long-term potassium balance depends on renal excretion of ingested potassium.
  - Renal adaptive mechanisms allow the kidneys to maintain potassium homeostasis until GFR < 15-20 mL/min.

HYPOKALEMIA

- Defined as serum K^+ < 3.5 mEq/L
- It may be an absolute deficiency or redistribution into ICF.
- Hypokalemia may occur with normal, low, or high total body potassium.
- A decrease in the serum K+ from 3.5 to 3.0 mEq/L implies a 5% reduction (~175 mEq) in total body potassium stores.
- A decline from 3.0 to 2.0 mEq/L implies an additional 200- 400-mEq deficit.

CASE SCENARIO-3

A healthy 23-year-old gravid woman at 32 weeks of gestation with preterm premature rupture of membranes received two doses of 12-mg betamethasone intramuscular (IM) 24 hours apart to accelerate fetal lung maturation. She developed significant proximal muscle weakness within 16 hours after the initial dose. Her serum potassium was 1.6 mEq/L.[8]

Comment: Hypokalemic periodic paralysis, a rare cause of weakness, may be induced by betamethasone injections during pregnancy and is reversible with low-risk interventions.

Differential Diagnosis

Consider all possible causes of hyperkalemia (Table 40.8)

Table 40.8: Causes of hypokalemia		
1.	Reduced intake	• Anorexia nervosa, starvation, alcoholism • Primary and secondary hyperaldosteronism
2.	GIT losses	• Vomiting, diarrhea, villous adenoma
3.	Renal losses	• Excess mineralocorticoids or diuretics • Barter's syndrome • Antibiotics (carbenicillin, penicillin, nafcillin, ticarcillin) • Renal tubular acidosis • Hypomagnesemia • Myelomonocytic leukemia
4.	Potassium shifts from ECF to ICF	• Acute alkalosis • Hypokalemic periodic paralysis • Insulin therapy • Vitamin B_{12} therapy • Lithium overdose • Hypokalemic periodic paralysis • $β_2$-agonists - stress-related catecholamine activity, exogenous catecholamines, isoproterenol, terbutaline, epinephrine and ritodrine. Includes pregnant patients receiving tocolytic therapy or respiratory treatment with $β_2$-agonists and critically ill patients requiring pharmacologic cardiovascular support (can acutely lower serum K^+ by 0.5-1 mEq/L).

Diagnostic Approach

1. Begin with a medical history and physical examination.[9]
   Symptoms of hypokalemia:
   Mild hypokalemia - often asymptomatic
   Symptoms in moderate or severe hypokalemia (Table 40.9):
   Acute redistribution of K^+ from the ECF to ICF, substantially changes resting membrane potentials; in chronic hypokalemia, the ratio of intracellular to extracellular K^+ remains relatively stable, so it is better tolerated.
2. Check other serum electrolytes (serum Mg)
3. EKG changes (serum K^+—2 to 2.5 mEq/L) - ST segment sagging, depression of T wave, U waves and cardiac dysrrhythmias - atrial fibrillation, premature ventricular beats.
4. If cause of hypokalemia not obvious check urinary K^+ excretion and ABG analysis. Correct alkalemia.
5. Hypokalemia with paralysis may be seen in hyperthyroidism or in familial or sporadic periodic paralysis.
6. In absence of severe polyuria, "spot" urinary $K^+ < 20$ mEq/L suggests renal K^+ conservation.
7. Random $U_K : U_{Cr}$ (mmol/g) > 1.5 suggests a renal cause of hypokalemia whereas a ratio < 1.5 suggests nonrenal cause of hypokalemia (Table 40.10).
8. Check digoxin level if the patient is on a digitalis preparation.

Treatment of Hypokalemia

- Treat the underlying cause
- Mild hypokalemia → May not need any K^+ replacement, correct cause
- Mild/ moderate hypokalemia (potassium level of 2.5-3.5 mEq/L) → Oral K^+ therapy
- Severe hypokalemia(Serum $K^+ < 2.5$ mEq/L/ cardiac arrhythmias/ significant symptoms → both intravenous and oral replacement
- Place patient on cardiac monitor, establish intravenous access, and assess respiratory status.

Table 40.9: Symptoms in moderate or severe hypokalemia	
GIT symptoms	Constipation, nausea or vomiting, abdominal cramping
Renal symptoms	Polyuria, nocturia, or polydipsia
	K^+ depletion → defects in renal concentrating ability → polyuria, reduction in GFR.
Musculoskeletal symptoms	Skeletal muscle weakness, cramping, paralysis, paresthesias.
Cardiac symptoms	Palpitations
Increase in digoxin toxicity	By increasing myocardial digoxin binding and pharmacologic effectiveness.
CNS symptoms	Psychosis, delirium, hallucinations, depression

Table 40.10: Renal and Non renal causes of hypokalemia	
Metabolic acidosis	
$U_K : U_{Cr} < 1.5$ (nonrenal)	Lower GIT losses, diarrhea or laxative abuse
$U_K : U_{Cr} > 1.5$ (renal)	Diabetic ketoacidosis (DKA), type 1 or 2 distal renal tubular acidosis (RTA)
Metabolic alkalosis	
$U_K : U_{Cr} < 1.5$ & normal BP (nonrenal)	Surreptitious vomiting
$U_K : U_{Cr} > 1.5$ & normal BP (renal)	Diuretic use, Bartter's syndrome, Gitelman syndrome
High $U_K : U_{Cr}$ & hypertension (renal)	Primary hyperaldosteronism, Cushing syndrome, congenital adrenal hyperplasia, renal artery stenosis, apparent mineralocorticoid excess/Liddle syndrome.

Oral Therapy

- For patients with mild hypokalemia and minimal symptoms
- Easy to administer, safe, inexpensive, readily absorbed from GIT
- Syrup KCl elevates concentrations within 1-2 hrs; bitter taste; tolerated poorly in doses > 25- 50 mEq.

Intravenous Therapy

- Intravenous K^+ dosages up to 40 mEq/hour have been advocated but typically patients should receive no more than 20 mEq/hr IV to avoid cardiac side effects
- Perioperative therapy → IV KCl 0.5 mEq/kg/hr (typically 10- 20 mEq/hr for a normal adult with constant EKG monitoring).
- Should never be given as an IV bolus; administer as a dilute solution.
- Higher concentrations of IV KCl are damaging to smaller peripheral veins.
- Replace S. Mg if low.

HYPERKALEMIA

Hyperkalemia (>5.5 mEq/L) can occur in response to drugs that diminish renal potassium excretion or after sudden transcellular shifts of potassium from the ICF to ECF.

CASE SCENARIO-4

A 37-year-lady at 26 weeks of gestation was admitted with abdominal pain. One day prior to admission, the patient had noticed a loss of fetal movement. The patient was diagnosed with hypertension 20 years ago. She had a history of CKD stage 4 (GFR 30 mL/min). Pertinent findings on examination were a distended and tender abdomen on palpation. Fetal movement or FHS were not appreciated. S. Na$^+$ was 131 mEq/L and S.K$^+$ was 6.1 mEq/L; EKG showed sinus tachycardia, peaked T-waves, and Q waves in inferior leads. Transabdominal ultrasonography revealed no identifiable heart motion and 9.1 and 9.7 cm echogenic kidneys without hydronephrosis, consistent with medical renal disease. Despite medical management the serum K$^+$ increased to 7.5 mmol/L within 6 hours.

Rhabdomyolysis, hemolysis, and lactic acidosis were ruled out by serum chemistry. Cesarean section revealed a dead fetus with peeling skin after which the patient's S. K$^+$ normalized without further medical intervention. The worsening hyperkalemia in this patient with advanced CKD may have been due to potassium leak from intrauterine fetal demise into the maternal circulation.[10]

> **Comments:** Patients with advanced CKD have impaired renal mechanisms to compensate for acute changes in fluid, electrolyte, and acid base changes.

Diagnostic Approach

1. Take complete history to rule out possible causes (Table 40.11).
   Hyperkalemia can be separated into acute and chronic processes. Acute hyperkalemia is more poorly tolerated than chronic hyperkalemia.
2. Evaluate for symptoms and signs of hyperkalemia:
   - Tingling, paraesthesia, weakness, flaccid paralysis, hypotension and bradycardia.
   - Alterations in cardiac conduction → increased automaticity and enhanced repolarization →. life-threatening cardiac arrhythmias
3. EKG:
   - 6 to 7 mEq/L → peaked T waves
   - 10 to 12 mEq/L → prolonged P–R interval, QRS widening, deep S-wave → sine wave → VF/asystole.
4. Renal function tests, ABG, appropriate lab tests

Table 40.11: Causes of hyperkalemia	
Pseudohyperkalemia	• Technical problems- sample lysis, fist clenching on sampling
	• Thrombocytosis
Altered internal K+ balance	• Acidosis
	• Insulin deficiency
	• Hypoaldosteronism
	• Malignant hyperthermia
	• Periodic paralysis
	• Cell necrosis
	• Drugs (succinylcholine, digitalis, nonselective β-blockers)
Altered external K+ balance	• Replacement therapy
	• Transfusions
	• Antibiotics containing potassium salts
	• Renal disease
	• Hypoaldosteronism
	• Drugs (heparin, K+ sparing diuretics, NSAIDs, ACE inhibitors, ARB's, EACA)
During anesthesia	• Reperfusion after period of ischemia (usually > 4 hours)
	• Tumor lysis syndrome (lymphoma, leukemia, large tumors)

Treatment of Hyperkalemia

Directed at the underlying cause and guided by ECG changes:[11,12]
- Evaluate for potential toxicities:
  - ECG for cardiotoxicity
  - Physiologic antagonist (Ca); stabilizes heart from effects of K+;
    In an adult 10 mL of 10% Ca chloride IV or 2-3 ampoules of calcium gluconate are given over 5-10 minutes. This has a rapid onset of action (3-5 minutes) which lasts for about 1 hour.
- Decrease K+ intake:
  - Discontinue oral and parenteral K supplements.
  - Examine the patient's diet
- Increase K+ uptake into cells:
  - Glucose/insulin—Regular insulin 5 - 10 U IV with dextrose 25 to 50 g (50 mL 50% glucose) reduces serum K within 10 to 20 minutes and effects last for 4 -6 hours
  - Hyperventilation,
  - Bicarbonate (1 mEq/kg over 5-10 minutes)
  - β-adrenergic agonists—Albuterol 10 to 20 mg inhaled over 10 minutes lowers serum K+ by 0.5 to 1.5 mEq/L; peak effect is seen in 90 minutes.
- Increase K+ excretion:
  - Discontinue K+ sparing diuretics, ACE inhibitors, ARBs, etc
  - Sodium polystyrene sulfonate (Kayexalate); binding resin given orally / enema; Ca resonium 15 g TDS
  - Loop diuretics—Furosemide 20-40 mg IV
  - Aldosterone agonists – Fludrocortisones
  - Dialysis—Serum K+ decreases 1.0- 1.5 mEq/L for each hour of dialysis

CALCIUM PHYSIOLOGY

Calcium is the key component that mediates muscle contraction, exocrine, endocrine, and neurocrine secretion, cell growth and the transport and secretion of fluids and electrolytes. A 70-kg adult contains approximately 1300 g of calcium, 99 percent of which is in the bones and teeth. The kidneys are the major organ which regulate plasma calcium between 4.5 - 5 mEq/L (8.5- 10.5 mg/dL).

Circulating Calcium Exists in Three Forms

- Bound to plasma proteins (primarily albumin) - 40 to 50 percent
- Ionized, physiologically active—50 percent (2 - 2.5 mEq/L)
- Nonionized and chelated with phosphate, sulfate, and citrate—10 percent.

Calcium Homeostasis

- Parathormone from the parathyroid glands increases calcium reabsorption in the thick ascending limb and distal tubule, decreasing calcium excretion.
- Calcitonin, decreases renal reabsorption of calcium acutely, but has little effect on long-term calcium homeostasis.
- Vitamin D increases absorption of calcium from the gastrointestinal tract, and its action is potentiated by parathyroid hormone.
- Acute acidemia increases and acute alkalemia decreases ionized calcium.

HYPOCALCEMIA

Hypocalcemia is defined as serum calcium < 4.5 mEq/L

CASE SCENARIOS

CASE 5: A 25-year-old gravida presented at 33 weeks' gestation with advanced preterm labor. She received magnesium sulfate followed by nifedipine and experienced bilateral hand contractures 12 hours after discontinuation of magnesium sulfate. Total serum calcium was 5.4 mg/dL.[13]

CASE 6: A 35-year-old gravida presented at 26 weeks' gestation with ruptured membranes and received magnesium sulfate until it was discontinued prematurely because of pulmonary edema. Twenty hours later she experienced bilateral hand contractures; total serum calcium was 5.9 mg/dL.[13]

Diagnostic Approach

1. Medical history and examination- establish cause
   Consider all possible causes of hypocalcemia which may be associated with low or high S.PTH (Table 40.12)
2. Check symptoms and signs of hypocalcemia:

Symptoms of Hypocalcemia

Chronic moderate hypocalcemia may be completely asymptomatic.
Moderate-to-severe hypocalcemia causes:
- Neuromuscular irritability:
  Perioral numbness and tingling muscle cramps in limbs → tetany (seen in severe hypocalcemia with ionized Ca+ < 1.1 mmol/L)
- Neuropsychiatric symptoms
  Irritability, impaired intellectual capacity, depression, personality changes, seizures, dementia, anxiety, extrapyramidal symptoms, calcification of basal ganglia
- Autonomic symptoms
  Biliary colic, laryngospasm, bronchospasm, diaphoresis, smooth muscle spasm → abdominal cramping and urinary frequency

Table 40.12: Causes of hypocalcemia	
Low PTH (Hypoparathyroidism)	*High PTH (Secondary Hyperparathyroidism)*
Parathyroid agenesis • Isolated • Di George syndrome	Vitamin D deficiency/ impaired 1,25 $(OH)_2$ D production/action • Nutritional Vitamin D deficiency • Vitamin D resistance • Renal insufficiency
Parathyroid destruction • Postoperative • Radiation • Infiltration by metastasis/malignancy • Autoimmune	PTH resistance syndromes • PTH receptor mutations • Pseudohypoparathyroidism (G protein mutations)
Reduced parathyroid function • Hypomagnesemia • Activating CaSR mutations	Drugs • Calcium chelators • Inhibitors of bone resorption (bisphosphonates, plicamycin) • Altered Vit D metabolism (phenytoin, ketoconazole)
Massive rapid blood transfusion • Citrated blood rate > 1.5 mL/kg/min leads to ionized hypocalcemia	Miscellaneous causes • Acute pancreatitis • Acute rhabdomyolysis • Hungry bone syndrome (post-parathyroidectomy) • Osteoblastic metastases (Ca prostate)
Acute hyperventilation Low albumin level • Low plasma Ca with normal ionized Ca	

Signs of Hypocalcemia

CVS
• Dysrrhythmias, digitalis insensitivity, heart failure, hypotension, impaired β-adrenergic action
Neuromuscular
• Tetany, muscle spasm, papilloedema, seizures, weakness, hyperreflexia
• Trousseaus sign (carpopedal spasm) seen on inflating BP cuff 20 mm Hg above systolic pressure for 3 mins → ischemia of radial and ulnar nerves → carpal spasm
• Chvostek's sign - Twitching of the ipsilateral facial musculature (perioral, nasal, and eye muscles) by tapping over cranial nerve VII at the ear. Contraction at the oral angle alone is seen in 10 to 25% of the normal population.
Respiratory
• Apnea, laryngeal spasm, bronchospasm, stridor - prolonged contraction of the respiratory and laryngeal muscles; can cause cyanosis.
  Others
• Cataracts, dry coarse skin, dermatitis, hyperpigmentation, eczema, steatorrhea, gastric achlorhydria
• EKG – prolonged QT interval, heart block, ST-T changes
3. Measure S. Calcium and albumin.
   • Each 1 g/dL reduction in serum albumin lowers total calcium by approx. 0.8 mg/dL without affecting the ionized Ca^{++} concentration (thus without producing any symptoms or signs of hypocalcemia).
   E.g. In a patient with a S. Alb 2 g/dL (ie. 2 g/dL below normal), if the measured serum total Ca is 8 mg/dL, corrected value will be 8 + 0.8 x 2 = is 9.6 mg/dL (which is normal).

4. Obtain phosphate levels and evaluate renal function; see if hypocalcemia is acute or chronic.
   - Low or normal phosphate → Vitamin D or Mg deficiency.
   - High phosphate → renal failure or hypoparathyroidism.
   - Chronic hypocalcemia & otherwise healthy patient → hypoparathyroidism.
   - Chronically ill adult with hypocalcemia → malabsorption, osteomalacia, or osteoblastic metastases.
5. Determine PTH level
   - Low PTH level with hypocalcemia → hypoparathyroidism.
   - High PTH level (secondary hyperparathyroidism) → Vitamin D axis likely cause
6. Determine S. Mg levels
   - Hypomagnesemia → PTH resistance or deficiency.
   - Tissue magnesium deficiency (chronic malabsorption or alcoholism) → Mg responsive hypocalcemia with normal S. Mg

Treatment of Hypocalcemia

1. Depends on severity of hypocalcemia, rapidity of development, accompanying complications.
2. Calcium replacement
   - Patients with acute symptomatic hypocalcemia (total Ca < 7.0 mg/dL, ionized Ca < 0.8 mmol/L) should be treated promptly with IV calcium.
   - Ca gluconate is preferred over Ca chloride - causes less tissue necrosis if extravasated.
   - 10% Ca gluconate, 10 mL (90 mg elemental Ca) diluted in 50 mL 5 % dextrose/ 0.9% NaCl , given iv over 10 mins.
   - Followed by constant iv infusion - typically 10 ampoules of Ca gluconate in 1 L of 5% dextrose/ 0.9% NaCl given over 24 hrs or elemental Ca 0.3–2.0 mg/kg/hr
   - Continue Ca infusion until patient is receiving effective doses of oral calcium & Vit D
3. Remove any offending drugs
4. Measure K^+ and other electrolytes and correct any abnormalities
5. Correct coexisting hypomagnesemia (Take care in patients with renal insufficiency who cannot excrete excess Mg) .
   - Mg infusion as 2 g (16 mEq) Mg sulfate over 10 to 15 minutes, followed by 1 g/hr.
   - Hypocalcemia resolves soon after restoration of normal S. Mg if hypomagnesemia was the cause of the hypocalcemia.
6. Correct hyperphosphatemia (tumor lysis syndrome, rhabdomyolysis, CRF).
   - Acute hyperphosphatemia usually resolves in patients with intact renal function.
   - Phosphate excretion may be aided by:
     - saline infusion (caution—this can lead to worsening of hypocalcemia)
     - acetazolamide, a carbonic anhydrase inhibitor, 10 to 15 mg/kg every 3- 4 hours.
   - Chronic hyperphosphatemia → low-phosphate diet/use of phosphate binders.
7. Hemodialysis- In patients with symptomatic hypocalcemia and hyperphosphatemia, especially if renal function is impaired.
8. Chronic hypocalcemia (hypoparathyroidism) - Oral Ca/Vitamin D; target S. Ca to about 8.0 mg/dL.
9. Further elevation → hypercalciuria (lack of PTH effect on the renal tubules). Chronic hypercalciuria → nephrocalcinosis, nephrolithiasis, renal impairment.

HYPERCALCEMIA

Defined as total serum calcium > 5.0 mEq/L or 10.5 mg/dL, or ionized Ca^{2+} >1.5 mmol/L

CASE SCENARIOS

CASE 7: A 32 year gravid woman with a large leiomyoma presented at 33 weeks of gestation with critical hypercalcemia requiring intensive care. Postpartum myomectomy cured her

Table 40.13: Causes of hypercalcemia	
Increased PTH	Primary hyperparathyroidism (adenoma, hyperplasia, carcinoma)
	Tertiary hyperparathyroidism (renal insufficiency)
	Ectopic PTH secretion (very rare)
	Inactivating mutations in the CaSR (FHH)
	Alterations in CaSR function (lithium therapy)
Excessive 1,25(OH)$_2$D production	Granulomatous diseases (sarcoidosis, tuberculosis, silicosis)
	Lymphomas
	Vitamin D intoxication
Primary increase in bone resorption	Hyperthyroidism
	Immobilization
Malignancy related	Overproduction of PTHrP (many solid tumors)
	Lytic skeletal metastases (breast, myeloma)
Excessive calcium intake	Milk-alkali syndrome
	Total parenteral nutrition
Other causes	Endocrine disorders (adrenal insufficiency, pheochromocytoma, VIPoma)
	Medications (thiazides, vitamin A, antiestrogens)

hypercalcemia, which was driven by parathyroid hormone-related protein (PTHrP) produced by the tumor.[14]

CASE 8: A 28 years pregnant woman developed hypercalcemic crisis after normal delivery of an infant. On the first postpartum day, the corrected serum calcium concentration increased to 19.4 mg/dL with a markedly increased serum level of PTHrP. After administration of saline and pamidronate, the serum levels of calcium and PTHrP rapidly normalized. Extensive examination revealed no malignant lesion, suggesting that the placenta may have been producing an excessive amount of PTHrP (humoral hypercalcemia of pregnancy).[15]

Diagnostic Approach

1. Consider all possible causes or hypercalcemia: (Table 40.13)
2. Check for signs and symptoms:
   - Mild hypercalcemia (S. Ca <11.5 mg/dL) - usually asymptomatic.
   - Moderate hypercalcemia (S. Ca—11.5 to 13 mg/dL) - lethargy, anorexia, nausea, polyuria.
   - Severe hypercalcemia (S. Ca >13 mg/dL) - more severe manifestations
     - Neuromyopathic—Irritability, ataxia, lethargy, depression, impaired memory, emotional lability or confusion preceding coma, muscle weakness
     - CVS—Hypertension, arrhythmias, heart block, cardiac arrest, digitalis sensitivity.
     - Skeletal-Multiple fractures
     - Others-Vomiting, polyuria, renal calculi, oliguric renal failure
       OR
       Remember rhyme ; Bones (osteopenia, pathologic fractures), Stones (kidney stones, polyuria), Groans (abdominal pain, anorexia, constipation, ileus, nausea, vomiting), Psychiatric overtones (depression, psychosis, delirium/confusion).
   - EKG—Short ST segment and shortened QT.

Treatment of Hypercalcemia

Severe hypercalcemia > 14 mg/dL is a medical emergency.
1. Correction of underlying cause
2. Supportive treatment
   - Hydration; 0.9% saline infusion
     - Dilutes S. Ca, promotes renal excretion, can reduce total S.Ca by 1.5 to 3 mg/dL.
     - Maintain urine output at 200 to 300 mL/hr

- Furosemide—Enhances Ca excretion
- Removal of offending drugs
- Dietary calcium restriction
- Correct dyselectrolytemia
- Increased physical activity
3. Drug treatment
    - Bisphosphonates
        - Inhibit osteoclast function and viability; in hypercalcemia mediated by osteoclastic bone resorption
    - Calcitonin
        - Secondary treatment for life-threatening hypercalcemia
        - Lowers S Ca within 24 to 48 hours by 1 -2 mg/dL.
    - Hydrocortisone/ mithramycin
        - In lymphatic malignancies, Vit D/ A intoxication
        - Associated with production by tumor or granulomas of 1,25(OH)2D or osteoclast-activating factor

MAGNESIUM PHYSIOLOGY

Total-body magnesium is approximately 2000 mEq and is essential for the production and functioning of ATP, DNA, RNA, and protein synthesis. It is an essential regulator of calcium access into the cell and of the actions of calcium within the cell and may be regarded as a natural physiologic calcium antagonist.

CLINICAL USES OF MAGNESIUM

Used in many clinical problems in patients who are not hypomagnesemic
- Premature labor, pre-eclampsia, eclampsia.
- Reduces effects of catecholamine excess in patients with tetanus and pheochromocytoma.
- May significantly reverse hypocoagulability in patients awaiting liver transplantation.
- Exerts analgesic effect on postoperative pain.
- Role in antivasospasm regimen following subarachnoid hemorrhage.
- Anti arrhythmic action in torsades de pointes, even in normomagnesemic patients.

HYPOMAGNESEMIA

Defined as $Mg^{2+} < 1.8$ mg/dL; is common in critically ill hospitalized patients; manifests similarly to hypocalcemia.

CASE SCENARIO-9

A woman with Gitelman syndrome presented to hospital with hyperemesis. After admission, IV potassium and magnesium supplementation was commenced to counter the observed hypokalemia and hypomagnesemia. Hyperemesis receded and although S. K^+ remained low, she became asymptomatic. Oral potassium and magnesium supplementation was administered throughout pregnancy and biweekly ion level measurements were scheduled. Despite the intensive replacement, ion levels remained constantly low. She delivered a healthy female baby at 38 weeks by an elective LSCS. Neonatal electrolyte profile was normal.[16]

Gitelman syndrome is also referred to as familial hypokalemia-hypomagnesemia. Diagnosis is based on the clinical symptoms and biochemical abnormalities (hypokalemia, metabolic alkalosis, hypomagnesemia and hypocalciuria). Lifelong supplementation of magnesium (magnesium-oxide and magnesium-sulfate) is recommended. Cardiac work-up should be offered to screen for risk factors of cardiac arrhythmias. All these patients are encouraged to maintain a high-sodium and high potassium diet.

Diagnostic Approach

1. Consider all the causes of low serum magnesium (Table 40.14):
2. Check for signs and symptoms of hypomagnesemia (Table 40.15):
   These are similar to those in hypocalcemia and characterized by increased neuronal irritability and tetany.
   Symptoms are rare when the serum Mg^{2+} is between 1.5 and 1.7 mg/dL
   In most symptomatic patients serum Mg^{2+} is < 1.2 mg/dL
   Attempts to correct hypokalemia with K^+ replacement therapy alone may not be successful without simultaneous Mg therapy. The interrelationships of Mg and K in cardiac tissue have probably the greatest clinical relevance in terms of dysrhythmias, digoxin toxicity, and myocardial infarction.
3. Send investigations:
   • Check S. Mg levels. Signs and symptoms depend on the serum magnesium levels (Table 40.16)

Table 40.14: Causes of hypomagnesemia	
Inadequate intake	
Excessive GIT losses	Chronic diarrhea, prolonged NG suction, GIT/biliary fistulae, intestinal drains.
Excessive renal losses	Polyuria
	Inability of the renal tubules to conserve Mg in a variety of systemic and renal diseases, genetic or acquired renal disorders
	Chronic alcohol ingestion
Drugs	Aminoglycosides, cis-platinum, cardiac glycosides, diuretics
Intracellular Mg shifts	Thyroid hormone/ insulin administration
Physiological	Athletes, hypermetabolic states (pregnancy), cold acclimatization

Table 40.15: Signs and symptoms of hypomagnesemia	
Nervous system	Weakness, lethargy, muscle spasms, paresthesias, depression. Diminished respiratory muscle power CNS irritability- seizures, hyperreflexia (Chvostek's sign), skeletal muscle spasm (Trousseau's sign). When severe - seizures, confusion, and coma.
CVS	Coronary artery spasm, cardiac failure, dysrhythmias, hypotension, aggravation of digoxin toxicity and CHF
Endocrine	Both severe hypomagnesemia and hypermagnesemia suppress PTH secretion and can cause hypocalcemia. Severe hypomagnesemia may also impair end-organ response to PTH.
Electrolyte abnormalities	Hypokalemia, hyponatremia, hypophosphatemia, and hypocalcemia.

Table 40.16: Clinical manifestations at various serum magnesium levels[9]	
Mg level(mEq/L)	*Clinical Manifestation*
<1	Tetany, seizures, arrhythmias
1-1.5	Neuromuscular irritability, hypocalcemia, hypokalemia
1.5-2.1	Normal
2.1-4.2	Typically asymptomatic
4.2–5.8	Lethargy, drowsiness, flushing, nausea, vomiting, diminished deep tendon reflexes
5.8–10	Somnolence, loss of deep tendon reflexes, hypotension, ECG changes
>10	Complete heart block, cardiac arrest, apnea, paralysis, coma

- Check 24-hour urinary Mg excretion
  The renal response to Mg deficiency due to increased GIT loss is to lower fractional excretion of Mg to < 2%.
  A fractional excretion > 2% with normal kidney function indicates renal Mg wasting.
- Hypomagnesemia is associated with hypokalemia, hyponatremia, hypophosphatemia, and hypocalcemia.

Treatment of Hypomagnesemia

- Mild deficiencies; treat with diet alone. Add replacement to daily Mg requirements (0.3 to 0.4 mEq/kg/day)
- Mg can be given orally, usually 60 to 90 mEq/day of magnesium oxide
- Symptomatic/severe hypomagnesemia (Mg^{2+} < 1.0 mg/dL); parenteral Mg therapy.
  Intravenous; 1–2 g $MgSO_4$ bolus over 1 hr, followed by 2–4 mEq/hr (250–500 mg/hr $MgSO_4$) as continuous infusion
  Intramuscular Mg: 10 mEq 4–6 hrly
  ($MgSO_4$: 1 g = 8 mEq , $MgCl_2$: 1 g = 10 mEq).
- Therapy should be guided subsequently by the serum Mg level.
- Rate of infusion should not exceed 1 mEq/min, even in emergency situations, and the patient should receive continuous cardiac monitoring to detect cardiotoxicity.
- Patellar reflexes should be monitored frequently and Mg withheld if suppressed.
- Patients with renal insufficiency require careful monitoring during therapy.
- Repletion of systemic Mg stores usually requires 5 to 7 days of therapy, after which daily maintenance doses of Mg should be provided.
- For acute arrhythmias, 1 to 2 g (8–16 mEq) magnesium sulfate is given over approximately 5 minutes intravenously with close monitoring of BP & HR.

HYPERMAGNESEMIA

Defined as serum magnesium level > 2.5 mEq/L

Causes of Hypermagnesemia

- Iatrogenic
- Excessive use of magnesium containing antacids or laxatives, total parenteral nutrition (TPN)
- Kidney failure

CASE SCENARIO-10

A pregnant woman with acute renal failure, caused by aggravation of HELLP syndrome, developed coma induced by overdose of continuous magnesium sulfate administration for eclampsia. Before examination of serum concentration of magnesium, coma was suspected to be the result of brain vascular problem or brain infarction. Patient was treated in ICU and hemodialysis was started, and she recovered fully from abnormal neurological symptoms.[17]

Comment: Hypermagnesemia should be considered in differential diagnosis in a pregnant woman with coma.

The clinical signs and symptoms in a case of hypermagnesemia are summarized in Table 40.17.

Treatment of Hypermagnesemia

- Stop all magnesium containing preparations
- Increase urinary excretion of magnesium   → expand ECV(NS infusion)
                                         → induce diuresis (furosemide)
- Temporary reversal of neuromuscular and cardiac toxicity → IV calcium therapy.
- Emergency/ renal failure → dialysis

Table 40.17: Signs and symptoms of hypermagnesemia	
Nervous system	CNS- depression
	Peripheral nervous system - interferes with release of neurotransmitters
CVS	Direct myocardial depressant
	Vasodilation - direct action on blood vessels & interference with vasoconstrictors Reduces peripheral vascular tone- sympathetic blockade & inhibition of catecholamine release
Respiratory	Bronchodilatation
Renal	Renal vasodilatation, diuresis
NMJ	Antagonizes release and effect of Ach at the NMJ - depressed skeletal muscle function & NM blockade.
	Potentiates action of nondepolarizing muscle relaxants and decreases potassium release in response to succinylcholine
Obstetrics	At supraphysiologic concentrations, magnesium is a powerful tocolytic (Used to prevent patients with pre-eclampsia from developing seizures)

KEY POINTS

- Precise perioperative management of acid-base status, fluids, and electrolytes may limit perioperative morbidity and mortality.
- Acidemia/ alkalemia refer to H^+ state or pH.
- Acidosis/ alkalosis are pathologic processes that tend to accumulate acid or alkali but do not necessarily produce a pH change.
- All acid-base abnormalities result from alterations in the dissociation of water; only three factors independently affect acid-base balance; $PaCO_2$, Strong ion difference (SID), total concentration of weak acids (A_{TOT}).
- Compensation for pH changes depends upon proper functioning of lungs, kidneys and the severity of the acid base disturbance; acute compensation takes 6-24 hrs and chronic compensation takes 1-4 days; respiratory compensation is faster than metabolic.
- Compensation in Respiratory Disorders;
  The **1 for 10** Rule for acute respiratory acidosis
      Acute 10 mm Hg ↑ $PaCO_2$ → 1 mmol/L ↑ in HCO_3
  The **4 for 10** Rule for chronic respiratory acidosis
      Chronic 10 mm Hg ↓ $PaCO_2$ → 4 mmol/L ↑ in HCO_3
  The **2 for 10** Rule for acute respiratory alkalosis
      Acute 10 mm Hg ↓ $PaCO_2$ → 2 mmol/L ↓ in HCO_3
  The **5 for 10** Rule for a chronic respiratory alkalosis
      Chronic 10 mm Hg ↓ $PaCO_2$ → 5 mmol/L ↓ in HCO_3^-
- SID is the absolute difference between completely disassociated anions and cations.
- Metabolic Acidosis is due to accumulation of an acid in the body other than CO_2, buffering of endogenous or exogenous acid loads by bicarbonate, an abnormal external loss of bicarbonate.
- Anything that decreases the SID acidifies the solution.
- Anything that increases the SID alkalinizes the solution.
- The Anion Gap is the contribution to electric neutrality ascribed to weak acids (PO_4 and albumin) and unmeasured anions ; $AG = Na^+ + K^+ - (Cl^- + HCO_3^-) = 12 \pm 4$.
- The pathophysiology of metabolic alkalosis is divided into generating and maintenance factors. Maintenance of metabolic alkalosis depends on a continued stimulus, such as renal hypoperfusion, hypokalemia, hypochloremia, or hypovolemia.
- The addition of iatrogenic respiratory alkalosis to metabolic alkalosis can produce severe alkalemia.
- The "Gap-Gap" or Delta Anion Gap is useful to detect a mixed disorder.

- Compensation in metabolic disorders
  The **One & a Half plus 8** Rule for Metabolic Acidosis
  Expected $PaCO_2 = (1.5 \times HCO_3^-) + (8 +/- 2)$
  The **Point Seven plus Twenty Rule** for Metabolic Alkalosis
  Expected $PaCO_2 = (0.7 \times HCO_3^-) + (21 +/- 2)$
- Total body water (TBW) represents about 60% of total body weight or about 42 L. It is divided into intracellular (2/3 TBW) and extracellular (1/3 TBW) fluid compartments.
- Sodium is the most abundant positive ion of the ECF compartment and is crucial in determining the extracellular and intracellular osmolality.
- Disorders of sodium depend on TBW concentration and can lead to neurologic dysfunction.
- Potassium is the most abundant cation in the human body and regulates intracellular enzyme function and neuromuscular excitability.
- Calcium mediates muscle contraction, exocrine, endocrine, and neurocrine secretion, cell growth and the transport and secretion of fluids and electrolytes.
- Magnesium is essential for many biochemical reactions and may be regarded as a natural physiologic calcium antagonist.
- Calcium, phosphorus, and magnesium are all essential for maintenance and function of the cardiovascular system.

REFERENCES

1. Miller RD, Eriksson LI, Fleisher LA, Wiener-Kronish JP, Young WL (eds.). Millers Anaesthesia. 7th edn. Philadelphia: Churchill Livingstone, 2010.
2. Sood P, Paul G, Puri S. Interpretation of arterial blood gas. Indian J Crit Care Med 2010;14:57-64.
3. Das B. Acid-Base Disorders. IJA 2003;47:373-9.
4. Barash PG, Cullen BF, Stoelting RK, Cahalan M, Stock MC (eds.). Clinical Anaesthesia. 6th edn. Philadelphia: Lippincott Williams & Wilkins, 2009.
5. Rudolph EH, Pendergraft III WF, Lerma EV. Common Electrolyte Disorders: Hyponatremia. Hospital Physician 2009;45:23-32.
6. Shannon G. Severe hyponatraemia – recognition and management. Aust Prescr 2011;34:42-5.
7. Sherer DM, Cutler J, Santoso P, Angus S, Abulafia O. Severe hypernatremia after cesarean delivery secondary to transient diabetes insipidus of pregnancy. Obstet Gynecol 2003;102:1166-8.
8. Teagarden CM, Picardo CW. Betamethasone-induced hypokalemic periodic paralysis in pregnancy. Obstet Gynecol 2011;117:433-5.
9. Assadi F, Diagnosis of Hypokalemia – A problem solving approach to clinical cases. Iran J Kidney Dis 2008;2:115-22.
10. Naderi AS, Palmer BF. An unusual case of acute hyperkalemia during pregnancy. Am J Obstet Gynecol 2007;197:e7-8.
11. Marino PL, Sutin KM (ed.). The ICU Book. 3rd edn. Philadelphia: Lippincott Williams & Wilkins, 2007.
12. Bersten AD, Soni N (eds.). Oh's Intensive Care Manual. 6th edn. Philadelphia: Elsevier Limited, 2009.
13. Koontz SL, Friedman SA, Schwartz ML. Symptomatic hypocalcemia after tocolytic therapy with magnesium sulfate and nifedipine. Am J Obstet Gynecol 2004;90:1773-6.
14. Tarnawa E, Sullivan S, Underwood P, Richardson M, Spruill L. Severe hypercalcemia associated with uterine leiomyoma in pregnancy. Obstet Gynecol 2011;117:473-6.
15. Sato K. Hypercalcemia during pregnancy, puerperium, and lactation: review and a case report of hypercalcemic crisis after delivery due to excessive production of PTH-related protein (PTHrP) without malignancy (humoral hypercalcemia of pregnancy). Endocr J 2008;55:959-66.
16. Daskalakis G, Marinopoulos S, Mousiolis A, Mesogitis S, Papantoniou N, Antsaklis A. Gitelman syndrome-associated severe hypokalemia and hypomagnesemia: case report and review of the literature. J Matern Fetal Neonatal Med 2010;23:1301-4.
17. Hayashi K, Oshiro M, Takara I, Iha H, Sugahara K. Coma caused by hypermagnesemia in a pregnant woman complicated with HELLP syndrome. Masui 2003;52:783-5.

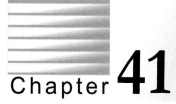

Chapter **41**

Rational use of Blood Components in Hemorrhage and Disseminated Intravascular Coagulation

Devender Kumar, Asmita Patil

INTRODUCTION

Blood transfusions are life-saving in modern intensive care, obstetric hemorrhage, cancer, hemolytic anemias, coagulation disorders, trauma and transplant recipients. In 1628, English physician William Harvey discovered the circulation of blood.[1] The first well-documented and successful human-to-human transfusion was performed in 1818 by James Blundell, a British obstetrician. He performed the first successful transfusion of human blood to a patient for the treatment of postpartum hemorrhage (using the patient's husband as a donor).[1]

Around 93 million units of blood are donated annually by all types of blood donors. Fifty percent of all blood donations are collected in developed countries (20% of the world's population).[2] Twenty percent of the world population living in developed countries have access to 60 percent of the world's blood supply. Eighty percent of world population living in developing countries have access to only 20 percent of the world's blood supply of safe and tested blood.[2] If 1 percent of a country's population donates blood, it would be sufficient to meet the country's basic requirement of blood for transfusion. But donation rates are still less than 1 percent of the population in 77 developing and transitional countries.[3] During the last five decades, the main emphasis has been on storage and safety of blood using better anticoagulants and testing for diseases like HIV, HBV, HCV, malaria etc.

Use of Blood Products is Common in the following Obstetric Conditions

- Anemia
- Obstetric hemorrhage
  - Abortions
  - Antepartum hemorrhage
    - Placental causes
      - ◆ Abruption
      - ◆ Placenta previa
  - Non placental causes
  - Post-partum hemorrhage
    - Atonic
    - Traumatic
- HELLP Syndrome
- Sepsis
- Disseminated intravascular coagulation (DIC)

WHOLE BLOOD

Whole blood is a living tissue that circulates through the heart, arteries, veins, and capillaries carrying nourishment, electrolytes, hormones, vitamins, antibodies, heat, and oxygen to the body's tissues. Whole blood contains red blood cells, white blood cells, and platelets suspended in fluid called plasma (Figures 41.1 and 41.2A and B).

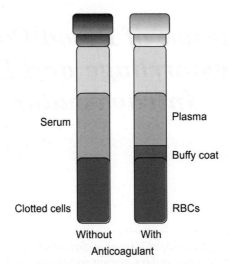

Figure 41.1: Whole blood (with and without anticoagulant)

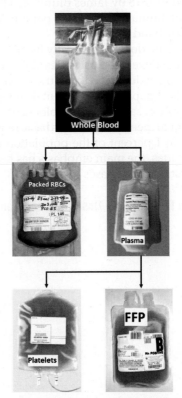

Figure 41.2A: Separated blood components (*For color version, see Plate 1*)

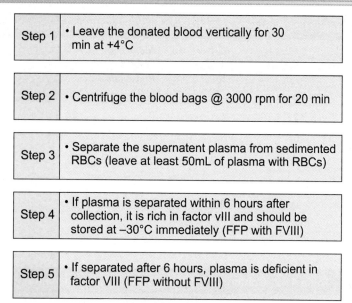

Step 1	• Leave the donated blood vertically for 30 min at +4°C
Step 2	• Centrifuge the blood bags @ 3000 rpm for 20 min
Step 3	• Separate the supernatent plasma from sedimented RBCs (leave at least 50mL of plasma with RBCs)
Step 4	• If plasma is separated within 6 hours after collection, it is rich in factor vIII and should be stored at −30°C immediately (FFP with FVIII)
Step 5	• If separated after 6 hours, plasma is deficient in factor VIII (FFP without FVIII)

Figure 41.2B: Steps for component separation

Types of Blood Components

- Packed red cells
- Leukocyte depleted red blood cells
- Fresh frozen plasma (FFP)
- Frozen or stored plasma
- Platelets concentrate
- Cryoprecipitate.

PACKED RED BLOOD CELLS[4,5,6,8,9,10]

Red blood cells (RBC) contain hemoglobin, a complex iron-containing protein that carries oxygen throughout the body and give blood its red color. Average life of RBC is 120 days. The percentage of blood volume composed of red blood cells is called the "hematocrit." The average hematocrit (hct) in an adult female is 36 to 47 percent.

Preparation of Packed Red Blood Cells

- RBCs are prepared from whole blood by removing the plasma, or the liquid portion of the blood. It has a hematocrit of 65 to 80 percent and a usual volume between 225 mL and 350 mL.
- Depending on the preservative – anticoagulant system used (Table 41.1), the hematocrit of Red Blood Cells ranges from about 50-65% (e.g., AS-1, AS-3, AS-5) to about 65-80% (e.g., CPDA-1, CPD, CP2D).
- Extended storage preservative-anticoagulant preparations such as AS-1 and AS-3 are appropriate for nearly all patient types (Table 41.2). Physicians concerned about preservative-anticoagulant in neonates may elect to use a different preparation (e.g., CPD or CPDA-1)
- Each unit contains approximately 42.5-80 g of hemoglobin or 128-240 mL of pure red cells, depending on the hemoglobin level of the donor, the starting whole blood collection volume, and the collection methodology or further processing.

Calculation for Packed Cell Transfusion Volume (mL)

- Estimated blood volume of patient (EBV) × (Hct desired – Hct observed)/Hct of packed cell unit

Table 41.1: Contents of Anticoagulant-Preservative Solutions

Anticoagulant preservative	Trisodium Citrate (g/L)	Citric acid (g/L)	Monobasic Sodium Phosphate (g/L)	Dextrose (g/L)	Adenine (g/L)	Shelf life (Days)
Citrate – dextrose A	22	8	0	24.5	0	21
Citrate – phosphate – dextrose (CPD)	26.3	3.27	2.22	25.5	0	21
Citrate – phosphate – dextrose (double dose) (CP2D)	26.3	3.27	2.22	51.1	0	21
Citrate – phosphate – dextrose – Adenine (CPDA - 1)	26.3	3.27	2.22	31.9	0.275	35

Table 41.2: Content of additive solutions (in mg/100ml)

Additive solution (mg/100 mL)	Dextrose	Adenine	Monobasic Sodium Phosphate	Mannitol	Sodium Chloride	Sodium Citrate	Citric Acid	Shelf life (days)
AS – 1 (Adsol)	2200	27	0	750	900	0	0	42
AS – 3 (Nutricel)	1100	30	276	0	410	588	42	42
AS – 5 (Optisol)	900	30	0	525	877	0	0	42

- EBV is 70 – 75 mL/kg
- e.g. for a 50 kg patient with hematocrit (Hct) 18: 50 × 70 × (32 – 18)/40 = 1225 mL
- An easier formula to calculate PCV required = wt (kg) × Hb (gm%) rise × 6
  - e.g. a 50 kg patient with Hb 6 gm% will require 1200 mL (50 × 4 × 6) of packed cell to raise Hb to 10 gm%.
- One unit of compatible RBCs will increase the hemoglobin level in an average sized adult (who is not bleeding or having hemolysis) by approximately 1g/dL or hct by 3 percent.[4]

Storage Conditions

- Red cells and whole blood must always be stored at a temperature between +2°C to +6 °C in a blood bank refrigerator. Blood bank refrigerators have in built temperature monitoring, alarm devices and a cooling fan to ensure even distribution of cold air throughout the equipment. Maintenance of above storage temp is essential to maintain the oxygen carrying ability of blood.
- The upper limit of +6°C is essential to minimize the growth of any bacterial contamination in the unit of blood. Below +2°C red cells get hemolyzed. So they must never be allowed to freeze.
- Hemolyzed cells if transfused can cause renal failure and fatal bleeding problems.

Shelf Life

- RBCs have a shelf life of 42 days and the effect of storage on pure RBCs (PRBC) includes decreased levels of 2, 3-diphosphoglycerate with a resultant increase in oxygen affinity and a decrease in the ability of hemoglobin to offload oxygen.
- Morphological changes in erythrocytes may result in increased fragility, decreased viability, and decreased deformability of the cells as well as the release of a number of substances resulting

in adverse systemic responses such as fever, cellular injury, alterations in regional and global blood flow, and organ dysfunction.

- Transfusion with PRBCs that have been stored for long periods is associated with poorer oxygen delivery than is transfusion with fresh cells. Evidence also suggests that the transfusion of older blood (stored >14 days) is an independent risk factor for the development of multiple organ failure.

Transportation of Blood and Blood Products from one Institution to another

Blood transport boxes should be used whenever blood is moved from the blood center to patient bed side or operation theatre. It is important to use clean and sturdy transport boxes that maintain optimum temperature required for blood during transport. Boxes should keep the temperature ≤+10 °C. The cross match compatibility form and serological tests report should be enclosed with box indicating the patient name and hospital number and blood bag number clearly.

Blood and Blood Component use in Hemorrhage and Anemia

- "Fresh blood" transfusion was considered useful in cases of acute hemorrhage with bleeding diathesis. In the present time, it is not recommended as damage caused by foreign immunoglobulin transfusion is more than benefits. In the present time, always consider packed cells with FFP (± cryoprecipitate) transfusion. The proper prior testing of blood for transmissible diseases will make it safe and absence of anti-immunoglobulins will generate less of post-transfusion inflammatory response
- In cases of anemia, pure RBCs transfusion (preferably leucodepleted) is recommended. The transfusion should begin slowly in chronic cases (to avoid sudden circulatory load) and frusemide in low doses may be used
- Always check serum calcium levels of the patient if transfusion volume is more than 3 units. Correct the serum calcium if required
- Always evaluate the need for transfusion with benefits and harmful effects. As far as possible avoid if any other alternative is available.

Risks of PCV Transfusion

RBCs are capable of transmitting viral, bacterial and parasitic infection and causing febrile, nonhemolytic reactions. For recipients at particular risk from these transfusion related complications, use of gamma-irradiated and leukoreduced preparations with serological tests should be considered.

PLATELETS[4,5,6,8,9,10]

Platelets are derived from megakaryocytes. The average lifespan of a platelet is normally just 5 to 9 days.

Platelet Collection for Transfusion

Platelets for transfusion are collected in two ways
- From the pooled buffy coats of the whole blood donated by four donors to make one unit. To obtain platelets, the platelet-rich plasma is centrifuged, causing the platelets to settle at the bottom of the bag. Plasma and platelets are then separated and made available for transfusion
- Individual donor apheresis (from a previously tested donor) can yield up to three units. In this process, blood is drawn from the donor into an apheresis instrument, which, using centrifugation, separates the blood into its components, retains the platelets, and returns the remainder of the blood to the donor. The resulting component contains about six times as many platelets as a unit of platelets obtained from whole blood.

Storage and Shelf Life

The optimal time is 5 days after its preparation. Most of the time, it is prepared on the same day. Platelets are stored in an incubator with agitator at a temperature of 20 to 24 °C. The agitator is to prevent clumping. The laminar flow while processing and gammma irradiation prevents infection. Platelets should be inspected prior to infusion. Packs must be rejected, or referred for further opinion, if there is any unexpected appearance such as discoloration or flocculation (i.e. large clumps of white debris).

Indications for Platelet Transfusion

The main reason for platelet transfusion is bleeding due to consumption or lack of platelets. This can occur in following conditions
- HELLP Syndrome
- DIC
- Prolonged bleeding
- Massive transfusion
- Pancytopenia

The Critical Platelet Count when one Needs to Transfuse Platelets

- In case of life threatening or severe/critical hemorrhage, platelet transfusion should be given to maintain a count above 1, 00,000/µl. Else a target platelet count of 50,000/µl is adequate.
- Prophylactic platelet transfusions are justified in very severe thrombocytopenia, <10,000/µl
- Platelet transfusions are not of much value in states of accelerated destruction, e.g. immune thrombocytopenic purpura (ITP) and are not used in thrombotic states like hemolytic uremic syndrome (HUS)/thrombotic thrombocytopenic purpura (TTP).

Increase in Count after Platelet Transfusion

Platelet count as well as platelet survival after transfusion is related to the dose of platelets infused and to the patient's body surface area (BSA). Usually these values are less than what would be expected.
- Corrected platelet count increment (CCI) = platelet increment at one hr x BSA (m^2)/platelets infused x 10^{11}
- Expected platelet increase (per µL) = platelets infused x CCI/BSA (m^2)
- The theoretical value of the CCI is 20,000/µL but clinically, the value is closer to 10,000/µL. If the CCI is less than 5,000/µL, patients are said to have "refractoriness" to platelet transfusion.
- Practically each unit of platelet increase the count by approximately 7-10,000/µL.

Precautions for Platelet Transfusion

- Platelets should be ABO-identical with the recipient when possible. Rh-negative recipients should receive Rh-negative platelets when possible, particularly in women of childbearing potential. Consider administering Rh immune globulin if Rh-positive platelets need to be administered.
- Do not use in patients with autoimmune thrombocytopenia or thrombotic thrombocytopenic purpura except for life-threatening hemorrhage.
- Single unit transfusion has no clinical benefits.

FRESH FROZEN PLASMA[4,5,6,8,9,10]

Plasma is the liquid portion of the blood – a protein-salt solution in which RBCs, WBCs and platelets are suspended. Plasma is 90 percent water and constitutes about 55 percent of blood volume. It contains albumin, fibrinogen, globulins (including antibodies) and other clotting proteins. Plasma serves a variety of functions, from maintaining a satisfactory blood pressure and volume to supplying critical proteins for blood clotting and immunity. It also serves as the medium of exchange for vital minerals such as sodium and potassium, thus helping maintain a proper balance in the body, which is critical to cell function.

Preparation of FFP

- Plasma is obtained by separating the liquid portion of blood from the cells (Figure 41.2B). Plasma is usually not used for transfusion purpose but is fractionated (separated) into specific products such as albumin, specific clotting factor concentrates and intravenous immune globulin (IVIG).
- FFP is plasma frozen within 6 hours after donation in order to preserve clotting factors and thawed before it is transfused.

Storage and Shelf Life

FFP which is prepared within hours of collection are rich in factor VIII and other clotting factors. Collected plasma is stored below -30°C and if stored properly it can be kept for many months (3 years). Thawed FFP is best used immediately but may be stored at +4°C and infused within 24 hours. Once FFP is thawed it should not be refrozen as it looses its benefits.

Indications for FFP Transfusion

It is most often used to treat certain bleeding disorders where a clotting factor or multiple factors are deficient and no factor-specific concentrate is available. FFP is used as empirical treatment of the acquired coagulopathy with prolonged prothrombin time (PT) and INR/activated partial thromboplastin time (APTT) not due to warfarin or heparin therapy. The dose is 12 to 15 ml/kg.

FFP should not be used for

- Increasing blood volume or albumin concentration
- Coagulopathy that can be corrected with administration of vitamin K
- Normalizing abnormal coagulation screen results, in the absence of bleeding.

CRYOPRECIPITATED ANTIHEMOPHILIC FACTOR (AHF)

It is the portion of plasma that is rich in certain clotting factors, including Factor VIII, fibrinogen, von Willebrand factor, and Factor XIII.

Preparation of Cryoprecipitated AHF

Cryoprecipitated AHF is removed from plasma by freezing and then slowly thawing the plasma. When the plasma which is frozen at - 80° C, is thawed to -40° C, a cryoglobulin remains as a precipitate which is called cryoprecipitate. It contains mainly F-VIII and fibrinogen.

Storage and Shelf Life

Shelf life depends on how quickly the cryoprecipitate is obtained and stored in the recommended conditions. It can be stored up to 3 years or more if temperature is less than - 30° C. The shelf life reduces to 12 months if stored at - 18° C. Product is frozen relatively quickly in an attempt to preserve the "labile coagulation factors" (primarily factors V and VIII) as much as possible.

Indications for using Cryoprecipitated AHF

It is used to prevent or control bleeding in individuals with hemophilia and von Willebrand's disease, which are common, inherited major coagulation abnormalities. Each unit of cryoprecipitate approximately contain 80 IU factor VIII in 5 to 20 ml of frozen sample.

FIBRINOGEN

Fibrinogen, also called Factor I, is a blood plasma protein produced by the liver that plays an important role in blood coagulation. Blood coagulation is a process in which several components of the blood form a clot. When blood escapes from a rupture in a blood vessel, coagulation is triggered. Several proteins, called coagulation factors, go into action to produce thrombin. The thrombin then converts fibrinogen to fibrin. Fibrin produced from fibrinogen is the main protein in a blood clot. Each unit of cryoprecipitate contains 150 mg of fibrinogen in 5 to 20 mL of frozen sample.

DISSEMINATED INTRAVASCULAR COAGULATION

Disseminated intravascular coagulation (DIC) is a complex systemic thrombohemorrhagic disorder involving the generation of intravascular fibrin and the consumption of procoagulants and platelets. The resultant clinical condition is characterized by intravascular coagulation and hemorrhage. DIC is the complication or progression of underlying disease(s). DIC has several components including exposure of blood to procoagulant substances, activation of intravascular coagulation, fibrin deposition in the microvasculature, depletion of clotting factors, and end-organ damage.

Mechanism of DIC

Four different mechanisms are primarily responsible for the hematologic derangements seen in DIC[12]
1. Increased thrombin generation,
2. Suppression of anticoagulant pathways,
3. Impaired fibrinolysis
4. Inflammatory activation.
    Exposure to tissue factor in the circulation occurs via endothelial disruption, tissue damage, or inflammatory or tumor cell expression of procoagulant molecules, including tissue factor. Tissue factor activates coagulation by the extrinsic pathway involving factor VIIa. Factor VIIa has been implicated as the central mediator of intravascular coagulation in sepsis.

Obstetric and Gynecological Conditions which may Lead to DIC

- Amniotic fluid embolism
- Abruptio placenta
- Puerperal and postabortal sepsis
- Hemorrhage (massive)
- Severe sepsis and cancer

Diagnostic Criteria for DIC include the following

- Thrombocytopenia(< 100,000 plat/μL)
- Prolongation of PT and APTT (>3 seconds difference between test and control sample or INR> 1.5 times)
- A low fibrinogen concentration(< 150 mg%)
- Increased levels of fibrin degradation products (FDP) (normal value = < 10 μg/mL)

Blood Components used for Correction of DIC

- Anticoagulants are rarely used when thrombus formation is likely to lead to imminent death (such as in coronary artery thrombosis or cerebrovascular thrombosis).
- Platelets may be transfused if counts are less than 10,000/cmm or required level if any intervention is planned (<50,000 for vaginal delivery and <90,000 for cesarean) and massive hemorrhage is occurring.

- FFP may be administered in an attempt to replenish coagulation factors and anti-thrombotic factors, although these are only temporizing measures and may result in the increased development of thrombosis.
- Components therapy is used when blood volume loss is significant despite surgical control during the operative period.
- Emergency use of blood components requires concurrent assessment of hemostasis.
- The on-going requirement for component therapy in the postoperative period will only be effective if all surgical causes of bleeding have been rectified.
- There is a high incidence of transfusion-related acute lung injury (TRALI) associated with platelet transfusions. This is usually due to an interaction between leukocyte antibodies in donor plasma and the corresponding antigen in the patient.

MASSIVE BLOOD TRANSFUSION

Massive blood transfusion is the replacement of blood loss equivalent to or greater than the patient's total blood volume (70mL/kg in adults) in less than 24 hrs.[7] It is often the underlying cause, and the end result of major hemorrhage, that cause complications, rather than the transfusion itself.

Complications of Massive Blood/Blood Components Transfusions

- Acidosis is more likely to be the result of inadequate treatment of hypovolemia than the effects of transfusion. The routine use of bicarbonate or alkalinizing agents based on the number of units transfused is unnecessary.
- Hyperkalemia (rare)
- Citrate toxicity and hypocalcemia. Citrate toxicity is rare, except in large volume, rapid transfusion of whole blood. Hypocalcemia particularly in combination with hypothermia and acidosis can cause a reduction in cardiac output, bradycardia and other arrhythmias.
- Hypothermia (with rapid transfusions)
- Depletion of fibrinogen and coagulation factors—Massive or large volume transfusions can therefore result in disorders of coagulation. ABO—compatible fresh frozen plasma (15mL/kg) and pure RBC should be the choice instead of whole blood. If APTT is also prolonged, Cryoprecipitate (Factor VII/fibrinogen concentrate) is recommended in addition to FFP.
- Depletion of platelets
- DIC may develop during massive blood transfusion although its cause is less likely to be due to the transfusion than to the underlying reason for transfusion, such as hypovolemia, trauma or obstetric complications.

AUTOLOGOUS TRANSFUSION

For elective surgeries in obstetrics and gynecology, autologus blood for transfusion can be considered. Five categories are recognized for autologous transfusion.
1. Preoperative autologous blood donation (3 - 4 weeks before elective surgery) and transfusion at time of surgery.
2. Intraoperative hemodilution - Just before surgery, some amount of blood is withdrawn and replaced with appropriate intravenous solution. Finally stored blood is reinfused after surgery.
3. Intraoperative blood salvaged from the surgical area during surgery and reinfused during or after the surgery.
4. Postoperative blood salvage after the completion of surgery by drainage of the operative area and reinfused
5. Autologous stored blood - Blood is preserved in frozen state for use at a later time. The safest blood you can receive is your own.

GENERAL INSTRUCTION FOR BLOOD/BLOOD PRODUCTS TRANSFUSION[10,11]

- The blood should be stored under appropriate condition
- Confirm the cross-match, indication for transfusion and any clinical contraindications. Check the patient's identification, blood group & type, expiry date and serological tests on the bag
- Aseptic technique must be employed and check the integrity of the pack, the component expires after 4 hours if maintained at room temperature
- All blood components must be transfused through a filter designed to remove clots and aggregates (generally a standard 170- to 260-micron filter)
- Blood and blood components must be inspected before use. Blood and blood components should be mixed thoroughly before use
- Don't infuse any other solution or medication through the same tubing
- Lactated Ringer's, Injection (USP) or other solutions containing calcium should never be added to or infused through the same tubing with blood or blood components containing citrate
- Blood components should be brought to room temperature before transfusion. Warming may cause hemolysis.
- Some life-threatening reactions occur after the infusion of only a small volume of blood or blood components. Therefore, the rate of infusion initially (up to 15 to 20 minutes) should be slow (8 to 10 drops per minute)
- Periodic observation and recording of vital signs should occur during and after the transfusion to identify suspected adverse reactions. If a transfusion reaction occurs, the transfusion must be discontinued immediately and appropriate therapy (Protocol) initiated.

SIDE EFFECTS OF BLOOD/BLOOD PRODUCTS TRANSFUSION

1. *Immunologic Complications (Immediate)*
   - Hemolytic transfusion reaction
   - Immune-mediated platelet destruction
   - Febrile non-hemolytic reaction
   - Allergic reactions
   - Anaphylactoid/anaphylactic reactions
   - Transfusion-related acute lung injury (TRALI). In addition to hypoxemia, criteria for diagnosis include the presence of bilateral infiltrates on frontal chest radiographs and the exclusion of transfusion-associated circulatory overload (TACO), or pre-existing acute lung injury.
2. *Immunologic Complications (Delayed)*
   - Delayed hemolytic reaction
   - Alloimmunization
   - Posttransfusion purpura (PTP)
   - Transfusion-associated graft-vs-host disease (TA-GVHD).
3. *Nonimmunologic Complications*
   - Because whole blood and blood components are made from human blood, they may carry a risk of transmitting infectious agents
   - Cytomegalovirus (CMV)
   - Bacterial sepsis
   - TACO, leading to pulmonary edema, can occur after transfusion of excessive volumes or at excessively rapid rates. This is a particular risk in the very young and the elderly and in patients with chronic severe anemia in whom low red cell mass is associated with high plasma volume.
   - Pulmonary edema should be promptly and aggressively treated
   - Hypothermia
   - Metabolic complications

- Citrate "toxicity" reflects a depression of ionized calcium caused by the presence in the circulation of large quantities of citrate anticoagulant.
- Hyper or hypokalemia.

4. *Fatal Transfusion Reaction*

KEY POINTS

- Separation of blood components has definite advantage and many patients may get benefit from one blood unit.
- Blood components particularly plasma components can be stored longer under specified conditions.
- Blood/blood components have inherited risk of infection transmission. Even stringent conditions of tests cannot pick up the disease in window period. So avoid transfusion if possible.
- Blood transfusion is also associated with reaction (minors or majors). These can complicate the clinical disease.
- Always identify the patient, blood group – type, serological tests of unit, indication/ contraindications (if any) for transfusion before initiation of transfusion. Complications should not outweigh the benefits.
- Always begin the transfusion at a slower rate and monitor the case for reactions.
- Match the blood group and type or use anti-D as some amount of RBCs may be present in plasma or platelets.
- Universal precautions and aseptic techniques should always be followed.

REFERENCES

1. Phil L. A Short History of Blood Transfusion [Internet]. 2006. Leeds Blood Centre. Available from: http://www.sld.cu/galerias/pdf/sitios/anestesiologia/history_of_transfusion.pdf
2. WHO. Global Blood Safety and Availability Key facts and figures. 2010 [Internet]. World Health Organization, Geneva. Available from: http://www.who.int/worldblooddonorday/media/Global_Blood_Safety_and_Availability_Key_facts_figures_2010.pdf
3. WHO. Universal access to safe blood transfusion [Internet]. 2008. WHO Press, Switzerland. Available from: http://www.who.int/bloodsafety/publications/UniversalAccesstoSafeBT.pdf
4. Ritchard C, Brian C, Linda C, et al. Practice guidelines for blood transfusion: A Compilation from Recent Peer-Reviewed Literature [Internet]. American Red Cross; 2007 April. Available from: http://www.redcrossmichigan.org/pdf/Practice%20Guidelines%20for%20Blood%20Transfusion.pdf
5. McClelland DBL. Handbook of transfusion medicine 4th edn [Internet]. United Kingdom Blood Services, London; 2007. Available from: http://www.transfusionguidelines.org.uk/docs/pdfs/htm_edition-4_all-pages.pdf
6. Circular of information for the use of human blood and blood components [Internet]. 2010. Available from: http://www.aabb.org/resources/bct/Documents/coi0809r.pdf
7. Dzik WH, Kirkley SA. Citrate toxicity during massive blood transfusion. Transfus Med Rev 1988;2:76-94.
8. Gould S, Cimino MJ, Gerber DR. Packed red blood cell transfusion in the intensive care unit: Limitations and consequences. Am J Crit Care 2007;16:39-48.
9. British Committee for Standards in Haematology, Blood Transfusion Task Force. Guidelines for the use of platelet transfusions. Br J Haematol 2003;122:10-23.
10. Blood transfusion and the anaesthetist: blood component therapy [Internet]. 2005. The Association of Anaesthetists of Great Britain and Ireland, London. Available from: http://www.aagbi.org/sites/default/files/bloodtransfusion06.pdf
11. MOHFW. National Blood Policy [Internet]. 2007. National Aids Control Organization, New Delhi. Available from: http://www.who.int/bloodsafety/transfusion_services/IndiaNationalBloodPolicy2007.pdf

Chapter **42**

Medicolegal and Ethical Issues in Obstetric and Gynecological Emergencies

Asmita M Rathore, Deepti Verma, P K Rathore

INTRODUCTION

The significance of medicolegal and ethical issues in obstetric and gynecological emergencies is manifold. The critical condition of the patient makes medical care a priority over other formalities and paperwork. The emergent situation makes time a limiting factor. The possibility of adverse outcome is more by virtue of severity of illness and suboptimal availability of resources and expertise in emergency hours. The patient and relatives are under stress not only because of severity of medical condition but also due to emergency nature and logistic problems, thus making these situations more vulnerable for patient dissatisfaction and resultant litigation. It is very important for every medical practitioner to be not only aware but well versed with the medicolegal and ethical issues and their applications in day to day clinical practice, more so in emergency situations when time may not permit consultation with books or experts. Some of these common problems faced in obstetrical and gynecological emergencies are discussed in this chapter.

There are two distinct aspects of law-medicine relationship:

- *Medical jurisprudence* dealing with legal responsibilities of the physician with particular reference to doctor patient relationship e.g. consent, medical negligence and
- *Forensic medicine* which deals with application of medical knowledge to aid in administration of justice e.g. sexual offence, medicolegal cases.

Medical ethics are the guiding principles which decide the correctness of medical actions.

Medical Jurisprudence (Law Applicable to Medical Care)

- Issues related to consent:
  - Unconscious patient
  - Minor patient
  - Extension of surgical procedure beyond the consent
  - Consent during labor
  - Refusal of consent.
- Death of the patient.
- Off-label use of Drugs.
- Issues related to quality of care-
  - Nonavailability of resources like blood, ICU bed etc.
  - Communication with patients and relatives
  - Patient not accompanied by close relative.

Legal/Forensic Medicine (Application of Medical Knowledge for Administration of Justice)

- Sexual offence
- Unnatural death
- Medicolegal cases.

Medical Ethics

- Patients wishes in contradiction with standard medical care.
- Rights of fetus as patient
- Contraception in teenager.

MEDICAL JURISPRUDENCE

ISSUES RELATED TO CONSENT

Consent means voluntary agreement of two or more persons and signifies acceptance by a person of consequences of act that is being carried out. Valid consent must be given after understanding what it is given for and of risks involved. The consent should be free, voluntary, clear, informed, direct and personal. Prerequisites for free consent have 6 components- Capacity to consent (e.g.- age more than 18 years), Act should not be forbidden by law, and there should be no undue influence, fraud, misrepresentation, mistake.[1]

Consent is essential for examination, treatment and any intervention. Generally implied consent vide making of OPD slip of doctor/hospital is considered adequate for examination but any procedure beyond routine physical examination needs written informed consent which should be taken before the act.[2] Consent given for committing a crime or an illegal act e.g. criminal abortion is invalid.

Advance directive is an informed consent which has been taken in advance during the regular visits of the patient.[3]

Consent in an Unconscious Patient

An unconscious patient lacks capacity to consent. An emergency is defined as a medical situation, such as to render immediate treatment advisable to save life or to safeguard health.[4] In case of emergency, the law implies the consent.

CASE SCENARIO-1

An unbooked G3P2L2 with eclampsia, previous 2 lower segment cesarean sections (LSCS), 8 months amenorrhea and with heavy bleeding per vaginum was brought to gyne casualty in unconscious state by her neighbor. After analyzing the situation the decision for urgent cesarean section (CS) was made. When the patient's neighbor was called for the consent of urgent CS, she was unavailable even after repeated announcements and calls.

It is a case scenario of an emergency where prompt actions have to be taken.
- In this emergency case, the patient is unable to give consent due to unconsciousness. The substitute decision maker (the husband or any other accompanying person) in such cases should be approached, but such a person is also not available.
- According to the Royal College of Obstetricians and Gynaecologists (RCOG) guidelines,[5] medical treatment can be undertaken in an emergency even when the patient lacks the capacity to consent.
- The obstetrician should act in what he/she considers to be in the best interests of the woman.[4] Now it is the duty of the doctor to do what is immediately necessary without consent. **The doctor has every right to start the treatment as per protocol or convention without waiting for the consent from appropriate sources.[4]**
- In such circumstances, where the treatment is given without the consent, a note must be made in the medical records explaining the reasons for considering the patient to be incompetent and

why the treatment is necessary. **The written advice of senior colleagues is sought at the earliest opportunity and documented. The police officer available in the emergency department should be informed if no attendant is available.**

CASE SCENARIO-1 (CONTINUED)

Emergency CS was done after the consent being signed by the two doctors and informing the administrative authorities (Chief medical officer in this case). On laparotomy, diagnosis of rupture uterus is made and after delivery of fetus and placenta, rent repair was performed. Should we do bilateral tubal ligation in this case, as the patient is grand multigravida and rupture uterus poses increased risks in future pregnancy?

- In this case, tubal ligation could be performed only when the patient has consented to it during pregnancy (advance directive).
- As per the RCOG guidelines, medical treatment undertaken in an emergency when the patient lacks the capacity to consent **must be limited to that which is a necessity in the best interests of the patient.**[4] Any lifesaving procedures like hysterectomy can be performed but prophylactic procedures like tubal ligation should be avoided.
- Risk of legal problem is more when sterilization is done in an emergency condition without adequate counseling prior to sterilization.[6]

Consent in a Minor

Legal age for consent is 18 years and a child under this age cannot give valid consent. In such situation consent is to be obtained from parents or legal guardians. In case of emergency when parents and guardians are not available, consent is to be taken from person in charge of child at that point of time.

Extension of Procedure Beyond the Scope of Consent

If in the course of an operation to which patient has consented, the physician discovers conditions that had not been anticipated before the operation and which would endanger the life or health of the patient if not corrected, the doctor would be justified in extending the operation to correct them, even though no express consent was obtained. The extension of procedure beyond scope of consent should be justified by "doctrine of necessity". A doctor may extend a procedure beyond the scope of consent to treat an emergency like resection anastomosis of gut following injury occurring during surgery.

CASE SCENARIO-2

A 35-year-old woman undergoes a cesarean section for breech presentation. During surgery, it was discovered that there is an ovarian dermoid tumor on the right side. The patient also had rudimentary horn of the uterus. How should we manage the case?

In this case even though there is no consent, the ovarian tumor should be removed as it may endanger health of woman but removal of rudimentary horn should not be performed as its effect on health of women are doubtful.

Consent by Husband

The consent of husband is not necessary for treatment or operation of wife. A husband has no right to refuse consent to any operation including gynecological operation which is required to safeguard the health of the woman. It is advisable to take consent of the spouse if the operation involves impact on sexual or reproductive function (e.g. contraceptive sterilization) but it is not legally mandatory.

Consent During Labor

In order to obtain valid consent, the patient should be competent[7] and the competence of woman to consent during labor is a controversial issue. It has been suggested that a woman in labor, often under the influence of pain, fatigue and analgesic drug is not competent and the decision making ability is compromised. However, general consensus is that labor alone does not limit the competence, and women in labor are considered sufficiently competent in law to consent or refuse elements of treatment (e.g. cesarean section, epidural analgesia). Affleck *et al* determined the ability of parturients to recall the risks of epidural analgesia from a discussion performed during active labor and found that laboring patients have a similar ability to recall information as other patients and the level of discomfort did not affect this ability.[8] The other argument against informed consent during labor is that a patient in pain does not want to hear a discussion regarding the risks of the proposed pain treatment but literature does not support such an authoritarian approach. Keel *et al* surveyed parturients within 24 h of delivery regarding the information provided about epidural analgesia. The majority of respondents appreciated the information and wanted the opportunity to discuss options with an anesthesiologist.[9]

Thus informed consent should be obtained from all laboring patients. In an attempt to overcome the issue of competence during labor, obtaining formal consent in advance has been suggested. All pregnant women should be educated during pregnancy about the possibility of anticipated problems like emergency CS, instrumental delivery and such counseling should be documented in case records. The consent for planned procedures like elective CS or sterilization can be obtained in advance. But all the consents have to be confirmed again before the procedure.

Refusal of Consent

If a patient does not want a recommended intervention, if competent, she has the right to refuse even if it harms her. In such situations inform senior person; seek advice through legal, administrative channels if necessary. Make detailed notes and respect patient's wishes.

CASE SCENARIO-3

A 45-year-old woman who is a known case of ovarian cancer stage III treated with surgery and chemotherapy presents to gynae casualty with clinical features suggestive of intestinal obstruction which was supported by imaging investigations. The conservative management was planned but after 48 hrs of conservative management, patient deteriorated and decision for surgery was made and explained to the woman. The woman refused surgery. Discussed with relatives but they could not convince the patient and she insisted on not getting operated. Patient was explained about the risk of mortality but persisted with decision.

- In this scenario, first of all it should be judged whether the patient has the capacity to give consent and refuse the recommended treatment.
- If the patient has the capacity, then she should be informed in detail about the situation and the risks and consequences involved in case of refusing the treatment. The discussion should be documented in case records. The next of kin should be informed.
- In spite of competence and full information if she refuses treatment, her wishes must be honored and informed refusal documented.

  Informed refusal: The physician has a duty to disclose adequately and appropriately to the patient and next kin the risks and possible consequences of refusal to undergo a test or treatment. After understanding all the facts, the patient can refuse a treatment or an operation.[10]

DEATH OF THE PATIENT

The death of a patient is a serious event, and unexpected death is more significant. Managing situations around death and communicating this bad news to the relatives is an important skill.

Certifying Death

While certifying the death, keep following points in mind:
- Examine the patient completely. Confirm death.
- Never declare death instantly but in a staged manner.
- Carry out resuscitatory measures. Document resuscitation procedures.
- Go through patient's case sheet and correct any discrepancies if noted. Prepare death summary and write final cause of death. If there is any controversy about cause of death, discuss with seniors.
- Breaking news of death to relatives should be done sympathetically and diligently. Break the news to a few close relatives in a room privately taking adequate time, compassionately and reviewing clinical information. Allow time for their emotions to be expressed and take help of counselor if needed. Avoid loose talks or blame game, use minimum words.
- Inform them about the procedures that are likely to be followed after this.
- Give the certificate to the close relative and take his signature. Make photocopy of certificate and keep it in records.
- In the event of death of a patient where diagnosis is not clear, the case should be discussed with senior most clinician so as to arrive at the possible cause of death and if no conclusion is arrived at, autopsy should be offered. If relatives refuse autopsy, refusal should be documented in case records.

In cases of sterilization or MTP death information should be sent in writing to District Health Officer within 24 hours and to additional Director Family Welfare within one week.

Patient Brought Dead

- Call for help, take quick history and examination. Get necessary information from a responsible person in writing.
- Start resuscitation—Intubation/ambu ventilation, chest compressions, IV line, IV or intratracheal atropine, adrenaline. Call anesthetist/medicine specialist if available.
- Declare dead if pupils dilated fixed or straight line on ECG after adequate resuscitation.
- Make notes on casualty paper.
- If fully satisfied from history and medical records about the cause of death and that the death is natural, make entry in casualty register, note details of relative who brought the case and issue the death certificate.

In case of person not under your care where cause cannot be ascertained or if there is a suspicion of foul play- make medicolegal case (MLC). Inform the CMO. Send the body to mortuary along with death summary and MLC sheet after informing the police constable on duty.

OFF-LABEL USE OF DRUGS

Drugs are sometimes prescribed in clinical practice for indications that have not been approved by appropriate authorities (US Food & Drug Administration/Drug Controller of India). This is called the off-label use of drugs. Off-label use of drugs is legal but following points should be kept in mind.
- A proper informed consent should be taken from the patient before prescribing these drugs. The doctor must ensure that the patient fully understands the relative risks and benefits of the treatment offered through off- label drug use, that a licensed alternative is available and the reasons why the particular course of action was chosen.
- When an off-label drug causes harm, the responsibility lies with the doctor and the doctor could be exposed to claim of negligence solely for using the off-license drug if harm was caused and if a licensed alternative was available.

The lack of approval for an off-label use can be due to many factors like, manufacturer's lack of interest due to commercial or financial reasons or the lack of randomized controlled trials confirming the efficacy, quality and safety of drugs in pregnant women.[11]

Sensible prescribing is the key to managing the risks of using off-label drugs. Whenever possible, licensed drugs should be used in preference to the off-license, particularly when both are equivalent in efficacy and no additional benefits are associated with the off-license drug. Off-label uses appear in a number of compendia that use expert committees to review approved and unapproved uses.[12] Some of these compendia have been recognized and can be consulted for use.

QUALITY OF CARE ISSUES

It is the responsibility of health care providers to provide quality care and substandard medical care or deficiency of service can be a basis of litigation under consumer protection act. Emergency situation is not an excuse to compromise on quality and all efforts should be done to maintain quality of care in terms of facilities as well as standards of medical care.

Medical Care

It is useful to have written standard operating procedures (SOPS) or protocols for management of common emergency situations and adhering to them will not only help in maintaining quality of care but also help in the event of litigations. Involvement of senior consultant and proper documentation is important.

Nonavailability of Resources

It is the responsibility of hospital to provide appropriate facilities and maintain standards of care. However it is possible that the facilities are not available at a particular time when patient reports, due to shortage or non functionality. In such situation, maximum efforts should be made to mobilize the resources required in the same institution. However if it is not possible to arrange the resources, patient should be informed of the facts. Suitable place should be identified where patient can be referred for proper care. Transfer of the patient should be done as per policies and procedures of the hospital and after discussing with seniors. Seriously ill patients may need transfer in an appropriately equipped ambulance and an accompanying doctor during transfer. Proper transfer summary detailing the care given and condition of the patient at the time of discharge should be given to the patient.

Patient not Accompanied by Close Relative

Generally it is recommended that patient should be accompanied by responsible relative when an invasive intervention like surgery is performed. However, nonavailability of close relatives is not unusual in emergency situations. Patient may be brought to hospital by acquaintances, neighbors or sometimes by unknown people like in road accidents who might be unwilling to take any responsibility of care. In such situation, it should be ensured that medical care is not affected by nonavailabiltiy of relatives. All emergency care should be provided as per standard protocol and life saving surgeries should not be delayed for this reason. The consents are taken from the patient herself. The efforts should be made to inform patient's relatives by means of telephone, phonogram etc as per the policy of institution, if patient is not in a condition to do so, and necessary documentation should be done. Help of hospital social worker should be taken if required.

Communication with Patient and Relatives

It is important to involve the relatives or other care givers in decision making. The patient and relatives should be kept regularly informed about the condition of patient and plan of care during emergency.

FORENSIC/LEGAL MEDICINE

Every medical practitioner is duty bound to help in delivery of justice. It is important to have a reasonable knowledge of laws as applicable to our specialty and the list is given in Table 42.1. Any

Table 42.1: Informational websites	
Act	*Website*
PCPNDT Act	http://mohfw.nic.in 2. http://pndt.gov.in/
MTP Act	mohfw.nic.in/MTP.htm
Domestic Violence Act	wcd.nic.in/wdvact.pdf
	mahilaayog.maharashtra.gov,in/../pdf/domestic_violence_act_05.pdf
Consumer Protection Act	ncdrc.nic.in/1_1html
	india.gov.in/sectors/consumer_/consumer_protection.php

clinical situation likely to involve any of these laws should be tackled carefully and special emphasis is given on documentation.

SEXUAL ASSAULT

Rape is a serious crime. The female survivor of assault may report in emergency and examination should be performed on demand of police, survivor, her guardian or other law enforcing agencies. Every doctor on duty should be aware of protocols and the authorized person should be called. First priority should be to give emergency care if required and once stabilized; the woman should be managed as per protocols without any delay.

The Goals of Management

- Medical assessment - treatment of injuries and prophylactic treatment
- Documentation and collection of forensic evidences
- Psychological support.

Management of a Sexual Assault Victim

- Attend immediate health needs
- Privacy, written informed consent
- Police involvement—Note the name and no. of accompanying constable
- Detailed history, head-to-toe examination
- Documentation—entries in MLC register
- Samples as per guidelines (available in all emergency departments), proper labeling and requisition form
- Prophylactic treatment-
  - Postexposure prophylaxis (PEP) for HIV
  - Infection prophylaxis—for *Gonorrhorea, Chlamydia*
  - Emergency contraception
  - Tetanus immunization
- Psychological support.

UNNATURAL DEATH

In case of unnatural death, local police should be informed through appropriate authorities in the hospital and the body should be sent for postmortem examination.

Do not give death certificate in following situations:

- Medicolegal cases (MLC)
- Unknown person
- Person not under your care

- Sudden death of a married lady within 7 years from date of her marriage
- Suspicion of unnatural death
- Death due to administration of injection—anaphylaxis.

MEDICOLEGAL CASES

Medicolegal cases are referred to casualty for examination and treatment and may be accompanied by police constable.

When dealing with these cases the following points should be kept in mind:
- Give MLC number and make entry in MLC register
- Note identification marks, address, take consent
- Thorough history, examination done maintaining privacy and confidentiality and treatment given.
- Complete documentation done.

In some situations, patients may come on their own to emergency department for medical care where there is suspicion of violations of law like illegal abortion, domestic violence etc. In these situations, MLC should be made as per institutional protocols after consent of the patient. If she refuses to make MLC, signed refusal should be documented in case record. The clinician should be aware of possibility of future litigation in such cases and documentation should be complete. The responsibility of clinician is mainly to provide appropriate medical care and senior clinician and administrator should be informed.

ISSUES RELATED TO MEDICAL ETHICS

The knowledge of main ethical principles of medical practice i.e. beneficence (in the best interest of the patient), nonmaleficence (do no harm), autonomy (patient's right to make decision regarding care) and justice form basic foundation of decision making in medicine and every medical practitioner must be well aware of these. In clinical judgments these principles are usually in harmony but in some circumstances they may conflict with each other making the decisions difficult and controversial. Their differences must be negotiated to determine which management strategies protect and promote the patients interests. The common controversial situations pertaining to emergency situations include patient's wishes in contradiction with standard medical practices, conflict of interest between pregnant woman and the fetus and social concerns like abortion, teenage contraception.

WHEN PATIENT'S WISHES ARE IN CONTRADICTION WITH STANDARD MEDICAL CARE

Sometimes there is a conflict between autonomy and nonmaleficence and patient may request an intervention which informed medical opinion suggests is not in her best interest e.g. CS on demand. In such situation, woman should be counselled in detail and if she insists even after thorough discussions, her wishes may be respected. Although woman has a right to choose treatment, the differentiation between positive and negative rights is important. The physician also has the right to decline to do something for which he or she has strong ethical or moral objection and cannot be forced to practice 'bad medicine'. In such situation, the woman should be referred to another physician.

Cesarean on Demand

Maternal request for CS during or before labor without obstetrical indication is common. The specific reasons for the request should be explored, discussed and recorded. When a woman requests a CS in the absence of an identifiable reason, the overall benefits and risks of CS compared with vaginal birth should be discussed and recorded. When a woman requests a CS because she has a fear of childbirth, she should be offered counseling (such as cognitive behavioral therapy) to help her to address her fears in a supportive manner.

An individual clinician has the right to decline a request for CS in the absence of an identifiable reason. However the woman's decision should be respected and she should be offered referral for a second opinion.[13]

RIGHTS OF THE FETUS

The conflict between maternal autonomy and fetal beneficence is an issue of debate in obstetric care. Most pregnant women make the decision that is in the best interest of the fetus but sometimes there may be conflict. The obstetrician's duty is to respect the mother's wishes as fetus has no legal rights. The rights of fetus are established only after it is born.[14]

CASE SCENARIO-4

A G2P1L1 with term pregnancy in first stage of labor was detected to have persistent drop in fetal heart rate to 90/min. Patient was informed about the situation and the need for emergency cesarean section. She refused to give the consent for the cesarean section.

- If the patient has the capacity to give consent and is refusing recommended treatment, then she should be informed in detail about the situation and the risks and consequences involved in case of refusing the treatment.
- Even after explaining about the risk of morbidity and mortality of her fetus, if she refuses for the cesarean section, then meticulous notes should be made in patient's record sheet. These must record:
  – The unequivocal assurance from the patient that the refusal represents an informed decision.
  – That she understands the nature and reasons for the proposed treatment, and the risks and likely outcome involved in the decision to refuse it.
- If the patient is unwilling to sign, an indication of this refusal too must be noted in writing.
  An obstetrician who complied with the mother's refusal of consent to the cesarean section would not incur legal liability towards the child, even if it suffered the harm.[5]

CONTRACEPTION IN A TEENAGER

Adolescent health and sex education has been a topic of hot debate in society. The implications of sexual activity and knowledge about sexually transmitted diseases (STD) and HIV has paramount importance in adolescents.[15]

CASE SCENARIO-5

A 14-year-old girl reports to gyne casualty along with her boyfriend for emergency contraception after having unprotected sexual intercourse. She insists that the information should not be disclosed to anybody including her parents.

- Assessment should be made whether the girl understands the implications of her actions.
- She should be examined after consent with sympathy.
- She should be given appropriate treatment along with proper contraceptive counseling and knowledge about safe sex practices.
- The girl should be encouraged to take parents in confidence.

CASE SCENARIO-5 (CONTINUED)

After appropriate evaluation, she chose emergency contraceptive pills along with regular oral contraception. After 1 week her mother discovers your prescription and complains to hospital authorities that her minor girl was treated without the consent of the guardian.

Legally, minors are not considered autonomous decision makers as they may not have ability to fully understand what is in their best interest. However provision of contraceptive services to adolescent is a special issue that needs consideration beyond realms of law. It is in the best interest of an adolescent to have knowledge of safe sex and contraception than the risk of unwanted pregnancy. The patient, who understands the consequences of her actions, should be given contraceptive advice she is seeking. Another issue is her right of confidentiality and not disclosing the information to parents. As far as possible it should be respected but if the girl is indulging in high-risk behavior which may be detrimental to her health, the option of disclosing the information to parents after informing her can be considered. Documentation of all the issues is necessary, as the possibility that parents or insurance company of girl may sue doctor/hospital exists. However interventions should not be done without consent of parents as informed consent of minor is not valid.

DISCLOSURE OF INFORMATION

The medical practitioner is under obligation to his patient to preserve confidentiality. The nature of illness of a patient should not be disclosed to any third party without the consent of the patient.[16] The controversial issues are disclosure of STD and HIV infection to other partner which patient should be encouraged do herself or should be done after informing patient.

Sometimes family may ask that patient should not be told about the truth of her illness, e.g. diagnosis of cancer, but such request should not be conceded and truth should always be told to the patient in an appropriate way and not concealed from her. Your primary duty is to the patient and not to the family.

CONCLUSION

In conclusion, it is important for clinician to be aware of potential medicolegal and ethical problems while managing obstetrical and gynecological emergencies. The doctor should learn to look at cases, that are likely to become a matter of judicial investigation, from a medicolegal viewpoint , acquire the habit of making careful note of all the facts observed and draw the conclusions logically and correctly. Needless to say, the medicolegal aspects of any case must always be secondary to the lifesaving treatment of the patient. The physician should keep in mind ethical principles and patient's best interest while making medical decisions.

KEY POINTS

- It is very important for every medical practitioner to be well versed with medical ethics and laws and their applications in day-to-day clinical practice, more so in emergency situations when time may not permit consultation with books or experts.
- The critical condition of the patient in the emergency conditions makes medical care priority over the formalities and paperwork.
- The doctor should learn to look from medicolegal standpoint upon the cases that are likely to become subject matter of judicial investigation and acquire the habit of making careful note of all the facts observed by him.
- Informed consent is essential for treatment and intervention.
- The appropriate medical treatment can be undertaken in an emergency even when the patient lacks the capacity to consent, although the **treatment given must be limited to that which is a necessity in the best interests of the patient.**
- The "doctrine of necessity" should be kept in mind when extending the procedure beyond scope of consent.
- Informed consent should be obtained from all laboring patients and it is advisable to obtain formal consent in advance for anticipated procedures like sterilization or cesarean which has to be confirmed again before the procedure.

- Informed consent should be taken from the patient before prescribing any off-label drug.
- The patient can refuse treatment or an operation after understanding all the facts.
- Every doctor on duty should be aware of various sexual offences and authorized person only should manage them as per protocols.
- The conflict in ethical principles should be managed keeping in mind patient's best interest.

Acknowledgments

Authors acknowledge inputs by Dr S Batra, Director Professor and Head, Dept of Obstetrics and Gynecology, Maulana Azad Medical College, New Delhi.

References

1. Alderson P, Goodey C. Theories of consent. BMJ 1998;317:1313-15.
2. Moreno J, Caplan AL, Wolpe PR. Updating protections for human subjects involved in resonant project of informed consent. Human Research Ethics Group: JAMA 1998;280:1951-58.
3. Jones AR, Siegler M, Winslade WJ (eds). Clinical ethics: A practical approach to ethical decisions in clinical medicine.4th edn. New York: McGraw-Hill. 1998.
4. Purandare CN, Patel MA, Purandare N, et al. Patient's rights and responsibilities. In: Mukherjee GG, Malhotra N (eds). Medicolegal Aspects in Obstetrics & Gynecology. 2nd edn. FOGSI: Jaypee. 2008. pp. 36-53.
5. Ethics Committee Guideline no.1. RCOG guidelines, September 2006. (www.annals.edu.sg/pdf/40VolNo1Jan2011/V40N1p43.pdf)
6. Biswas SC, Bal R, Adhikary S, et al. Potential areas of litigation in Gynecology. In: Mukherjee GG, Malhotra N (eds). Medicolegal Aspects in Obstetrics & Gynecology. 2nd edn. FOGSI: Jaypee. 2008. pp. 247-56.
7. Grisso T, Appelbaum PS. Assessing competence to consent to treatment: A guide for physicians and other health professionals. New York: Oxford University Press. 1998.
8. Affleck PJ, Waisel DB, Cusick JM, Van Decar T. Recall of risks following labor epidural analgesia. J Clin Anesth 1998;10:141-44.
9. Keel M, Jackson I, Madej T, Wheatley R. Adequacy of information and acceptability of pain relief as assessed by a postpartum questionnaire. Int J Obstet Anaesth. 1997;6:247-49.
10. Ethical decision making in obstetrics and gynecology. ACOG committee on Ethics 2003-2004. (issuu.com/olinad_2005/docs/guidelines_eco_acog)
11. Nightingale SL. Use of drugs for unlabelled indication. Am Fam Physician 1986;34:269.
12. Fernel RE. Prescribing licenced drugs for unlicenced indication. Pesc J; 36: 73-8.
13. National Collaborating Centre for Women's and Children's Health (UK). Caesarean Section. London: RCOG Press; 2004 Apr. (NICE Clinical Guidelines, No. 13.)
14. Fasouliotis SJ, Schenker JG. Maternal fetal conflict. Eur J Obstet Gynecol Reprod Biol 2000;89:101-7.
15. Edmonds DK. Sexual Activity in Adolescents. In: Edmonds DK (ed). Dewhurst's Practical Pediatrics and Adolescent Gynecology. 2nd edn. London: Butter Worth. 1989.
16. American College of Obstetrician and Gynecologists. Human Resources. In: Guidelines for woman health care. 2nd edn. Washington DC: ACOG. 2002. pp. 13-31.

Chapter 43

Emergency Laboratory Investigations and Basic Medical Devices

Rashmi Jain Gupta, Reena

INTRODUCTION

There are several medical and non-medical emergency condition associated with pregnancy. In addition to clinical and radiological findings, some routine and simple laboratory tests may help to clinch the diagnosis. Therefore, an early and specific treatment can be given to reduce the maternal morbidity and mortality. To obtain early and more accurate test results, proper collection of samples is very important.

COLLECTION OF BLOOD SAMPLE

1. For hemoglobin (Hb), hematocrit (Hct), TLC, DLC, platelet count, reticulocyte count, red cell indices, ESR and peripheral blood smear, 2 mL blood sample is collected in EDTA vial or vacutainer (purple cap). After collection of blood sample, blood should be properly mixed with EDTA by inverting tube 2 to 3 times to prevent formation of clots. EDTA acts by its chelating effect on the calcium. Required concentration of EDTA is 1.2 mg anhydrous salt per mL.
2. For coagulation studies, blood is collected in a vial containing 3.8 percent sodium citrate solution in proportion of 9:1(0.5 ml of sodium citrate and 4.5 mL of blood).Sodium citrate also acts by its chelating effect on the calcium.
3. For liver function test, kidney function test, serum electrolytes (sodium, potassium, chloride etc.)- 4 to 5 mL blood is collected in plain vial/vacutainer (red cap). Blood is clotted; serum is separated for various tests.
4. For blood sugar—2 mL blood is taken in sugar vial/vacutainer (grey cap) containing sodium fluoride as anti-coagulant, which also acts to destroy glycolytic enzymes.
   Note: If the sample is collected from syringe and needle, then after collection of blood, first detach the needle and then transfer the blood in different vials to prevent hemolysis of blood and distortion of morphology of blood cells.

COLLECTION OF URINE SAMPLE

1. For physical, chemical and microscopic examination of urine—First morning urine sample is collected in a clean container.
2. For bacteriological examination—A "clean catch" midstream urine sample is collected in a sterile container.

3. For 24-hour urine protein estimation, instructions are given to patient to collect the urine sample. Ask the patient to discard the first morning sample and to note the time. After that to collect all subsequent urine samples till the same time next day.

Effects of Storage on Blood Cell Morphology

The quality of peripheral smear, if prepared within one hour of collection of blood, is as good as prepared from freshly withdrawn blood sample. By three hours mild changes and by 12 to 18 hours marked changes may occur.[1] Therefore, the blood samples should be transported to the laboratory as soon as possible, preferably, with in one hour of collection.

Reference Ranges in Hematology[1]

1.	Hemoglobin	Males	– 13-17 gm%
		Female	– 12-15 gm%
2.	Packed cell volume (PCV)/ Hematocrit (Hct)		
		Male	– 40-50%
		Female	– 36-46%
3.	Red blood cell count	Male	– 4.5- 5.0 million/cumm.
		Female	– 3.8- 4.8 million/cumm.
4.	Mean corpuscular volume (MCV)		– 83-101 fL.
5.	Mean cell hemoglobin (MCH)		– 27- 32 pg.
6.	Mean cell hemoglobin concentration (MCHC)		– 31.5- 34.5%
7.	Red cell distribution width (RDW)	RDW-CV	– 11.6- 14%
		RDW-SD	– 39-46 fL
8.	White blood cell count (TLC)		– 4,000-10,000/cumm.
9.	Differential white cell count(DLC)		
		Neutrophils	– 2.0-7.0 x 10^9/L (40-80%)
		Lymphocytes	– 1.0-3.0 x 10^9/L (20-40%)
		Monocytes	– 0.2-1.0 x 10^9/L (2-10%)
		Eosinophils	– 0.02- 0.5x 10^9/L (1-6%)
		Basophils	– 0.02- 0.1x 10^9/L
10.	Platelet count		– 1.5- 4.0 lakh/cu mm.
11.	Bleeding time	Ivy's	– 2-7 minutes
		Template	– 2.5-9.5 minutes.
12.	Prothrombin time		– 11-16 seconds.
13.	Partial thromboplastin time (APTT)		– 30-40 seconds.
14.	Thrombin time		– 15- 19 seconds.
15.	Plasma fibrinogen		– 2.0-4.0 g/L.
16.	Reticulocyte count		– 0.5-2.5%

Reference Ranges in Clinical Biochemistry in Normal Adult Female[2]

1.	Serum alanine aminotransferase (ALT, SGPT)	< 34 U/L
2.	Serum aspartate aminotransferase (AST, SGOT)	< 31 U/L
3.	Total serum protein	6.4-8.3 g/dL
4.	Serum albumin	3.5-5.2 g/dL
5.	Serum alkaline phosphatase	52-98 U/L
6.	Total serum bilirubin	0-2 mg/dL
7.	Serum amylase	28-100 U/L
8.	Serum creatinine	0.6- 1.1 mg/dL

9.	Serum C-Reactive Protein	< 0.5 mg/dL
10.	Serum Sodium	136-145 mEq/L
11.	Serum Potassium	3.5- 5.1 mEq/ L
12.	Serum Chloride	98-107 mEq/L
13.	Serum Phosphate	2.5-4.5 mg/dL
14.	Serum Uric acid	2.3-6.6 mg/dL
15.	pH (whole blood, arterial)	7.31-7.42 ph units
16.	Serum Lactate dehydrogenase (LDH)	180-360 U/L
17.	Fasting S.Glucose	74-100 mg/dL
18.	HbA1C (% total Hb) (Whole blood)	4.0-6.0%

THE SI UNITS OF MEASUREMENT

In 1960, the General Convention on Weights and Measures adopted the International System of Units (le Système International d'Unites), with the international abbreviation SI International (SI), to bring about uniformity in reporting various measurement.[3,4]

The common laboratory tests with their conventional units, conversion factors and SI units are given in Table 43.1.[2,3-8]

Table 43.1: Common laboratory tests with their conventional units, conversion factors and SI units

S. No.	Component	Conventional Unit	Conversion Factor	SI Unit
1.	Alanine aminotransferase (ALT)	units/L	1.0	U/L
2.	Albumin	g/dL	10	g/L
3.	Alkaline phosphatase	units/L	1.0	U/L
4.	Amylase	units/L	1.0	U/L
5.	Anion gap	mEq/L	1.0	mmol/L
6.	Aspartate aminotransferase (AST)	units/L	1.0	U/L
7.	Bicarbonate	mEq/L	1.0	mmol/L
8.	Bilirubin	mg/dL	17.1	µmol/L
	Blood gases (arterial)-ABG:			
9.	$PaCo_2$	mm Hg	1.0	mm Hg
10.	pH	pH units	1.0	pH units
11.	PaO_2	mm Hg	1.0	mm Hg
12.	Calcium	mg/dL	0.25	mmol/L
		mEq/L	0.50	mmol/L
13.	Carbon dioxide	mEq/L	1.0	mmoI/L
14.	Chloride	mEq/L	1.0	mmol/L
15.	Cholesterol	mg/dL	0.0259	mmol/L
16.	Creatinine	mg/dL	88.4	µmol/L
17.	Creatinine clearance	mL/min	0.0167	mL/s
18.	Digoxin	ng/mL	1.281	nmol/L
19.	Epinephrine	pg/mL	5.46	pmol/L
20.	Erythrocyte sedimentation rate	mm/h	1.0	mm/h
21.	Fibrinogen	mg/dL	0.0294	µmol/L
22.	Glucose	mg/dL	0.0555	mmol/L
23.	Hematocrit	%	0.01	Proportion of 1.0
24.	Hemoglobin	g/dL	10.0	g/L
25.	Human chorionic gonadotropin (HCG)	mlU/mL	1.0	IU/L
26.	Insulin	µIU/mL	6.945	pmol/L
27.	Iron, total	µg/dL	0.179	µmol/L

Contd...

Contd...

28.	Iron binding capacity, total	µg/dL	0.179	µmol/L
29.	Lactate (lactic acid)	mg/dL	0.111	mmol/L
30.	Lactate dehydrogenase	units/L	1	U/L
31.	Lipids (total)	mg/dL	0.01	g/L
32.	Low-density lipoprotein cholesterol (LDL-C)	mg/dL	0.0259	mmol/L
33.	Magnesium	mg/dL	0.411	mmol/L
		mEq/L	0.50	mmol/L
34.	Nitrogen, nonprotein	mg/dL	0.714	mmol/L
35.	Norepinephrine	pg/mL	0.00591	nmol/L
36.	Osmolality	mOsm/kg	1.0	mmol/kg
37.	Phosphorus	mg/dL	0.323	mmol/L
38.	Platelets	$\times 10^3/\mu L$	1.0	$\times 10^9/L$
39.	Potassium	mEq/L	1.0	mmol/L
40.	Protein, total	g/dL	10.0	g/L
41.	Prothrombin time (PT)	s	1.0	s
42.	Red blood cell count	$\times 10^6/\mu L$	1.0	$\times 10^{12}/L$
43.	Sodium	mEq/L	1.0	mmol/L
44.	Thyroid-stimulating hormone (TSH)	mIU/L	1.0	mIU/L
45.	Thyroxine, free (T_4)	ng/dL	12.87	pmol/L
46.	Thyroxine, total (T_4)	µg/dL	12.87	nmol/L
47.	Transferrin	mg/dL	0.01	g/L
48.	Triglycerides	mg/dL	0.0113	mmol/L
49.	Triiodothyronine			
50.	Free (T_3)	pg/dL	0.0154	pmol/L
51.	Total (T_3)	ng/dL	0.0154	nmol/L
52.	Troponin I (cardiac)	ng/mL	1.0	µg/L
53.	Troponin T (cardiac)	ng/mL	1.0	µg/L
54.	Urea nitrogen	mg/dL	0.357	mmol/L
55.	Uric acid	mg/dL	59.48	µmol/L
56.	White blood cell count	$\times 10^3/\mu L$	1.0	$\times 10^9/L$
57.	White blood cell differentialcount (number fraction)	%	0.01	Proportion of 1.0

Multiples or fractions of these units are indicated by prefixes, e.g. mega (10^6), kilo (10^3), milli (10^{-3}), and micro (10^{-6}). One will note that the prefixes are conventionally the powers of 10 divisible by 3.

However conventional units are still familiar and commonly used in clinical practice.

Some examples of conventional measurement are:

- Sodium is administered intravenously as "Normal saline" or "0.9 percent NaCl" which contains 154 mmol NaCl per liter and is chemically a 0.154 normal solution.
- Dissolved substances are variously measured in milligrams per deciliter, "grams percent," or as ratios, e.g. 1:100,000
- A few drugs particularly the ones used in resuscitation are traditionally given as a dilution or percentage concentration, e.g. adrenaline 1:1000 and sodium bicarbonate 8.4 percent solution

LAB INVESTIGATIONS IN SOME COMMON OBSTETRIC CONDITIONS

Hyperemesis Gravidarum

In hyperemesis gravidarum there is hemoconcentration resulting in raised Hb%, RBC count and hematocrit value. Loss of water and salts results in fall in plasma sodium, potassium and chlorides. Blood urea and uric acid may rise. There may be hypoglycemia and hypoproteinemia.

Disseminated Intravascular Coagulation (DIC)

The most important obstetric emergency condition in which hematological investigations play an important role in diagnosis is disseminated intravascular coagulation (DIC) and related disorders which give rise to microangiopathic hemolytic anemia (MAHA). A large number of individuals with DIC are obstetric patients having complications of pregnancy. In general, patient with acute DIC in association with obstetric complication usually presents with bleeding disorder. DIC may occur in association with abruptio placentae, retained dead fetus, septic abortion, amniotic fluid embolism, toxemia.[9] DIC is characterized by formation of microthrombi throughout the microcirculation of the body. There is consumption of platelets, fibrin and coagulation factors and activation of the fibrinolytic mechanism. Therefore, DIC is also termed as "consumption coagulopathy".[9]

No single test establishes the diagnosis of DIC. Lab investigations should include coagulation tests, markers of fibrin degradation, red cell and platelet count and a study of peripheral blood smear for red cell morphology. These tests should be repeated over 6 to 8 hours.

Fibrin-related markers are fibrin and fibrinogen degradation products (FDPs), D-dimer, and soluble fibrin. *The most sensitive test for DIC is FDP*. DIC is unlikely in presence of normal FDP levels.[10] Low-grade DIC may occur in presence of dead retained fetus and is characterized by raised FDP levels but normal clotting profile.[11] D-dimer levels have also been used as a predicting factor for DIC following single twin death.[12]

Laboratory Findings in DIC

- Hemoglobin and platelet count are reduced
- Reticulocyte count is increased
- Peripheral blood smear (PS) examination reveals features of microangiopathic hemolytic anemia with thrombocytopenia. PS shows presence of fragmented red cells (Helmet cells or schistocytes), increased number of polychromatophils, presence of nucleated red cells and few spherocytes.[13]
- As a result of consumption of platelets and clotting factors bleeding time (BT), clotting time (CT), prothrombin time (PT) and partial thromboplastin time (aPTT) are prolonged
- There is activation of plasminogen to plasmin, which cleaves fibrin and also digests factor V and VIII. As a result, there is increased concentration of fibrin degradation products (FDP). Normal level of FDP in blood is 0-5 μg/mL.

A related condition called thrombotic thrombocytopenic purpura(TTP) may be associated with pregnancy.[14] PS in TTP also shows features of MAHA with thrombocytopenia but results of screening tests of coagulation are usually normal without increased levels of FDP.[15]

Proteinuria in Pregnancy

- The common causes of proteinuria in pregnant women are pre-eclampsia and eclampsia, urinary tract infection (UTI), chronic nephritis and nephritic syndrome, essential hypertension and orthostatic
- Protein in urine may be tested by heat and acetic acid test, sulphosalicylic acid test or by strip method
- UTI is indicated by presence of proteinuria and presence of pus cells on chemical and microscopic examination and positive urine culture report. If proteinuria is associated with presence of pus cells, casts and RBC with negative urine culture report, then possibility of renal parenchymal lesion should be excluded
- More than 10^5/mL bacterial count in midstream urine sample on two occasions, without any symptom of UTI is termed as "asymptomatic bacteriuria". Counts less than 10^4/mL indicate contamination of urine.

Measuring Units for Medical Equipments

French Sizing

Joseph-Frédéric-Benoɪt Charrière, a 19th century Parisian maker of surgical instruments, developed a uniform, standard gauge specifically designed for use in medical equipment. Unlike the gauge system adopted by the British for measurement of needles and intravenous catheters, this system has uniform increments between gauge sizes (1/3 of a millimeter), is easily calculated in terms of its metric equivalent, and has no arbitrary upper end point. This system is commonly referred to as French sizing.[17,18]

The French scale is most correctly abbreviated as Fr, but also often abbreviated as FR or F. It is used to measure the size (outside diameter) of a catheter, drain, probe and endoscopic equipment.

1 Fr = 0.33 mm, thus the diameter of the catheter in millimeters can be determined by dividing the French size by 3, e.g. if the French size is 12, the diameter is 4 mm.

An increasing French size corresponds to a larger-diameter catheter. This is contrary to needle-gauge size, where the diameter is 1/gauge, and where the larger the gauge, the narrower the bore of the needle.

Gauge Numbers

The gauge, formally known as the Stubs Iron Wire Gauge, was developed in early 19th century England. Developed initially for use in wire manufacture, each gauge size arbitrarily correlates to multiples of .0010 inches. It was first used to measure needle sizes in the early 20th century. Today it is used in medicine to measure not only needles, but also intravenous catheters and suture wires.[19,20]

Size steps between gauges range from 0.001inches between high gauge numbers to 0.046 inches between the two lowest gauge numbers and do not correspond to a particular mathematical pattern, although for the most part the steps get smaller with increasing gauge number.

In medicine, the gauge specifies the outside diameter of hypodermic needles, catheters, and suture wires.

Hypodermic Needles

Hypodermic needles are available in a wide variety of outer diameters described by gauge numbers. Smaller gauge numbers indicate larger outer diameters. Inner diameter depends on both gauge and wall thickness.

Various needle lengths are available for any given gauge. Needles in common medical use range from 7 gauge (the largest) to 33 (the smallest) on the Stubs scale (Table 43.2).

21-gauge needles are most commonly used for drawing blood for testing purposes, and 16- or 17-gauge needles are most commonly used for blood donation, as they are wide enough to allow red blood cells to pass through the needle without rupturing (this also allows more blood to be

Table 43.2: Color coding of Hypodermic Needles		
Color	*Size*	*Outer diameter (mm)*
Grey	27G	0.4
Brown	26G	0.45
Orange	25G	0.5
Purple	24 G	0.55
Blue	23 G	0.6
Black	22G	0.7
Green	21G	0.8
Yellow	20G	0.9
White/Cream	19G	1.1
Pink	18G	1.2

Table 43.3. Color coding of Intravenous cannulae	
Color	*Size (Gauge)*
Yellow	24
Blue	22
Pink	20
Green	18
White	17
Grey	16
Orange	14

Table 43.4: Color coding of the connecting piece of adult size Foley's catheter			
Color	*Size (French)*	*Size (millimeter)*	*Balloon volume (mL)*
Grey	10	3.3	30
White	12	4.0	30
Green	14	4.7	30
Orange	16	5.3	30
Red	18	6.0	30
Yellow	20	6.7	30
Purple	22	7.3	30
Blue	24	8.0	30

collected in a shorter time). Larger-gauge needles (with smaller diameter) will rupture the red blood cells, and if this occurs, the blood is useless for the patient receiving it.

Intravenous Cannula

Color-coded casing cap allows for easier identification of catheter size (Table 43.3).

Foley's Catheter

Catheter diameters are measured in French. The color of the connecting piece or the filling opening of the balloon in Foleys catheters represents a color-code and designates the diameter of the catheter (Table 43.4). International color-coded connectors are useful for easy and rapid size identification in clinical practice. Sizes 6 to 10 are used for children and larger sizes are used for adults.

KEY POINTS

- When sending the investigations in emergency conditions it is important to collect the blood samples correctly making sure the adequacy of the sample and timely transport to the lab in correct preservative chemicals/vacutainers (which are color coded).
- When instructing the patient for 24 hour urinary collection and for obtaining sample for urine culture, one must explain the correct procedure for collection in order to get correct results.
- A delay in transportation of the sample may distort the red blood cell morphology.
- It is worthwhile to be aware of the conventional and SI units of various investigations and when checking the results from different labs one should always check the units and interpret the results accordingly.
- The medical personnel dealing with emergency situations should be well aware of the color coding of the basic medical equipments for rapid identification of their correct size.

REFERENCES

1. Dacie JV, Lewis M (eds.). Practical Haematology, 8th edn. Edinburgh: Churchill Livingstone. 1994.pp -4, 12.
2. Roberts WL, McMillin GA, Burtis CA. Reference information for the clinical laboratory. In: Burtis CA, Ashwood ER, Bruns DE (eds.).Tietz textbook of clinical chemistry and molecular diagnostics. 4th edn. St. Louis: Elsevier. 2006.pp. 2251-303.
3. van Assendelft OW. The international system of units (SI) in historical perspective. Am J Public Health. 1987;77:1400-3.
4. Clark DE, Laeseke PF. Système International in the ICU in the United States. Chest 2010;137:932-7.
5. Iverson C, Flanagin A, Fontanarosa PB, et al. American Medical Association Manual of Style: A Guide for Authors and Editors. 9th edn. Baltimore: Williams & Wilkins. 1998.
6. Jacobs DS, Demott WR, Grady HJ, et al (eds.). Laboratory Test Handbook. 4th edn. Hudson, Ohio: Lexi-Comp Inc. 1996.
7. Young DS, Huth EJ. SI Units for Clinical Measurement. Philadelphia, Pa: American College of Physicians; 1998.
8. Kratz A, Lewandrowski KB. Normal reference laboratory values. N Engl J Med 1998;339:1036-42.
9. Aster JC. Red blood cell and Bleeding disorders. In: Kumar V, Fausto N, Abbas AK (eds.). Robbins and Cotran Pathologic Basis of Disease. 7th edn. Elsevier. 2004.pp.656-58.
10. Horan JT, Francis CW. Fibrin degradation products, fibrin monomer and soluble fibrin in disseminated intravascular coagulation. Semin Thromb Hemost 2001;27:657-66.
11. Arntda V, High KA. Coagulation disorders. In: Longo LD (ed.).Harrison's Hematology and Oncology. McGraw Hill. 2010.pp. 235-45.
12. Daniilidis A, Sardeli C, Tantanasis T, Dinas K, Mavromichali M, Tzafettas J.D-dimer levels as a predicting factor for DIC following single twin death: a case report and review of the literature. Clin Exp Obstet Gynecol 2010;37:67-8.
13. Jain R, Singh ZN, Gaiha M, Singh T. Thrombotic Thrombocytopenic purpura Classical presentation: a case report. Indian J Hematol Blood Transfus 2003;21:67-68.
14. Koyama T, Higuchi M, Nakajima T, Kakishita E, Nagai K, Ikeda Y, et al. Thrombotic thrombocytopenic purpura (TTP) associated with pregnancy. Report of a case. Rinsho Ketsueki 1985; 26:549-54.
15. Jaffe EA, Nachman RL, Mersky C. Thrombotic thrombocytopenic purpura- Coagulation parameters in twelve patients. Blood 1973;42:499.
16. Ridolfi RL, Bell WR. Thrombotic thrombocytopenic purpura. Report of 25 cases and review of the literature. Medicine 1981;60:413-28.
17. Iserson KV. J.-F.-B. Charrière: the man behind the "French" gauge. J Emerg Med 1987;5:545-8.
18. Casey RG, Quinlan D, Mulvin D, Lennon G. Joseph-Frédéric-Benoit Charrière: master cutler and instrument designer. Eur Urol 2003;43:320-2.
19. Iserson KV. The origins of the gauge system for medical equipment. J Emerg Med 1987;5:45-8.
20. Pöll JS. The story of the gauge. Anaesthesia 1999;54:575-81.

Index

Page numbers followed by *f* refer to figures and *t* refer to tables